Rehabilitation Interventions in the Patient with Obesity

Paolo Capodaglio
Editor

Rehabilitation Interventions in the Patient with Obesity

Springer

Editor
Paolo Capodaglio
Rehabilitation Unit
Istituto Auxologico Italiano
Piancavallo, Verbania
Italy

ISBN 978-3-030-32273-1 ISBN 978-3-030-32274-8 (eBook)
https://doi.org/10.1007/978-3-030-32274-8

This Springer imprint is published by the registered company Springer Nature Switzerland AG
The registered company address is: Gewerbestrasse 11, 6330 Cham, Switzerland

To Maggie and Joy

Foreword

It gives me great pleasure to write the foreword to this book on *Rehabilitation Interventions in the Patient with Obesity*, edited by Dr. Paolo Capodaglio. It is a very important book because it contributes to the field of obesity, presenting evidence-based rehabilitation protocols to rehabilitation professionals, as well as giving guidelines for effectively overcoming the difficult phase of obesity rehabilitation.

Also, it provides to the field of obesity management the dimension of Physical and Rehabilitation Medicine, necessary for tailoring individual multidisciplinary rehabilitation plans.

I would like to congratulate all the well-known (European and non-European) PRM physicians and other health professionals, who have contributed several chapters to this unique book on obesity rehabilitation. I would also like to extend my congratulations to the editorial team for their contribution to this educative book.

As President of the European Society of PRM, I encourage all the PRM physicians in Europe to use this very important resource in their daily practice, improving the therapeutic results of their work in obesity rehabilitation for the benefit of their patients.

Nicolas Christodoulou
European Society of Physical and Rehabilitation Medicine
Nicosia, Cyprus

Preface

While the age old advice to just "eat less and move more" is well known and often repeated to people living with obesity, the science of physical activity and its role in weight regulation and rehabilitation is still rather underdeveloped and often misunderstood. Thus, it is commendable that this volume brings together a stellar group of experts in the field, to discuss the current knowledge and knowledge gaps around the specific requirements and recommendations related to physical activity and rehabilitation for people living with obesity. The book covers a range of topics from the role of aerobic and strength training to the use of virtual reality and post-surgical rehabilitation to improve the health and well-being of people living with obesity. Thus, these pages should be of considerable interest to all researchers and health professionals working in the field of obesity medicine and bariatric care.

Walter Frontera
International Society of Physical and
Rehabilitation Medicine
San Juan, Puerto Rico

Contents

Introduction

Obesity is a global health crisis with detrimental effects on all organ systems leading to poor health status, rising health costs and disability. A significant twist may occur in the fight scenario against complicated obesity in the near future: the massive gap between lifestyle interventions and bariatric surgery could be bridged by newly released drugs. They provide hope for increasing the medicinal armoire against obesity with more effective treatment strategies. However, the present rates of the condition worldwide call for the immediate action of all of the health professionals involved. Those at the forefront and called upon to face the disabling functional consequences of comorbid obesity are physiotherapists, physical activity experts and physical medicine and rehabilitation physicians.

Decreased effort tolerance and respiratory capacity, pain and impaired function, reduced strength and balance, and increased risk of falling can *per se* lead to disability. Associated comorbidities can tip the balance of independence in patients who already have functional limitations or develop conditions (diabetes, cardiovascular conditions, nonalcoholic fatty liver disease, skin conditions, sarcopenia, sleep apnoea) where an abnormal metabolism of adipose tissue prevails. Nonetheless, the impact of obesity on individual capacities and rehabilitative outcomes is often neglected by physiotherapists and physical trainers alike. Rehabilitation units with optimal standards of care for normal-weight patients are often structurally, organizationally and technologically inadequate for patients with severe obesity. The number of disabled subjects who are also obese is now increasing worldwide, as is the rate of obese patients admitted to post-acute rehabilitation units. They require careful comprehensive assessment, appropriate therapeutic and rehabilitative protocols carried out by specially trained physiotherapists and physical activity experts in an ergonomically sound and safe environment.

This book has a unique focus on the physiotherapy techniques and training methods that are ideally suited to the patient with obesity. The aim of the present volume is to provide rehabilitation specialists an up-to-date practical guide to evidence-based exercise and rehabilitation protocols for patients with obesity with either post-acute or chronic disabling conditions. With this volume, we intend to fill the gap rehabilitation professionals may feel when treating patients with obesity, providing them with support while venturing out of the comfort zone of treating lean patients. With their multidisciplinary backgrounds, the volume's authors illustrate why multidisciplinarity is indeed the key approach. Two chapters review the existing physiological evidence on the effectiveness of strength and aerobic training modalities. The most recent adapted physical therapies—such as whole-body cryotherapy, whole-body vibration and repetitive transcranial magnetic stimulation—or rehabilitation strategies—such as motor control exercises, aquatic exercises, balance exercises, virtual reality, lymphatic drainage and mobile technologies—which have shown results, in some cases only preliminary, in patients with obesity are reviewed in other chapters by experts in the respective field. The relationship between nutrition and exercise, crucial to counteract obesity-related sarcopenia, and the clinical red flags in the post-acute neurological and orthopaedic patient with obesity are also discussed to promote a multidisciplinary and holistic approach.

Paolo Capodaglio
Istituto Auxologico Italiano
Piancavallo, Verbania, Italy

1 Physical Activity and Endurance Training Modalities: Evidences and Perspectives

Davide Malatesta, Paolo Fanari, Alberto Salvadori, and Stefano Lanzi

Key Points
- Daily physical activity and endurance training are crucially important for improving aerobic and metabolic fitness and health levels in individuals with obesity.
- Continuous moderate- and high-intensity exercise training are two complementary, rather than exclusive, training tools.
- Innovative training modalities as normobaric hypoxic training and noninvasive ventilation may be promising and useful training methodologies.
- Promotion of daily physical activity in any forms and accumulated in a minimum of 10-min bouts during the day should be encouraged rather than focusing solely on structured endurance exercise training.

Obesity has been recognized as one of the most important growing problems in our society, and its prevention and treatment are a public health priority [1]. Obesity is a manifestation of positive energy balance over an extended period of time: the daily energy intake is higher than the daily energy expenditure.

D. Malatesta (✉)
Institute of Sport Sciences of the University of Lausanne (ISSUL), University of Lausanne, Lausanne, Switzerland
e-mail: davide.malatesta@unil.ch

P. Fanari · A. Salvadori
Pulmonary Rehabilitation Department, San Giuseppe Hospital, Istituto Auxologico Italiano Piancavallo, Verbania, Italy

S. Lanzi
Division of Angiology, Heart and Vessel Department, Lausanne University Hospital (CHUV), Lausanne, Switzerland

P. Capodaglio (ed.), *Rehabilitation Interventions in the Patient with Obesity*,
https://doi.org/10.1007/978-3-030-32274-8_1

This is due to an increase in food energy supply, essentially due to an increase and simple food access [2], associated with an increase in sedentary activities and a decrease in physical activities, related to a reduction in movement at work, an increase in domestic mechanization of daily tasks, and an increase in passive transportation [3]. A global prevalence of insufficient physical activity of 27.5% has recently been reported in the world's population [3]. Although, based on this evidence, it seems intuitive that the rise of obesity prevalence in the world is attributable to decreased energy expenditure due to insufficient physical activity level. This relationship is not often confirmed and supported by scientific evidence in the literature. In fact, the energy balance is a complex and dynamic process and the physical activity influences different factors, which interact with each other and modify the energy balance independently of the energy expenditure spent during the physical activity [4]. Moreover, some recent meta-analyses reported that the impact of physical activity on weight loss is marginal with 0–2 kg of weight loss for aerobic/endurance exercise and it can be increased to 10 kg when the endurance training is combined with low-caloric restriction (1000–1500 kcal/day) [5–8] (Table 1.1). Therefore, as reported in the new physical activity recommendations of *American College of Sports Medicine* [5], to increase the effect of the physical activity on weight loss it seems important to increase the duration (volume) of physical activities performed at moderate-to-vigorous intensity from 150 min, for improving or maintaining health, to 300–400 min per week for promoting clinically significant weight loss [5, 7] (Table 1.2). However, independently of weight loss, the pivotal role of physical activity in the prevention and treatment of obesity is its well-known effect on the improvement of cardiorespiratory (aerobic) and metabolic fitness and health, decreasing the chronic disease and mortality risks associated with obesity [9, 10].

Table 1.1 Weight loss and clinically significant weight loss for the different training modalities (modified from Swift et al. [7])

Training modality	Weight loss (kg)	Clinically significant weight loss
Pedometer-based step goal	0–1	Unlikely
Endurance training	0–2	Possible, but only with extremely high exercise volume
Caloric restriction combined with endurance training	Range −9 to −13	Possible

Table 1.2 Recommendations for weekly physical activity duration according to the American College of Sports Medicine (ACSM [5]; Swift et al. [7])

• Maintaining and improving health	150 min
• Prevention of weight gain	150–250 min
• Promote clinically significant weight loss	225–420 min
• Prevention of weight gain after weight loss	200–300 min

1.1 Definition and Classification of Physical Activity

Physical activity is defined as "any bodily movement produced by skeletal muscles that results in energy expenditure" [11]. Physical activity can be classified across four domains, which can be grouped in two main categories. First is the daily physical activity: (1) physical activity to work, (2) physical activity in the household, and (3) physical activity for transport. Second is the physical activity during leisure time (i.e., sports and active recreation) also defined as "exercise" in the scientific literature and related to all structured and supervised training programs by physical trainers or clinical exercise physiologists or specialists in adapted physical activities. These two types of physical activity should be considered and used in weight management programs aiming to prevent and treat obesity.

1.2 Daily Physical Activity

Some authors have recently reported that the duration of the moderate-to-vigorous physical activity (MVPA) should exceed 10 min per bout to accumulate more time spent in "bouted MVPA" in order to reduce the risk of incident obesity [12]. For each 10-min increase in "bouted MVPA," the risk of obesity is reduced by 21%. On the contrary, this decreased obesity risk was not associated in accumulated time spent per day in "bouted MVPA" of less than 10-min duration [12]. These recent findings support the pivotal role of the accumulation and repetition of minimum 10-min MVPA bouts during the day. However, the posture time allocation of daily physical activity is different in obese than in lean sedentary individuals [13]. The former spends less time standing/ambulating (−152 min) and more time sitting (+164 min) than their lean counterparts. This induced a lower daily total energy expenditure (−350 kcal/day) in obese compared with lean individuals. Moreover, this different posture time allocation did not change when obese individuals lost weight or when lean individuals gained weight [13] highlighting the difficulty to change the daily physical activity behavior in obese or sedentary people. For this reason, it is important to develop strategies to increase the energy expenditure associated with daily physical activity without changing its posture time allocation. The use of commercially available unstable shoes, increasing the energy expenditure of standing and walking by 5–7% when compared with conventional shoes [14], may be a valuable solution to increase the non-exercise activity thermogenesis (NEAT, [15]). This could be complementary to the promotion of daily physical activity in any forms and accumulated in a minimum of 10-min bouts during the day that should be encouraged using and promoting options for the environments in which individuals may elect to engage in physical activity.

1.3 Endurance Training Modalities

Several studies have investigated different exercise training programs with different modalities, frequencies, intensities (moderate or high), and durations to evaluate the optimal dose-response relationship between endurance exercise training and health-related outcomes in overweight/obese individuals.

1.3.1 Moderate-Intensity Exercise Training

Continuous moderate exercise training (CMT) normally corresponds to 46–63% of the maximal oxygen uptake ($\dot{V}O_{2\max}$) (or 64–76% of the maximal heart rate (HR_{max})) (Table 1.3) [16]. CMT was initially adopted in sedentary and overweight/obese individuals because it is safe, feasible, and well tolerated. Moreover, because this training modality increases the reliance on fat oxidation rates during exercise, it was logically prescribed to this population.

Although previous observations reported successful weight and fat mass loss following CMT (without energy restriction) in sedentary overweight and obese men and women [17], others investigations found no significant changes across different CMT durations (i.e., 50%, 100%, 150% of public health recommendation) [18]. These findings suggest that exercise training is not necessarily accompanied by changes in body weight and/or fat mass in this population. This may be explained by compensatory mechanisms (physiological and behavioral) occurring during an exercise program [19]. Recently, Flack et al. [20] showed that similar energy compensation occurred following two moderate exercise training programs with distinct energy expenditures (1500 vs. 3000 kcal/week). Interestingly, percentage and kg of body fat decreased significantly only in the 3000 kcal/week group. These results suggest that compensatory responses are not proportional to exercise energy expenditure and that greater exercise volume may therefore overcome compensatory behavior limiting exercise-induced negative energy balance [20].

Concerning the effect of this type of training on aerobic and metabolic fitness and health in individuals with obesity, it has been shown that 8-week CMT at 65–70% $\dot{V}O_{2\max}$ may be effective to increase fat oxidation, which may, at least in part, provide a mechanism for the enhanced insulin sensitivity in obese individuals [21]. Indeed, the authors showed that the oxidative capacity increased after intervention, leading to an increased rate of mitochondrial fat oxidation [21]. This phenomenon was associated with a significant reduction of lipid intermediates, which was inversely correlated with glucose tolerance [21]. Finally, an increased $\dot{V}O_{2\max}$ has also been found after intervention. Consistent with these results, other studies [22, 23] have also shown that 16-week CMT at 60–70% HR_{max} may increase $\dot{V}O_{2\max}$ and insulin sensitivity in overweight/obese individuals and that the best predictor of improved insulin sensitivity is the increase in fat oxidation [22]. In contrast, it has also been indicated that the impact of muscle oxidative capacity and lipid oxidation on the regulation of insulin sensitivity remains controversial [24], suggesting that other mechanisms (such as the excessive plasma non-esterified fatty acid (NEFA) levels [25, 26] or flux [27]) are likely involved.

Table 1.3 Description of different exercise training modalities for practical implications

Exercise modality		Intensity	Duration (min)	Frequency (per week)	Exercise session example	Main adaptations
CMT		**HR_{max}:** 64–76% **HRR:** 40–59% **$\dot{V}O_{2max}$:** 46–63% **$\dot{V}O_2R$:** 40–59% **RPE:** 12–13	30–60	3–5×	30–60 min at ~70–75% HR_{max}	↓ Body weight and ↑ body composition + ↑ Aerobic fitness ++ ↑ Fat oxidation ++ ↑ Insulin sensitivity +++
Fat_{max} training		**HR_{max}:** 60–65% **HRR:** 35–55% **$\dot{V}O_{2max}$:** 45–50% **$\dot{V}O_2R$:** 35–55% **RPE:** 11–13	30–60	3–5×	30–60 min at ~60–65% HR_{max}	↓ Body weight and ↑ body composition + ↑ Aerobic fitness ++ ↑ Fat oxidation ++ ↑ Insulin sensitivity +++
HIIT	Short aerobic HIIT	**HR_{max}:** 80–95% **HRR:** 60–85% **$\dot{V}O_{2max}$:** 65–90% **$\dot{V}O_2R$:** 60–85% **RPE:** 14–17	10	2–3×	8–12 × 60 s at ~90% HR_{max} interspersed with 60 s of recovery or low intensity	↓ Body weight and ↑ body composition + ↑ Aerobic fitness +++ ↑ Fat oxidation ++ ↑ Insulin sensitivity ++
	Long aerobic HIIT		16	2–3×	4 × 4 min at ~90% HR_{max} interspersed with 3 min of recovery or low intensity	↓ Body weight and ↑ body composition + ↑ Aerobic fitness ++++ ↑ Fat oxidation ++ ↑ Insulin sensitivity ++
	Sprint interval training (SIT)	**Maximal intensity "all out"**	2–3	2–3×	4–6 × 30 s "all out" interspersed with 4–5 min of rest	↓ Body weight and ↑ body composition + ↑ Aerobic fitness ++ ↑ Fat oxidation + ↑ Insulin sensitivity +

CMT continuous moderate exercise training, *Fat_{max} training* exercise training intensity elicits maximal fat oxidation, *HIIT* high-intensity interval training, *SIT* sprint interval training, *HR_{max}* maximal heart rate, *HRR* HR reserve, $\dot{V}O_{2max}$ maximal oxygen uptake, $\dot{V}O_2R$ oxygen uptake reserve, *RPE* ratings of perceived exertion (6–20 RPE scale), ↓ decrease, ↑ increase or improvement

The level of adaptations is expressed as a function of the number of "+" symbols

Exercise intensities are adapted from Garber et al. [16]

1.3.2 Individualized Moderate-Intensity Exercise Training (Fat_{max} Training)

As the balance of substrates might be altered during exercise in metabolic diseases, it seems judicious to individualize the exercise training to consider the individual metabolic profile [28]. During submaximal incremental exercise, whole-body fat oxidation rates (calculated applying the classical stoichiometric equations of indirect calorimetry [29]) increase from low to moderate and decrease from moderate to high exercise intensities [28, 30–32], implying that exercise intensity (Fat_{max}) elicits maximal fat oxidation (MFO) [33]. Thus, a moderate exercise training program targeted at individualized Fat_{max} appears to be a good candidate [28, 34, 35]. In obese individuals, the training intensity that elicits MFO normally corresponds to ~45–50% $\dot{V}O_{2max}$ (60–65% HR_{max}) [36–39] (Table 1.3).

Bordenave et al. [40] showed no significant decrease in body mass (BM), body mass index (BMI), fasting plasma glucose, and insulin concentrations after a 10-week program of individualized Fat_{max} training in diabetic patients. However, these authors found a significant increase in Fat_{max} and MFO and a greater reliance to fat oxidation during exercise after intervention, which was related to an increase in muscle oxidative capacity [40]. The effects of individualized Fat_{max} training were also tested in overweight/obese adults. Consistent with previous studies, this training modality increases Fat_{max}, MFO, and the reliance on fat oxidation during exercise [41, 42] concomitant with changes in insulin sensitivity after 8 weeks of training [41]. However, resting plasma glucose and insulin concentrations, as well as lipid profile variables (total cholesterol (TC), triglycerides (TG), low-density lipoprotein (LDL), high-density lipoprotein (HDL)), were unchanged after intervention [41, 42]. In addition, it also has been recently shown that a shorter 4-week program of individualized Fat_{max} training may increase fat oxidation rates during exercise and insulin sensitivity in overweight/obese men [39].

1.3.3 High-Intensity Exercise Training

It is now well known that many people do not meet the minimum physical activity recommendations [3]. It seems that "lack of time" is one of the most commonly barriers to fail to achieve this goal. Therefore, it is of importance to develop more time-efficient training programs with regard to improving exercise training adherence. A good candidate to achieve this goal might be high-intensity interval training (HIIT). Indeed, although it has been suggested that this training modality may not be feasible and is associated with a low level of adherence in overweight/obese individuals [43], it has now been well established that HIIT rapidly induces adaptations that are linked to improved health-related outcomes in sedentary and overweight/obese individuals [44–46]. Moreover, this training intensity is perceived to be more enjoyable than CMT in obese individuals [47]. High-intensity exercise normally corresponds to 64–90% $\dot{V}O_{2max}$ (or 77–95% HR_{max}) [16] (Table 1.3). HIIT is composed of brief bursts of vigorous intensity interspersed with periods of rest or low-intensity exercise [45].

Because there are many factors (intensity, duration, and number of intervals and duration and nature of the recovery) that may describe this form of training, a HIIT classification based on the literature is needed. The HIIT mainly used in obese individuals, the aerobic HIIT, may be divided into two categories. First is short aerobic HIIT [48–50], which consists of 8–12 repetitions of 60 s at 85–95% HR_{max} interspersed with 60 s of recovery or low intensity. Second is long aerobic HIIT [51–54], which consists of four repetitions of 4 min at ~90% HR_{max} followed by 3 min of recovery. Additionally, another HIIT model intervention is the Wingate-based HIIT (or sprint interval training (SIT)), which consists of 4–6 repetitions of 30 s of "all out" cycling effort against a supramaximal workload interspersed with 4–5 min of rest [45]. However, although SIT (8–30 s of "all out") has been performed in individuals with metabolic diseases [47, 55–60], this type of HIIT may be unsuitable for some individuals. This highlights the importance of alternative HIIT strategies to adopt this training in clinical settings [45, 46, 48, 49, 52, 53, 61].

It was previously demonstrated that only 2 [60] or 4 [58] weeks of SIT (3 days/week; protocol involved ~35 min/session with only 2–3 min of exercise) was a sufficient stimulus to increase $\dot{V}O_{2\,max}$ in overweight/obese men [60] and in obese women [58]. However, less evidence has been found with regard to the effect of SIT on increased insulin sensitivity in obese individuals [62]. Whyte et al. [60] demonstrated an increase in insulin sensitivity after 24 h, but not after 72 h, after a 2-week SIT. Similarly, resting fat oxidation also increased only after 24 h but not after 72 h [60]. In addition, there were no differences in plasma NEFA concentrations or other lipid profile variables (e.g., TC, TG, HDL) after the intervention [60]. Recent investigations also showed no significant changes in insulin sensitivity after longer SIT training program (i.e., 12 weeks) [55]. In contrast, short aerobic HIIT (10 × 60 s at ~90% HR_{max} interspersed with 60 s of recovery for 3 days/week for 2 week) has been shown to simultaneously increase the oxidative capacity of muscle and insulin sensitivity in sedentary overweight/obese individuals [48] and improve 24-h blood glucose control in overweight/obese diabetic subjects [49]. Finally, it has previously been shown that a single exercise bout consisting of 4 min performed at 90% HR_{max} may increase $\dot{V}O_{2\,max}$ and reduce blood pressure and fasting glucose to a similar extent as 4 × 4 min performed at 90% HR_{max} for 10 weeks (3 times/week) in overweight individuals [63].

1.3.4 Comparison Between Moderate- and High-Intensity Exercise Training

Although both moderate- and high-intensity exercise training have been shown to improve health-related outcomes, to determine which training intensity is associated with additional risk reduction and well-being in clinical population, it is now imperative to compare these two training modalities. Despite the large amount of experimental studies, inconclusive and inconsistent results exist on the superiority, or not, of HIIT compared to CMT in individuals with obesity. It is important to note that energy expenditure has not always been matched among training groups, leading to difficulty interpreting the results.

Previous studies have initially compared the effects of different intensities at which CMT was performed in individuals with obesity. Van Aggel-Leijssen et al. [64] have shown that low-to-moderate exercise training (40% $\dot{V}O_{2max}$ for 57 min) for 12 weeks increases total fat oxidation during moderate-intensity exercise compared to moderate-to-high exercise training at 70% $\dot{V}O_{2max}$ (33 min duration, matched for energy expenditure) in overweight/obese individuals. This result was due to an increase in intramuscular triglyceride oxidation after intervention, which indicated that low-to-moderate exercise training might be an effective strategy to improve fat oxidation during exercise in this population. However, $\dot{V}O_{2max}$ was significantly increased in both groups after intervention (+11% and +15%, respectively). In addition, Salvadori et al. [65, 66] have recently shown that CMT (30 min at ventilatory threshold, ~70% HR_{max}) for 4 weeks increases insulin sensitivity, decreases β-cell function, and decreases plasma NEFA concentrations at rest and during exercise compared to a mixed exercise training program composed of 25 min at ventilatory threshold (~70% HR_{max}) followed by 5 min at 85% HR_{max} (intensity higher than ventilatory threshold) in severely obese individuals. However, this mixed exercise program promoted a higher fat mass loss associated with an increase in post-training plasma NEFA concentrations at rest and during exercise when compared to CMT alone. This phenomenon, probably driven by an increased flow of some lipolytic substances as growth hormone (GH), catecholamines, and others, may be linked to an excessive mobilization of NEFA from body fat without an equally concomitant NEFA utilization [65]. Although these two short training programs were not matched for energy expenditure (i.e., higher energy expenditure during mixed exercise training program) and both did not lead to significant changes in $\dot{V}O_{2max}$ after intervention, these findings may suggest that mixed exercise program with the final 5-min bout above the ventilatory threshold may be recommended to induce a larger fat mass loss in the initial training period [65, 66].

More recently, several studies have compared the effects of CMT versus HIIT on the aerobic and metabolic fitness and health in obese individuals. In a recent meta-analysis which includes experimental studies ≥4-week intervention, it has been shown that the improvements in aerobic fitness are similar after CMT or HIIT in obese individuals [67]. Interestingly, in a subgroup analysis, which differentiates the interval bout duration (i.e., ≥2 min or <2 min), the results showed that only HIIT performed with bouts of ≥2-min duration had greater effectiveness than CMT on improving aerobic fitness [67], highlighting the importance of the interval duration during HIIT with regard to increase in the cardiorespiratory fitness in this population. This is in line with recent observations showing that only 4 × 4 min performed at 90% HR_{max} for 6 weeks significantly improved $\dot{V}O_{2max}$ compared to 10 × 60 s at $\dot{V}O_{2max}$ load or CMT in overweight/obese adults [68]. In addition, it is also interesting to note that greater improvements in aerobic fitness after HIIT were found when the energy expenditure was similar to that of CMT [67].

Concerning glucose metabolism, this meta-analysis showed that there was no significant difference in improving fasting glucose and insulin levels, but also highlighted that the majority of the included individuals were adults without metabolic diseases [67]. Indeed, Tjonna et al. [52], when comparing CMT and long aerobic HIIT (16-week duration), showed that insulin sensitivity increased more after a long aerobic HIIT compared to a CMT intervention in individuals with metabolic syndrome. Moreover, peroxisome proliferator-activated receptor gamma coactivator 1-alpha (PGC-1α) levels increased only after long aerobic HIIT, suggesting a potential increase in mitochondrial biogenesis only after HIIT program.

Results from this meta-analysis also showed that both HIIT and CMT induce significant reduction in TC, but that only HIIT reduces LDL relative to CMT, highlighting the importance of HIIT in CV risk reduction and prevention of CV diseases [67]. Finally, it has also recently been shown that both CMT and HIIT are effective, in a similar extent, in body fat and waist circumference reductions (associated with no changes in body weight) in obese individuals [69].

It is interesting to note that recent studies also investigated the effect of very short HIIT and CMT training durations (i.e., ≤2 week) in obese individuals. Skleryk et al. [57] showed no significant metabolic or skeletal muscle adaptations after only 2 weeks of reduced-volume SIT (8–12 × 10-s "all out" sprints) or CMT (30 min at 65% $\dot{V}O_{2\max}$) in obese men. Indeed, no significant changes in $\dot{V}O_{2\max}$, plasma NEFA, insulin, glucose and insulin resistance, or protein expression of glucose transporter 4 (GLUT-4) were found after intervention. In contrast, Lanzi et al. [70] recently showed that 2 weeks of an individualized moderate-intensity continuous training (40–50 min at Fat_{max}) or short aerobic HIIT (10 × 60-s intervals at ~90% HR_{max} interspersed with 60-s recovery) were both effective for the improvement of aerobic fitness and fat oxidation rates during exercise in obese men with II and III class of obesity. Although there was no significant difference in increased $\dot{V}O_{2\max}$, HIIT had tendency toward promoting a more marked increase in $\dot{V}O_{2\max}$ compared to Fat_{max} training (+8% and 4%, respectively). On the other hand, fasting insulin and insulin resistance were reduced only after moderate-intensity training at Fat_{max}, suggesting the importance of exercise duration for improving insulin sensitivity in obese individuals [71].

Based on the above reported considerations, different endurance training modalities seem to be effective to improving health-related outcomes in overweight/obese individuals. With regard to the necessity of increasing exercise training adherence in a real-world setting [72], we suggest that continuous moderate- and high-intensity exercise training are two complementary, rather than exclusive, training tools which should be performed for improving aerobic and metabolic fitness and other health-related outcomes.

1.4 Innovative Training Modalities

1.4.1 Normobaric Intermittent Hypoxic Exercise Training

As already presented above, physical exercise training is an important lifestyle behavior for weight management, fitness, and health benefits. However, adherence to prescribed or spontaneous exercise remains low [73] and often declines over time in obese individuals inducing to a plateau in weight loss or partial or total recovery of lost weight 6 months after the beginning of intervention [74, 75]. Furthermore, obesity may increase joint stresses during walking, which likely modify gait pattern [76–81], and may contribute to lead eventually musculoskeletal pathologies (e.g., lower-extremity osteoarthritis, rheumatoid arthritis, and/or low back pain) [82]. This may increase the dropout during exercise training programs [83] and, thus, limit their beneficial effects in weight management interventions in obese individuals [84]. For this reason, it is imperative that alternative and innovative strategies are developed for individuals with obesity to increase variation, adherence, and effectiveness of exercise training programs to finally match current exercise recommendations [5].

Among these innovative strategies, normobaric hypoxic training is used and compared with equivalent normoxic training, to improve weight loss and cardiometabolic markers in individuals with obesity (see for review [74, 75, 85–87]). Normobaric hypoxia (i.e., simulated altitude (2500–3000 m) via a reduced inspired O_2 fraction (14–15 FiO_2) usually obtained using hypoxic chamber) is defined as a reduced O_2 supply to tissues caused by decreases in O_2 saturation of arterial blood with normal barometric pressure. Normobaric hypoxic training, which activates the hypoxia-inducible factor (HIF), may play a pivotal role in effective metabolism regulation (weight maintenance, glucose homeostasis, O_2 transport and satiety) and, thus, could be a useful tool to treat obesity. Recent systematic review and meta-analysis [74] supports this concept showing that, similar to normoxic training, normobaric hypoxic training results in significant decreases in body weight, fat mass, weight-to-hip ratio, waist circumference, and in several cardiometabolic markers (triglycerides, LDL, HDL, systolic and diastolic blood pressure). However, only the magnitude of reductions in triglycerides and higher muscle mass gain was greater in hypoxic than in normoxic training. Moreover, these mostly similar results between the two interventions may be obtained using lower exercise intensity in normobaric hypoxic than in normoxic training [88–90]. Fernandez Menendez et al. [91] recently reported that a 3-week normobaric hypoxic (3000 m) walking training program at slower preferred walking speed than in normoxia elicited similar responses in terms of body mass and composition, energetics and mechanics of walking, and metabolic risk markers in individuals with obesity. However, this slower walking speed in hypoxia may reduce joint loads and stresses and increase adherence to training compared to normoxic training performed at faster walking speed and, thus, with higher risk of orthopedic injury [90, 92] and dropout during intervention. According to recent practical applications and recommendations for normobaric hypoxic training [74], this training should start using low-to-moderate intensity and include the following features: 4–6 weeks of 2–3 sessions of 60–90 min at 55–65% of $\dot{V}O_{2max}$ or 60–70% of maximum heart rate at 13–14% of FiO_2. Then, HIIT in moderate level of hypoxia (FiO_2, 14–17.2%) should be added always in combination with other sessions of endurance training. HIIT sessions should include a duration of 30–60 min/session, using intervals of 8–30 s all-out followed by 3 min of active recovery at 55–65% of peak power output performed 3–4 times/week. This second part of HIIT hypoxic training could induce an additional effect in reducing fat and body mass and maximizing muscle growth [93–95]. It has also been suggested that, to optimize the effect of normobaric hypoxic training, saturation levels of 75–89% should be targeted and used to increase the hypoxic stress and stimulus [91].

1.4.2 Noninvasive Ventilation (NIV) and Proportional Assist Ventilation (PAV) During Physical Training

Noninvasive ventilation (NIV) is able to improve work capacity in individuals with obstructive pulmonary diseases as well as in patients with restrictive thoracic disorders [96, 97]. Obese individuals must overcome some peculiarities which alter respiratory mechanics like a reduced lung compliance, an increased chest wall resistance, antagonistic activity of respiratory muscles, and modified work on the abdominal viscera. They suffer from dyspnea even during mild exertion, partly by an increased oxygen cost of breathing [98].

Interesting results have been obtained in obese individuals with obstructive sleep apnea (OSA) already treated with continuous positive air pressure (CPAP) when adding NIV during physical training or respiratory muscle training (RMT – isocapnic hyperpnea). This latter is able to improve walking distance by increasing respiratory muscle endurance [99]. Aerobic fitness, assessed by $\dot{V}O_{2peak}$, significantly improved after 3 months of the combination of exercise plus RMT and exercise plus NIV when compared with exercise alone. Moreover, the use of NIV during exercise training produces a dramatic reduction in systolic as well in diastolic blood pressures versus exercise alone, with a likely protective effect on cardiovascular function, and a more important reduction of waist circumference at the end of the training period [100].

Another type of NIV is the proportional assist ventilation (PAV), which represents an extension of the activity of the patient's own respiratory muscles. PAV generates inspiratory pressures in proportion to inspired flow and inspired volume such that the ratio between airway pressure and instantaneous patient-generated pressure is approximately 1. This method gives some advantages like reduction of peak airway pressure required to sustain ventilation, less risk of overventilation, and preservation of homeostatic control mechanisms and patient's own reflex. On the whole, PAV is able to unload the resistive and elastic burdens of the ventilatory system [101]. During a cyclo-ergometer exercise, PAV has shown to increase the exercise endurance in more than 50% obese individuals [102]. Interestingly, in agreement with findings in patients affected by restrictive thoracic disorders, obese "responder" individuals have lung volumes that are lower than those of "nonresponders" [102].

1.5 Conclusions

Daily physical activity and endurance training are crucially important for improving aerobic and metabolic fitness and health levels. Their role in weight loss is marginal and this may become clinically significant only whether a higher exercise duration

(300–400 min/session) is used and/or exercise is combined with caloric restriction. In structured endurance training, the moderate-intensity continuous and high-intensity interval trainings seem to be both effective to improving health-related outcomes and increasing adherence and variation during training interventions and should be considered two complementary training tools in overweight/obese individuals. Moreover, innovative training modalities as normobaric hypoxic training and noninvasive ventilation may be promising and useful for improving fitness and health. However, "one approach that may be effective is to encourage the accumulation of moderate-to-vigorous physical activity throughout the day by increasing steps of ambulatory movement rather than focusing solely on structured periods of more traditional forms of exercise" [103].

Acknowledgment The authors thank Elsevier for the permission to reuse Figures and Tables of the manuscript of Swift et al. [7].

References

1. Collaboration NCDRF. Trends in adult body-mass index in 200 countries from 1975 to 2014: a pooled analysis of 1698 population-based measurement studies with 19.2 million participants. Lancet. 2016;387(10026):1377–96. https://doi.org/10.1016/S0140-6736(16)30054-X.
2. Swinburn B. Commentary: physical activity as a minor player in the obesity epidemic: what are the deep implications? Int J Epidemiol. 2013;42(6):1838–40. https://doi.org/10.1093/ije/dyt162.
3. Guthold R, Stevens GA, Riley LM, Bull FC. Worldwide trends in insufficient physical activity from 2001 to 2016: a pooled analysis of 358 population-based surveys with 1.9 million participants. Lancet Glob Health. 2018;6(10):e1077–86. https://doi.org/10.1016/S2214-109X(18)30357-7.
4. Blundell JE, Gibbons C, Caudwell P, Finlayson G, Hopkins M. Appetite control and energy balance: impact of exercise. Obes Rev. 2015;16(Suppl 1):67–76. https://doi.org/10.1111/obr.12257.
5. Donnelly JE, Blair SN, Jakicic JM, Manore MM, Rankin JW, Smith BK, American College of Sports Medicine. American College of Sports Medicine Position Stand. Appropriate physical activity intervention strategies for weight loss and prevention of weight regain for adults. Med Sci Sports Exerc. 2009;41(2):459–71. https://doi.org/10.1249/MSS.0b013e3181949333.
6. Shaw K, Gennat H, O'Rourke P, Del Mar C. Exercise for overweight or obesity. Cochrane Database Syst Rev. 2006;4:CD003817. https://doi.org/10.1002/14651858.CD003817.pub3.
7. Swift DL, Johannsen NM, Lavie CJ, Earnest CP, Church TS. The role of exercise and physical activity in weight loss and maintenance. Prog Cardiovasc Dis. 2014;56(4):441–7. https://doi.org/10.1016/j.pcad.2013.09.012.
8. Thorogood A, Mottillo S, Shimony A, Filion KB, Joseph L, Genest J, Pilote L, Poirier P, Schiffrin EL, Eisenberg MJ. Isolated aerobic exercise and weight loss: a systematic review and meta-analysis of randomized controlled trials. Am J Med. 2011;124(8):747–55. https://doi.org/10.1016/j.amjmed.2011.02.037.
9. Blair SN, Brodney S. Effects of physical inactivity and obesity on morbidity and mortality: current evidence and research issues. Med Sci Sports Exerc. 1999;31(11 Suppl):S646–62. https://doi.org/10.1097/00005768-199911001-00025.
10. Wei M, Kampert JB, Barlow CE, Nichaman MZ, Gibbons LW, Paffenbarger RS Jr, Blair SN. Relationship between low cardiorespiratory fitness and mortality in normal-weight, overweight, and obese men. JAMA. 1999;282(16):1547–53. https://doi.org/10.1001/jama.282.16.1547.

11. Caspersen CJ, Powell KE, Christenson GM. Physical activity, exercise, and physical fitness: definitions and distinctions for health-related research. Public Health Rep. 1985;100(2):126–31. https://www.ncbi.nlm.nih.gov/pmc/articles/PMC1424733/pdf/pubhealthrep00100-0016.pdf.
12. White DK, Gabriel KP, Kim Y, Lewis CE, Sternfeld B. Do short spurts of physical activity benefit cardiovascular health? The CARDIA study. Med Sci Sports Exerc. 2015;47(11):2353–8. https://doi.org/10.1249/MSS.0000000000000662.
13. Levine JA, Lanningham-Foster LM, McCrady SK, Krizan AC, Olson LR, Kane PH, Jensen MD, Clark MM. Interindividual variation in posture allocation: possible role in human obesity. Science. 2005;307(5709):584–6. https://doi.org/10.1126/science.1106561.
14. Maffiuletti NA, Malatesta D, Agosti F, Sartorio A. Unstable shoes increase energy expenditure of obese patients. Am J Med. 2012;125(5):513–6. https://doi.org/10.1016/j.amjmed.2012.01.001.
15. Levine JA, Eberhardt NL, Jensen MD. Role of nonexercise activity thermogenesis in resistance to fat gain in humans. Science. 1999;283(5399):212–4. https://doi.org/10.1126/science.283.5399.212.
16. Garber CE, Blissmer B, Deschenes MR, Franklin BA, Lamonte MJ, Lee IM, Nieman DC, Swain DP, American College of Sports M. American College of Sports Medicine position stand. Quantity and quality of exercise for developing and maintaining cardiorespiratory, musculoskeletal, and neuromotor fitness in apparently healthy adults: guidance for prescribing exercise. Med Sci Sports Exerc. 2011;43(7):1334–59. https://doi.org/10.1249/MSS.0b013e318213fefb.
17. Donnelly JE, Honas JJ, Smith BK, Mayo MS, Gibson CA, Sullivan DK, Lee J, Herrmann SD, Lambourne K, Washburn RA. Aerobic exercise alone results in clinically significant weight loss for men and women: midwest exercise trial 2. Obesity (Silver Spring). 2013;21(3):E219–28. https://doi.org/10.1002/oby.20145.
18. Church TS, Earnest CP, Skinner JS, Blair SN. Effects of different doses of physical activity on cardiorespiratory fitness among sedentary, overweight or obese postmenopausal women with elevated blood pressure: a randomized controlled trial. JAMA. 2007;297(19):2081–91. https://doi.org/10.1001/jama.297.19.2081.
19. Thomas DM, Kyle TK, Stanford FC. The gap between expectations and reality of exercise-induced weight loss is associated with discouragement. Prev Med. 2015;81:357–60. https://doi.org/10.1016/j.ypmed.2015.10.001.
20. Flack KD, Ufholz K, Johnson L, Fitzgerald JS, Roemmich JN. Energy compensation in response to aerobic exercise training in overweight adults. Am J Phys Regul Integr Comp Phys. 2018;315(4):R619–26. https://doi.org/10.1152/ajpregu.00071.2018.
21. Bruce CR, Thrush AB, Mertz VA, Bezaire V, Chabowski A, Heigenhauser GJ, Dyck DJ. Endurance training in obese humans improves glucose tolerance and mitochondrial fatty acid oxidation and alters muscle lipid content. Am J Physiol Endocrinol Metab. 2006;291(1):E99–E107. https://doi.org/10.1152/ajpendo.00587.2005.
22. Goodpaster BH, Katsiaras A, Kelley DE. Enhanced fat oxidation through physical activity is associated with improvements in insulin sensitivity in obesity. Diabetes. 2003;52(9):2191–7. https://doi.org/10.2337/diabetes.52.9.2191.
23. Menshikova EV, Ritov VB, Toledo FG, Ferrell RE, Goodpaster BH, Kelley DE. Effects of weight loss and physical activity on skeletal muscle mitochondrial function in obesity. Am J Physiol Endocrinol Metab. 2005;288(4):E818–25. https://doi.org/10.1152/ajpendo.00322.2004.
24. Turner N, Bruce CR, Beale SM, Hoehn KL, So T, Rolph MS, Cooney GJ. Excess lipid availability increases mitochondrial fatty acid oxidative capacity in muscle: evidence against a role for reduced fatty acid oxidation in lipid-induced insulin resistance in rodents. Diabetes. 2007;56(8):2085–92. https://doi.org/10.2337/db07-0093.
25. Bajaj M, Suraamornkul S, Romanelli A, Cline GW, Mandarino LJ, Shulman GI, DeFronzo RA. Effect of a sustained reduction in plasma free fatty acid concentration on intramuscular long-chain fatty Acyl-CoAs and insulin action in type 2 diabetic patients. Diabetes. 2005;54(11):3148–53. https://doi.org/10.2337/diabetes.54.11.3148.
26. Santomauro AT, Boden G, Silva ME, Rocha DM, Santos RF, Ursich MJ, Strassmann PG, Wajchenberg BL. Overnight lowering of free fatty acids with Acipimox improves insu-

lin resistance and glucose tolerance in obese diabetic and nondiabetic subjects. Diabetes. 1999;48(9):1836–41. https://doi.org/10.2337/diabetes.48.9.1836.
27. Schenk S, Harber MP, Shrivastava CR, Burant CF, Horowitz JF. Improved insulin sensitivity after weight loss and exercise training is mediated by a reduction in plasma fatty acid mobilization, not enhanced oxidative capacity. J Physiol. 2009;587(Pt 20):4949–61. https://doi.org/10.1113/jphysiol.2009.175489.
28. Brun JF, Romain AJ, Mercier J. Maximal lipid oxidation during exercise (Lipoxmax): from physiological measurements to clinical applications. Facts and uncertainties. Sci Sports. 2011;26:57–71. https://doi.org/10.1016/j.scispo.2011.02.001.
29. Frayn KN. Calculation of substrate oxidation rates in vivo from gaseous exchange. J Appl Physiol. 1983;55(2):628–34. https://doi.org/10.1152/jappl.1983.55.2.628.
30. Achten J, Jeukendrup AE. Maximal fat oxidation during exercise in trained men. Int J Sports Med. 2003;24(8):603–8. https://doi.org/10.1055/s-2003-43265.
31. Romijn JA, Coyle EF, Sidossis LS, Gastaldelli A, Horowitz JF, Endert E, Wolfe RR. Regulation of endogenous fat and carbohydrate metabolism in relation to exercise intensity and duration. Am J Phys. 1993;265(3 Pt 1):E380–91. https://doi.org/10.1152/ajpendo.1993.265.3.E380.
32. van Loon LJ. Use of intramuscular triacylglycerol as a substrate source during exercise in humans. J Appl Physiol. 2004;97(4):1170–87. https://doi.org/10.1152/japplphysiol.00368.2004.
33. Achten J, Gleeson M, Jeukendrup AE. Determinaion of the exercise intensity that elicits maximal fat oxidation. Med Sci Sports Exerc. 2002;34(1):92–7. https://doi.org/10.1152/japplphysiol.00368.2004.
34. Brun JF, Malatesta D, Sartorio A. Maximal lipid oxidation during exercise: a target for individualizing endurance training in obesity and diabetes? J Endocrinol Investig. 2012;35(7):686–91. https://doi.org/10.3275/8466.
35. Romain AJ, Carayol M, Desplan M, Fedou C, Ninot G, Mercier J, Avignon A, Brun JF. Physical activity targeted at maximal lipid oxidation: a meta-analysis. J Nutr Metab. 2012;2012:285395. https://doi.org/10.1155%2F2012%2F285395.
36. Ara I, Larsen S, Stallknecht B, Guerra B, Morales-Alamo D, Andersen JL, Ponce-Gonzalez JG, Guadalupe-Grau A, Galbo H, Calbet JA, Helge JW. Normal mitochondrial function and increased fat oxidation capacity in leg and arm muscles in obese humans. Int J Obes. 2011;35(1):99–108. https://doi.org/10.1038/ijo.2010.123.
37. Lanzi S, Codecasa F, Cornacchia M, Maestrini S, Salvadori A, Brunani A, Malatesta D. Fat oxidation, hormonal and plasma metabolite kinetics during a submaximal incremental test in lean and obese adults. PLoS One. 2014;9(2):e88707. https://doi.org/10.1371/journal.pone.0088707.
38. Larsen S, Ara I, Rabol R, Andersen JL, Boushel R, Dela F, Helge JW. Are substrate use during exercise and mitochondrial respiratory capacity decreased in arm and leg muscle in type 2 diabetes? Diabetologia. 2009;52(7):1400–8. https://doi.org/10.1007/s00125-009-1353-4.
39. Venables MC, Jeukendrup AE. Endurance training and obesity: effect on substrate metabolism and insulin sensitivity. Med Sci Sports Exerc. 2008;40(3):495–502. https://doi.org/10.1249/MSS.0b013e31815f256f.
40. Bordenave S, Metz L, Flavier S, Lambert K, Ghanassia E, Dupuy AM, Michel F, Puech-Cathala AM, Raynaud E, Brun JF, Mercier J. Training-induced improvement in lipid oxidation in type 2 diabetes mellitus is related to alterations in muscle mitochondrial activity. Effect of endurance training in type 2 diabetes. Diabetes Metab. 2008;34(2):162–8. https://doi.org/10.1016/j.diabet.2007.11.006.
41. Dumortier M, Brandou F, Perez-Martin A, Fedou C, Mercier J, Brun JF. Low intensity endurance exercise targeted for lipid oxidation improves body composition and insulin sensitivity in patients with the metabolic syndrome. Diabetes Metab. 2003;29(5):509–18. https://doi.org/10.1016/s1262-3636(07)70065-4.
42. Dumortier M, Perez-Martin A, Pierrisnard E, Mercier J, Brun JF. Regular exercise (3x45 min/wk) decreases plasma viscosity in sedentary obese, insulin resistant patients parallel to an improvement in fitness and a shift in substrate oxidation balance. Clin Hemorheol Microcirc. 2002;26(4):219–29. https://content.iospress.com/articles/clinical-hemorheology-and-microcirculation/ch497.

43. Ekkekakis P, Lind E, Vazou S. Affective responses to increasing levels of exercise intensity in normal-weight, overweight, and obese middle-aged women. Obesity (Silver Spring). 2010;18(1):79–85. https://doi.org/10.1038/oby.2009.204.
44. Campbell WW, Kraus WE, Powell KE, Haskell WL, Janz KF, Jakicic JM, Troiano RP, Sprow K, Torres A, Piercy KL, Bartlett DB, Physical Activity Guidelines Advisory Committee. High-intensity interval training for cardiometabolic disease prevention. Med Sci Sports Exerc. 2019;51(6):1220–6. https://doi.org/10.1249/MSS.0000000000001934.
45. Gibala MJ, Little JP, Macdonald MJ, Hawley JA. Physiological adaptations to low-volume, high-intensity interval training in health and disease. J Physiol. 2012;590(Pt 5):1077–84. https://doi.org/10.1113/jphysiol.2011.224725.
46. Weston KS, Wisloff U, Coombes JS. High-intensity interval training in patients with lifestyle-induced cardiometabolic disease: a systematic review and meta-analysis. Br J Sports Med. 2014;48(16):1227–34. https://doi.org/10.1136/bjsports-2013-092576.
47. Kong Z, Fan X, Sun S, Song L, Shi Q, Nie J. Comparison of high-intensity interval training and moderate-to-vigorous continuous training for cardiometabolic health and exercise enjoyment in obese young women: a randomized controlled trial. PLoS One. 2016;11(7):e0158589. https://doi.org/10.1371/journal.pone.0158589.
48. Hood MS, Little JP, Tarnopolsky MA, Myslik F, Gibala MJ. Low-volume interval training improves muscle oxidative capacity in sedentary adults. Med Sci Sports Exerc. 2011;43(10):1849–56. https://doi.org/10.1249/MSS.0b013e3182199834.
49. Little JP, Gillen JB, Percival ME, Safdar A, Tarnopolsky MA, Punthakee Z, Jung ME, Gibala MJ. Low-volume high-intensity interval training reduces hyperglycemia and increases muscle mitochondrial capacity in patients with type 2 diabetes. J Appl Physiol. 2011;111(6):1554–60. https://doi.org/10.1152/japplphysiol.00921.2011.
50. Sawyer BJ, Tucker WJ, Bhammar DM, Ryder JR, Sweazea KL, Gaesser GA. Effects of high-intensity interval training and moderate-intensity continuous training on endothelial function and cardiometabolic risk markers in obese adults. J Appl Physiol (1985). 2016;121(1):279–88. https://doi.org/10.1152/japplphysiol.00024.2016.
51. Gerosa-Neto J, Antunes BM, Campos EZ, Rodrigues J, Ferrari GD, Rosa Neto JC, Bueno CRJ, Lira FS. Impact of long-term high-intensity interval and moderate-intensity continuous training on subclinical inflammation in overweight/obese adults. J Exerc Rehabil. 2016;12(6):575–80. https://doi.org/10.12965/jer.1632770.385.
52. Tjonna AE, Lee SJ, Rognmo O, Stolen TO, Bye A, Haram PM, Loennechen JP, Al-Share QY, Skogvoll E, Slordahl SA, Kemi OJ, Najjar SM, Wisloff U. Aerobic interval training versus continuous moderate exercise as a treatment for the metabolic syndrome: a pilot study. Circulation. 2008;118(4):346–54. https://doi.org/10.1161/CIRCULATIONAHA.108.772822.
53. Tjonna AE, Stolen TO, Bye A, Volden M, Slordahl SA, Odegard R, Skogvoll E, Wisloff U. Aerobic interval training reduces cardiovascular risk factors more than a multitreatment approach in overweight adolescents. Clin Sci (Lond). 2009;116(4):317–26. https://doi.org/10.1042/CS20080249.
54. Zhang H, Tong TK, Qiu W, Zhang X, Zhou S, Liu Y, He Y. Comparable effects of high-intensity interval training and prolonged continuous exercise training on abdominal visceral fat reduction in obese young women. J Diabetes Res. 2017;2017:5071740. https://doi.org/10.1155/2017/5071740.
55. Martins C, Kazakova I, Ludviksen M, Mehus I, Wisloff U, Kulseng B, Morgan L, King N. High-intensity interval training and isocaloric moderate-intensity continuous training result in similar improvements in body composition and fitness in obese individuals. Int J Sport Nutr Exerc Metab. 2016;26(3):197–204. https://doi.org/10.1123/ijsnem.2015-0078.
56. Metcalfe RS, Babraj JA, Fawkner SG, Vollaard NB. Towards the minimal amount of exercise for improving metabolic health: beneficial effects of reduced-exertion high-intensity interval training. Eur J Appl Physiol. 2012;112(7):2767–75. https://doi.org/10.1007/s00421-011-2254-z.
57. Skleryk JR, Karagounis LG, Hawley JA, Sharman MJ, Laursen PB, Watson G. Two weeks of reduced-volume sprint interval or traditional exercise training does not improve metabolic functioning in sedentary obese men. Diabetes Obes Metab. 2013;15(12):1146–53. https://doi.org/10.1111/dom.12150.

58. Trilk JL, Singhal A, Bigelman KA, Cureton KJ. Effect of sprint interval training on circulatory function during exercise in sedentary, overweight/obese women. Eur J Appl Physiol. 2011;111(8):1591–7. https://doi.org/10.1007/s00421-010-1777-z.
59. Whyte LJ, Ferguson C, Wilson J, Scott RA, Gill JM. Effects of single bout of very high-intensity exercise on metabolic health biomarkers in overweight/obese sedentary men. Metabolism. 2013;62(2):212–9. https://doi.org/10.1016/j.metabol.2012.07.019.
60. Whyte LJ, Gill JM, Cathcart AJ. Effect of 2 weeks of sprint interval training on health-related outcomes in sedentary overweight/obese men. Metabolism. 2010;59(10):1421–8.
61. Kessler HS, Sisson SB, Short KR. The potential for high-intensity interval training to reduce cardiometabolic disease risk. Sports Med. 2012;42(6):489–509. https://doi.org/10.1016/j.metabol.2010.01.002.
62. Gibala MJ, Little JP. Just HIT it! A time-efficient exercise strategy to improve muscle insulin sensitivity. J Physiol. 2010;588(Pt 18):3341–2. https://doi.org/10.1113/jphysiol.2010.196303.
63. Tjonna AE, Leinan IM, Bartnes AT, Jenssen BM, Gibala MJ, Winett RA, Wisloff U. Low- and high-volume of intensive endurance training significantly improves maximal oxygen uptake after 10-weeks of training in healthy men. PLoS One. 2013;8(5):e65382. https://doi.org/10.1371/journal.pone.0065382.
64. van Aggel-Leijssen DP, Saris WH, Wagenmakers AJ, Senden JM, van Baak MA. Effect of exercise training at different intensities on fat metabolism of obese men. J Appl Physiol. 2002;92(3):1300–9. https://doi.org/10.1152/japplphysiol.00030.2001.
65. Salvadori A, Fanari P, Marzullo P, Codecasa F, Tovaglieri I, Cornacchia M, Brunani A, Luzi L, Longhini E. Short bouts of anaerobic exercise increase non-esterified fatty acids release in obesity. Eur J Nutr. 2014;53(1):243–9. https://doi.org/10.1007/s00394-013-0522-x.
66. Salvadori A, Fanari P, Marzullo P, Codecasa F, Tovaglieri I, Cornacchia M, Walker G, Brunani A, Longhini E. Dynamics of GH secretion during incremental exercise in obesity, before and after a short period of training at different work-loads. Clin Endocrinol. 2010;73(4):491–6. https://doi.org/10.1111/j.1365-2265.2010.03837.x.
67. Su L, Fu J, Sun S, Zhao G, Cheng W, Dou C, Quan M. Effects of HIIT and MICT on cardiovascular risk factors in adults with overweight and/or obesity: a meta-analysis. PLoS One. 2019;14(1):e0210644. https://doi.org/10.1371/journal.pone.0210644.
68. Baekkerud FH, Solberg F, Leinan IM, Wisloff U, Karlsen T, Rognmo O. Comparison of three popular exercise modalities on V O2max in overweight and obese. Med Sci Sports Exerc. 2016;48(3):491–8. https://doi.org/10.1249/MSS.0000000000000777.
69. Wewege M, van den Berg R, Ward RE, Keech A. The effects of high-intensity interval training vs. moderate-intensity continuous training on body composition in overweight and obese adults: a systematic review and meta-analysis. Obes Rev. 2017;18(6):635–46. https://doi.org/10.1111/obr.12532.
70. Lanzi S, Codecasa F, Cornacchia M, Maestrini S, Capodaglio P, Brunani A, Fanari P, Salvadori A, Malatesta D. Short-term HIIT and Fat max training increase aerobic and metabolic fitness in men with class II and III obesity. Obesity (Silver Spring). 2015;23(10):1987–94. https://doi.org/10.1002/oby.21206.
71. Houmard JA, Tanner CJ, Slentz CA, Duscha BD, McCartney JS, Kraus WE. Effect of the volume and intensity of exercise training on insulin sensitivity. J Appl Physiol. 2004;96(1):101–6. https://doi.org/10.1152/japplphysiol.00707.2003.
72. Lunt H, Draper N, Marshall HC, Logan FJ, Hamlin MJ, Shearman JP, Cotter JD, Kimber NE, Blackwell G, Frampton CM. High intensity interval training in a real world setting: a randomized controlled feasibility study in overweight inactive adults, measuring change in maximal oxygen uptake. PLoS One. 2014;9(1):e83256. https://doi.org/10.1371/journal.pone.0083256.
73. Dalle Grave R, Calugi S, Centis E, El Ghoch M, Marchesini G. Cognitive-behavioral strategies to increase the adherence to exercise in the management of obesity. J Obes. 2011;2011:348293. https://doi.org/10.1155/2011/348293.
74. Ramos-Campo DJ, Girard O, Perez A, Rubio-Arias JA. Additive stress of normobaric hypoxic conditioning to improve body mass loss and cardiometabolic markers in individuals with overweight or obesity: a systematic review and meta-analysis. Physiol Behav. 2019;207:28–40. https://doi.org/10.1016/j.physbeh.2019.04.027.

75. Urdampilleta A, Gonzalez-Muniesa P, Portillo MP, Martinez JA. Usefulness of combining intermittent hypoxia and physical exercise in the treatment of obesity. J Physiol Biochem. 2012;68(2):289–304. https://doi.org/10.1007/s13105-011-0115-1.
76. Browning RC. Locomotion mechanics in obese adults and children. Curr Obes Rep. 2012;1(3):152–9. https://doi.org/10.1007/s13679-012-0021-z.
77. Browning RC, McGowan CP, Kram R. Obesity does not increase external mechanical work per kilogram body mass during walking. J Biomech. 2009;42(14):2273–8. https://doi.org/10.1016/j.jbiomech.2009.06.046.
78. Fernandez Menendez A, Saubade M, Millet GP, Malatesta D. Energy-saving walking mechanisms in obese adults. J Appl Physiol (1985). 2019;126(5):1250–8. https://doi.org/10.1152/japplphysiol.00473.2018.
79. Malatesta D, Vismara L, Menegoni F, Galli M, Romei M, Capodaglio P. Mechanical external work and recovery at preferred walking speed in obese subjects. Med Sci Sports Exerc. 2009;41(2):426–34. https://doi.org/10.1249/MSS.0b013e31818606e7.
80. Malatesta D, Vismara L, Menegoni F, Grugni G, Capodaglio P. Effect of obesity onset on pendular energy transduction at spontaneous walking speed: Prader-Willi versus nonsyndromal obese individuals. Obesity (Silver Spring). 2013;21(12):E586–91. https://doi.org/10.1002/oby.20455.
81. Wearing SC, Hennig EM, Byrne NM, Steele JR, Hills AP. The biomechanics of restricted movement in adult obesity. Obes Rev. 2006;7(1):13–24. https://doi.org/10.1111/j.1467-789X.2006.00215.x.
82. Sheehan K, Gormley J. Gait and increased body weight (potential implications for musculoskeletal disease). Phys Ther Rev. 2012;17(2):91–8. https://doi.org/10.1179/1743288X11Y.0000000057.
83. Hootman JM, Macera CA, Ainsworth BE, Addy CL, Martin M, Blair SN. Epidemiology of musculoskeletal injuries among sedentary and physically active adults. Med Sci Sports Exerc. 2002;34(5):838–44. https://doi.org/10.1097/00005768-200205000-00017.
84. Girard O, Malatesta D, Millet GP. Walking in hypoxia: an efficient treatment to lessen mechanical constraints and improve health in obese individuals? Front Physiol. 2017;8:73. https://doi.org/10.3389/fphys.2017.00073.
85. Hobbins L, Hunter S, Gaoua N, Girard O. Normobaric hypoxic conditioning to maximize weight loss and ameliorate cardio-metabolic health in obese populations: a systematic review. Am J Phys Regul Integr Comp Phys. 2017;313(3):R251–64. https://doi.org/10.1152/ajpregu.00160.2017.
86. Kayser B, Verges S. Hypoxia, energy balance and obesity: from pathophysiological mechanisms to new treatment strategies. Obes Rev. 2013;14(7):579–92. https://doi.org/10.1111/obr.12034.
87. Navarrete-Opazo A, Mitchell GS. Therapeutic potential of intermittent hypoxia: a matter of dose. Am J Phys Regul Integr Comp Phys. 2014;307(10):R1181–97. https://doi.org/10.1152/ajpregu.00208.2014.
88. Kong Z, Zang Y, Hu Y. Normobaric hypoxia training causes more weight loss than normoxia training after a 4-week residential camp for obese young adults. Sleep Breath. 2014;18(3):591–7. https://doi.org/10.1007/s11325-013-0922-4.
89. Netzer NC, Chytra R, Küpper T. Low intense physical exercise in normobaric hypoxia leads to more weight loss in obese people than low intense physical exercise in normobaric sham hypoxia. Sleep Breath. 2008;12(2):129–34. https://doi.org/10.1007/s11325-007-0149-3.
90. Wiesner S, Haufe S, Engeli S, Mutschler H, Haas U, Luft FC, Jordan J. Influences of normobaric hypoxia training on physical fitness and metabolic risk markers in overweight to obese subjects. Obesity (Silver Spring). 2010;18(1):116–20. https://doi.org/10.1038/oby.2009.193.
91. Fernandez Menendez A, Saudan G, Sperisen L, Hans D, Saubade M, Millet GP, Malatesta D. Effects of short-term normobaric hypoxic walking training on energetics and mechanics of gait in adults with obesity. Obesity (Silver Spring). 2018;26(5):819–27. https://doi.org/10.1002/oby.22131.

92. Haufe S, Wiesner S, Engeli S, Luft FC, Jordan J. Influences of normobaric hypoxia training on metabolic risk markers in human subjects. Med Sci Sports Exerc. 2008;40(11):1939–44. https://doi.org/10.1249/MSS.0b013e31817f1988.
93. Camacho-Cardenosa A, Camacho-Cardenosa M, Brazo-Sayavera J, Burtscher M, Timon R, Olcina G. Effects of high-intensity interval training under normobaric hypoxia on cardiometabolic risk markers in overweight/obese women. High Alt Med Biol. 2018;19(4):356–66. https://doi.org/10.1089/ham.2018.0059.
94. Camacho-Cardenosa A, Camacho-Cardenosa M, Burtscher M, Martinez-Guardado I, Timon R, Brazo-Sayavera J, Olcina G. High-intensity interval training in normobaric hypoxia leads to greater body fat loss in overweight/obese women than high-intensity interval training in normoxia. Front Physiol. 2018;9:60. https://doi.org/10.3389/fphys.2018.00060.
95. Kong Z, Shi Q, Nie J, Tong TK, Song L, Yi L, Hu Y. High-intensity interval training in normobaric hypoxia improves cardiorespiratory fitness in overweight chinese young women. Front Physiol. 2017;8:175. https://doi.org/10.3389/fphys.2017.00175.
96. Borel JC, Wuyam B, Chouri-Pontarollo N, Deschaux C, Levy P, Pepin JL. During exercise noninvasive ventilation in chronic restrictive respiratory failure. Respir Med. 2008;102(5):711–9. https://doi.org/10.1016/j.rmed.2007.12.017.
97. van 't Hul A, Kwakkel G, Gosselink R. The acute effects of noninvasive ventilatory support during exercise on exercise endurance and dyspnea in patients with chronic obstructive pulmonary disease: a systematic review. J Cardpulm Rehabil. 2002;22(4):290–7. https://doi.org/10.1097/00008483-200207000-00013.
98. Babb TG, Ranasinghe KG, Comeau LA, Semon TL, Schwartz B. Dyspnea on exertion in obese women: association with an increased oxygen cost of breathing. Am J Respir Crit Care Med. 2008;178(2):116–23. https://doi.org/10.1164/rccm.200706-875OC.
99. Pepin JL, Tamisier R, Levy P. Obstructive sleep apnoea and metabolic syndrome: put CPAP efficacy in a more realistic perspective. Thorax. 2012;67(12):1025–7. https://doi.org/10.1136/thoraxjnl-2012-202807.
100. Vivodtzev I, Tamisier R, Croteau M, Borel JC, Grangier A, Wuyam B, Levy P, Minville C, Series F, Maltais F, Pepin JL. Ventilatory support or respiratory muscle training as adjuncts to exercise in obese CPAP-treated patients with obstructive sleep apnoea: a randomised controlled trial. Thorax. 2018; https://doi.org/10.1136/thoraxjnl-2017-211152.
101. Younes M. Proportional assist ventilation, a new approach to ventilatory support. Theory Am Rev Respir Dis. 1992;145(1):114–20. https://doi.org/10.1164/ajrccm/145.1.114.
102. Dreher M, Kabitz HJ, Burgardt V, Walterspacher S, Windisch W. Proportional assist ventilation improves exercise capacity in patients with obesity. Respiration. 2010;80(2):106–11. https://doi.org/10.1159/000245272.
103. Jakicic JM, Rogers RJ, Davis KK, Collins KA. Role of physical activity and exercise in treating patients with overweight and obesity. Clin Chem. 2018;64(1):99–107. https://doi.org/10.1373/clinchem.2017.272443.

2 Which Strength Training?

Damiano Formenti, Luca Cavaggioni, and Giampietro Alberti

Key Points

- Resistance training is a key element in the treatment of obesity.
- High-intensity resistance training should be used with caution; low-intensity resistance training should be preferred because of reduced mechanical stress on the joints.
- In particular, low-intensity, low-velocity resistance training is well tolerated and appears to provide evidence-based benefits in the obese population.
- The combination of low-intensity, low-velocity strength training with aerobic training and a supervised dietary plan lead to weight loss, improved function, postural control and independence in daily life activities.
- Low-velocity resistance training modalities need to be investigated for the obese population.

D. Formenti
Department of Biomedical Sciences for Health, Università degli Studi di Milano, Milan, Italy

Department of Biotechnology and Life Sciences, University of Insubria, Varese, Italy
e-mail: damiano.formenti@uninsubria.it

L. Cavaggioni (✉)
Department of Biomedical Sciences for Health, Università degli Studi di Milano, Milan, Italy

IRCCS Istituto Auxologico Italiano, Obesity Unit and Laboratory of Nutrition and Obesity Research, Department of Endocrine and Metabolic Diseases, Milan, Italy
e-mail: luca.cavaggioni@unimi.it

G. Alberti
Department of Biomedical Sciences for Health, Università degli Studi di Milano, Milan, Italy
e-mail: giampietro.alberti@unimi.it

P. Capodaglio (ed.), *Rehabilitation Interventions in the Patient with Obesity*,
https://doi.org/10.1007/978-3-030-32274-8_2

2.1 Strength Training in Obese Individuals

Strength training has been demonstrated to be beneficial in reducing cardiometabolic risk and disability in obese and overweight individuals. The inclusion of strength training within a multidimensional exercise therapy program (combined with both aerobic and neuromotor training) has been promoted by the scientific community over the last years. Scientific associations as the American College of Sports Medicine [1, 2] and the American Heart Association [3] provided recommendations for the use of resistance training in those populations. Several studies showed that muscle mass was negatively associated with an increased risk of mortality [4] and metabolic syndrome [5]. In this wake, the key role played by lean muscle mass and increased muscular strength for wellness and quality of life is evident.

It should be noted that obesity may be associated with sarcopenia. Sarcopenia is a condition characterized by progressive loss of muscle mass, strength and poor quality of life [6]. This condition of loss in muscle mass accompanied by an increase in body fat with a considerable weakness is defined as sarcopenic obesity. The presence of obesity combined with sarcopenia implies also many functional limitations in performing daily life physical activities requiring muscular strength [7]. Such limitations were shown by Rolland and colleagues, who compared difficulties in walking, climbing stairs and rising from a chair in a sample of 1308 women divided into four categories: healthy body composition, sarcopenic, obese and sarcopenic obese. The Authors showed that obese had a higher probability of having functional limitations, whereas the sarcopenic obese individuals were impaired in climbing stairs [7]. This showed how sarcopenia and obesity yield synergistic negative effects in daily life functional movements and quality of life. Overall, there is a clear association between increased fat mass, physical inactivity and loss of muscle mass/strength, suggesting that physical activity plays a protective role for the prevention but also the management of sarcopenic obesity and body composition.

Many lines of evidence suggest that strength training may be an appropriate modality for contrasting sarcopenia and metabolic risk factors, such as control of body weight and adipose tissue. In this perspective, this chapter aims to describe the potential of strength training in the treatment of obesity. From a practical point of view, we also wanted to provide indications for defining a strength training program. Particular emphasis was given to a non-conventional resistance training method based on the reduction of muscular action velocity particularly suited for obese individuals [8, 9]. Together with the practical recommendations for structuring a resistance training program, we should acknowledge the importance of enhancing self-awareness of obese individuals in engaging in resistance training and, more generally, in physical activity, focusing on the quality of movement [10] and postural control [11]. Increased awareness about the importance of physical activity is a requisite for successful treatment of obesity. A physical activity program should include aerobic and resistance training, as well as neuromotor

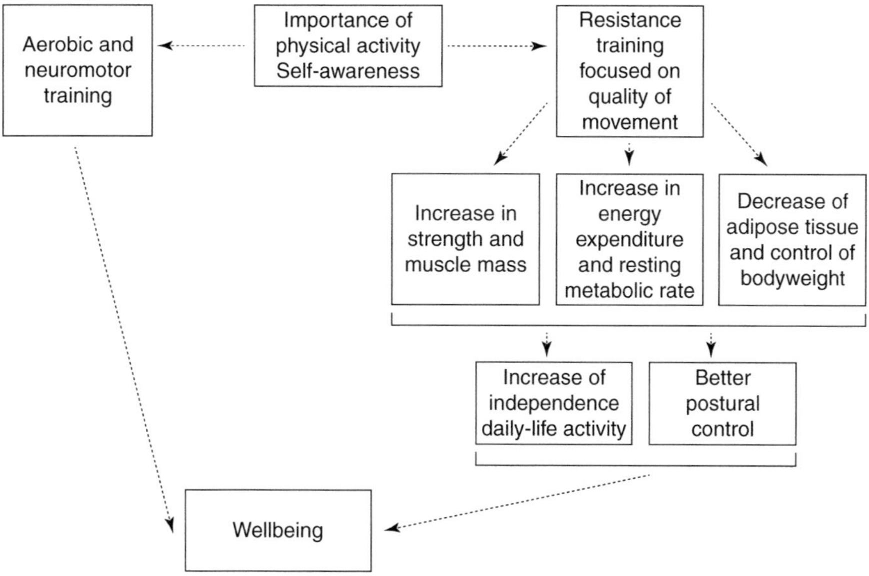

Fig. 2.1 Overview of the effects of resistance training for promoting well-being

training [12]. The latter should be focused on the quality of movement, because it has positive effects on muscle mass and strength, increasing energy expenditure and reducing adipose tissue leading to a better postural control and performance of daily life activities. The integration of all of these aspects is fundamental in reducing obesity-related disability (Fig. 2.1).

2.2 Metabolic Effects

It has been demonstrated that regular participation in a strength training program is beneficial for promoting weight loss [13]. However, a decrease in fat mass was found to be usually associated with an increase in lean body mass, thus inducing a small-to-null effect on the control of body weight [14, 15]. Taking part in a strength training program is not necessarily accompanied by a decrease in total body weight. Strength training, as other types of physical activities for obese patients, is usually prescribed together with a dietary restriction regimen. Indeed, Geliebter et al. demonstrated that an 8-week strength training program accompanied by a supervised nutritional counselling was beneficial for reducing fat-free mass [16].

In addition to a decrease in fat-free mass and an increase in lean body mass, beneficial effects were also present on energy expenditure, with an increase in resting metabolic rate. This process was found to be modulated by the muscle protein turnover [17], thanks to the requirement of elevated ATP level consumption during the whole-body protein synthesis.

In a study by Kraemer and colleagues, 35 overweight individuals were randomly assigned into four groups: a dietary group, a dietary group that performed aerobic training, a dietary group that performed both strength and aerobic training and a control group for 12 weeks [18]. The three experimental groups showed a significant reduction in weight loss, without significant differences in serum glucose, cortisol, testosterone and high-density lipoprotein (HDL) concentrations. This research demonstrated that a combination of resistance and aerobic training with a dietary regimen contributes to limit the physiological decrement in fat-free mass and muscular strength, as compared to diet only [18].

A further study on the potential effect of resistance training in overweight individuals was conducted with the aim of assessing whether increases in lean body mass and decreases in fat mass over 15 weeks of supervised resistance training could be preserved after 6 months of non-supervised training [19]. The body composition remained almost unchanged over the 6 months of non-supervised training. The authors concluded that supervised resistance training could be useful for improving body composition and that such improvements can be maintained over time also in a following period of non-supervised training. These findings lead to two important considerations. Firstly, a supervised resistance training program is beneficial for improving body composition in middle-aged women, thus laying the foundation for promoting resistance training in limiting and preventing age-associated fat gains. Secondly, it should be acknowledged that the immediate efficacy of a supervised program could be seen also when performing a consecutive non-supervised resistance training program. Individuals involved in a supervised training program were able to learn and practice correctly specific exercises under the guidance of an expert trainer, thus boosting compliance to home exercise. This point is of fundamental importance for individuals not so used to engage in regular physical activity.

Another study [20] investigated the effects of an 8-week resistance training program on body composition in obese individuals. Twenty-eight males were randomly assigned to a resistance training group or a control group. Outcome measures were body mass, percentage body fat, lean body mass, fat mass, waist-to-hip ratio and body mass index, assessed before and after the experimental period. Results indicated that the resistance training group was able to significantly improve body mass, percentage body fat and lean body mass with respect to the control group, thus supporting a relationship between resistance training and body composition.

Together with the positive effects on body composition, it is well known that physical exercise may positively affect also circulating blood lipid levels. Therefore, parallel to the assessment of body composition, outcome measures of studies on the effect of resistance training on obese individuals included also blood lipid levels. A longitudinal controlled trial [21] was conducted to investigate the effects of a 12-week strength and aerobic training on body mass index, weight, fat mass, serum lipid profile and insulin resistance in obese women who cannot follow any sort of restricted diets. Sixty obese women with eating disorders were enrolled and randomly divided into three groups: control group with no exercise, aerobic exercise group and strength exercise group. Results were that body mass index, waist and weight measurements, serum lipid profile, triglyceride and total cholesterol levels decreased significantly in each of the study groups. However, it is worth noticing that only the aerobic exercise group induced a reduction in low-density lipoprotein cholesterol level, fat mass and insulin resistance, as compared to the other two groups. Although outcomes of this controlled trial indicated that aerobic exercise seems to be superior as compared to strength exercise in reducing fat mass and insulin resistance, this study indicated that the two experimental groups (aerobic exercise and strength exercise) were able to ameliorate body fat composition with a concomitant metabolic effect also in patients with severe eating disorders. Overall, these experimental studies provide further evidence of the beneficial effects of resistance training for a better control of body weight and body composition in overweight individuals [18–21].

Considerations are also needed for the potential beneficial effects of strength training on the mobilization of visceral adipose tissue. Originally, body fat tissue is located into two main sections with various metabolic characteristics: subcutaneous adipose tissue and visceral adipose tissue. Abdominal obesity, which is characterised by an increased adipose tissue surrounding organs within the abdominal region, is also denoted as visceral obesity. Excessive visceral adipose tissue was found to be associated with dyslipidaemia, hypertension, insulin resistance, type 2 diabetes and cardiovascular diseases [22].

Numerous studies have investigated the potential role of resistance training to contrast visceral adipose tissue [23–26]. Ross et al. investigated the influence of diet in combination with aerobic or resistance training on adipose tissue distribution in 24 obese women. The combination of moderate energy restriction with resistance or aerobic exercise induced significant decrements in visceral adipose tissue and subcutaneous adipose tissue. Moreover, the same research group structured an almost identical study design by adding an experimental group which followed a diet-only program. The main results were that diet combined with aerobic training and diet combined with resistance training were superior for preserving skeletal muscle tissue and mobilizing subcutaneous adipose tissue from the abdominal region than diet-only group [24].

These studies emphasized the key role that the resistance training, associated with an energy restriction program, can play for determining the reduction of visceral adipose tissue. Overall, there is evidence supporting the notion that resistance training can effectively alter body composition in overweight individuals, regardless of dietary restriction by acting on visceral adipose tissue in abdominal region.

Strong evidence derived from epidemiological studies showed a relationship between obesity, cardiovascular diseases [27] and type 2 diabetes [28]. It is well known that factors such as cholesterol, elevated plasma glucose and blood pressure contribute to increase the risk for cardiovascular diseases [29]. Such risks may be reduced by an adequate physical activity program. The literature focused on the relationship between physical exercise and control of glycaemia in patients with type 2 diabetes [30].

An experimental study provided evidence for the positive effect of resistance training in the treatment of type 2 diabetes individuals [15]. The authors demonstrated that a resistance training program involving multiple exercises at high intensity induced a slight decrease in glycated haemoglobin. Another study by the same research group [31] investigated whether improvements in glycaemic control and body composition after 6 months of supervised resistance training could be maintained after an additional 6 months of home-based resistance training. Although glycaemic control was not maintained, muscular strength and lean body mass were preserved, demonstrating the effectiveness of home-based training.

2.3 Types of Strength

Resistance training can include different types of strength, each of which may be relevant for certain individuals and their own characteristics. For clarity, in the present chapter we provide a brief classification of the types of strength in terms of the type of muscle action, the qualities of strength and the force-velocity relationship. Our aim is to describe the strength-related variables that may be useful for practitioners for understanding, planning and structuring appropriate resistance training programs adapted for overweight individuals [12]. For simplicity, we have decided to refer also to the definitions provided in a distinguished recent book about strength training and periodization [32].

Before describing the different qualities of strength and the force-velocity relationship, it is worth providing a brief overview on the types of muscle action [33]. Three basic types of muscle action are recognized: concentric, eccentric and isometric. The term muscle action should be preferred than muscle contraction. This is because contraction means shortening, which does not appropriately define two of the three muscle actions. In concentric muscle action, as the contractile force is greater than the resistive force, the muscle shortens. The forces generated within the muscle to shorten it are greater than the external forces which act to stretch it. Typical concentric actions of quadriceps femoris are climbing stairs. In eccentric muscle action, as the contractile force is lower than the resistive force, the muscle lengthens. The forces generated within the muscle to shorten it are lower than the external forces which act to stretch it. Typical eccentric actions of quadriceps femoris are descending stairs. Contrary to what happens during concentric and eccentric, in isometric muscle action, the contractile force is equal to the resistive force, and therefore the muscle length does not change. The forces generated within the muscle which act to shorten it are of the same amount of the external forces acting at its tendons to stretch it. A typical isometric action can be found when the muscles of the hand and forearm grip an object. In this action, muscles generate enough force to prevent the falling of the object while the joints of the hand do not move. All these three types of muscle action can be present within a resistance exercise.

The desired effect of a strength training program may refer to one of the following three qualities of strength: maximum strength, muscular power and local muscular endurance. Maximum strength is the highest force applied by the neuromuscular system during a contraction. It can be increased through a combination of neural and structural adaptations. From a practical viewpoint, maximum strength refers to the heaviest overload that an individual can lift in one attempt and is usually expressed as 100% of maximum repetition (1RM). 1RM is a common measure of muscular strength and is defined as the value of resistance against which a given movement can be performed only once [34]. It is important to know the 1RM of individuals engaged in resistance training in each exercise for calculating loads (in percent of 1RM) to apply appropriately. Careful considerations should be done to determine the 1RM. Direct assessment of 1RM needs time and may increase risk of cardiovascular diseases, as well as of muscle-skeletal injuries. Therefore, an indirect assessment of 1RM should be preferred [34].

Muscular power is the ability to exert the highest force in the shortest time and depends on two abilities as strength and speed. Athletes have time constraints in the majority of sports and therefore should apply force as fast as possible. Training power and exerting the highest force in the shortest time require an almost perfect capacity of controlling the whole movement through the execution of the exercise. Being a peculiarity of sport disciplines, it can be considered very marginal for overweight and obese individuals, where training has the purpose of incrementing well-being and quality of life, rather than reaching the highest performance.

A strength ability which should be instead developed for obese is local muscular endurance. It is the ability of a muscle, or a group of muscles, to sustain a certain work as repeated contractions against a submaximal resistance for a prolonged period. Examples are performing numerous repetitions in specific exercises using a fixed load (such as overload with a percentage of 1RM or body weight).

Generally, muscular strength, power and hypertrophy are the main goals in resistance training; adequate training adaptations depend on the correct combination of numerous variables, such as external load, intensity, volume, exercise selection, exercise order, rest period and the velocity of muscle action [35]. A training variable which is quite often not considered, but essential in obtaining the desired strength responses, is the velocity of muscle action [36]. This variable is important because modifies the time under tension (TUT), muscle activation and hormonal and metabolic responses, which are key factors for strength and hypertrophy development [37].

Muscle force-velocity is an important relationship in the field of strength training. The force-velocity curve illustrates that the greater the amount muscular force generated, the slower the muscle shortening and the related movement velocity (and *vice versa*). Performing a 1RM involves slower movement velocities, the amount of force generated is maximum but power is low. Conversely, maximal power is produced at intermediate velocities by lifting light to moderate loads. As the speed increases, the force production would diminish due to number of actomyosin cross-bridges created: when the speed is high, the number of active cross-bridges is lower [38].

2.4 Improving Muscle Mass and Strength

Maximizing hypertrophic response to resistance training can be reached by manipulating exercise program variables, such as type and order of exercises, length of rest intervals, intensity of maximal load and training volume [39]. In overweight individuals, resistance training could be beneficial for many aspects previously mentioned. The available literature provides a wide range of parameters regarding strength training. As concern the load, there is a large consensus in using moderate-to-high loads

Table 2.1 Overview of some studies on resistance training in overweight individuals, (−) decrease, (+) increase, *reps* repetitions, *1RM* one maximal repetition

Authors	Participants	Resistance training variables	Main effects
Dunstan et al. [15]	Older adults	50–85% 1RM, 3 sets, 8–10 reps, 16 weeks	– Body weight – Fat mass + Lean mass
Maiorana et al. [40]	Middle-aged adults	55–65% 1RM, 3 sets, 15 reps, 8 weeks	+ Muscular strength – % fat mass – Waste/hip ratio
Castaneda et al. [41]	Middle-aged adults	60–80% 1RM, 3 sets, 16 weeks	+ Sodium-dependent glucose co-transporter system
Loimaala et al. [42]	Middle-aged adults	70–80% 1RM, 3 sets, 10–12 reps, 12 months	+ Muscular strength – Baroreflex sensitivity
Shaw and Shaw [20]	Males	60% 1RM, 3 sets, 8 weeks	– Body mass – % body fat + Lean mass
Rice et al. [43]	Middle-aged males	80% 1RM, 1 set, 8–12 reps, 16 weeks	– Body weight = Effects on lowering fasting insulin
Manning et al. [44]	Middle-aged women	60–70% 1RM, 3 sets, 6–8 reps, 12 weeks	+ Muscular strength = Lipid profiles
Vincent et al. [45]	Older adults	50–80% 1RM, 8–13 reps, 24 weeks	+ Muscular strength – Systemic oxidative stress levels
Lambers et al. [46]	Diabetes participants	60–85% 1RM, 3 sets, 10–15 reps, 12 weeks	+ Upper and lower body strength – Cholesterol and glycosylated haemoglobin
Comstock et al. [47]	Young men	85–95% 1RM, 3 set, 10 reps, one session	= Perceptual measures and muscle damage

for three sets performing a moderate number of repetitions. Table 2.1 shows the parameters commonly used in resistance training protocols of some of the previous studies published on the effect of resistance training in obese. It is possible to notice that the intensity is often superior than 50% of 1RM. Accordingly, to increase muscle mass and strength, high-intensity resistance training has been considered the most effective intervention [35].

It should be noted that high-intensity resistance training is based on relatively high load (~70–85% of 1RM) which induces large mechanical stress that would result in increased systolic blood pressure and increased risk of orthopaedic injuries [3, 48, 49]. Therefore, using a reduced load in resistance training appears of fundamental importance for those individuals who have not a correct technique of exercise execution and who cannot overload osteo-articular structures, such as obese.

Recently, particular attention has been devoted to repetition duration (the velocity of muscle action), which may have an impact on muscular adaptations [36]. Reducing the velocity of muscle action during both concentric and eccentric action phases permits to increase the TUT (i.e. the time the muscle is under tension).

Studies have reported that a combination of relatively low intensity (~30–60% of 1RM) with slow movement (reduced velocity of muscle action) during resistance training was able to significantly increase muscle size and strength in untrained young [50, 51] and old adults [52, 53]. One of the physiological mechanisms of muscle hypertrophy is the lowered peripheral muscular oxygenation occurring during exercise [54], which can be exhacerbated during resistance training with slow movement [51, 55]. Moreover, an increase in TUT results in an increment of levels of metabolic stress within muscle (as a result of the intramuscular environment with reduced oxygenation) [56], which in turn stimulates growth hormone (GH) secretion, cell swelling, production of reaction oxygen species and increased recruitment of fast-twitch fibres [57].

To the best of the authors' knowledge, there is only one study that investigated the effects of relatively low-intensity resistance training with slow movement on strength in obese [9]. Forty obese female patients were assigned randomly to a slow (ST) and a traditional (TT) resistance training groups. The ST was composed by five repetitions for five sets on the leg press and leg extension machines. The duration of each repetition (concentric and eccentric phases) was 6 s for leg press and 5 s for leg extension. The initial load was 50% of 1RM, which was gradually reduced by 20% of the previous load for each bout. The TT protocol included the same exercises with six repetitions for five bouts using an intensity of 80% of 1RM. Although the velocity of muscle action of the TT group was not specified in that manuscript, as named traditional training, we can assume that a normal velocity was presumably adopted (1–2 s for phases of repetition). Both groups performed ten training sessions. Similar improvements in isokinetic strength variables were observed for both groups, but a larger decrement in knee pain and perceived fatigue was found in ST with respect to TT group. This study provides support for the efficacy of relatively low-intensity resistance training with slow movement for obese patients as it can induce significant strength gains with a relatively lower load on the osteo-articular structures, together with a reduced perception of pain and fatigue [9].

Similar to the low-intensity resistance training with slow movement, another resistance training method (i.e. blood flow restriction resistance training) has been demonstrated to be efficacy for improving strength and muscle mass without the need of using high load [58]. Blood flow restriction resistance training, also denoted as Kaatsu training, implies a decreasing of muscular blood flow by applying devices such as blood pressure cuff or restrictive straps, thus inducing the pooling of blood with a consequent muscular deoxygenation [56]. Recently, the safety of blood flow restriction resistance training has been questioned [59] because of the increased blood pressure and potential undesired coagulation at sites of vascular damage or atherosclerosis. Obese and overweight individuals are known to be susceptible to vascular dysfunction [60]. Moreover, a decreased vasodilation capacity has been observed after resistance training with restricted venous blood flow [61].

With this in mind, a recent study tested the hypothesis that a 3-week training period of unilateral knee extension blood flow restriction exercise in overweight individuals would increase muscle strength and decrease vascular reactivity in both limbs [62]. Although strength increased, a decrease in endothelial function and vascular autoregulation was observed. These findings described the potential negative effects on the mechanisms of vascular regulation produced by blood flow restriction resistance training for overweight individuals, increasing risks for blood vessel dysfunction and remodelling, which are known to be risk factors for cardiovascular diseases. This suggests an impairment of vascular autoregulation that may exacerbate the endothelial dysfunction, which commonly occurs in overweight individuals [62].

On the same line, a systematic review investigated the effects of blood flow restriction exercise on blood haemostasis in healthy individuals and patients with known diseases (i.e. hypertension, diabetes, obesity, ischemic heart disease) [63]. Overall, the main finding was that blood flow restriction exercise seems not to exacerbate the activation of the coagulation system nor enhance fibrinolytic activity. However, the limited number of studies included in the review suggests the need for more randomized controlled trials to properly verify the safety of blood flow restriction resistance training on vasal regulation in individuals with increased risk for thromboembolic disorders, impaired fibrinolysis, diabetes and obesity [64]. It is worth noticing that, when blood flow restriction cannot be applied in individuals with potential risk factors (obese, diabetes, cardiovascular disease), the authors of this review proposed to prescribe low-intensity resistance training with slow movement [63]. This attributes increased value to such method that is proposed as safety and efficacy strength training with great potentialities for obese individuals.

2.5 Recommendations for Practitioners

Traditional resistance training programs, despite relatively low intensity (<50% of 1RM, as in the blood flow restriction and low-intensity resistance training with slow movement), are mainly based on the use of isotonic machines and free weights. When using external equipment, individuals should master a proper technique for a correct exercise execution. This requires time to learn the proper modality and an expert trainer who supervises the session. A key point is to focus on the quality of the movement patterns, rather than on the quantity (doing less but better). Obese patients usually show poor motor control and self-awareness, which are important prerequisites for a correct execution of the exercise movement [65, 66]. Therefore, trainers should firstly aim to improve postural control and increase self-awareness, defining appropriate progressive goals. Resistance training should begin after those goals have been achieved. In this phase, it is important to provide the correct cues, to pay attention to the patient's feedback and to establish a trustworthy relationship with the patient.

Only once the proper execution of the exercise movement has been achieved, patients should start the resistance training program, consistently supervised by expert trainers. Low-intensity, low-velocity resistance training is to be preferred. Reducing the velocity of muscle action in both phases (eccentric and concentric), in fact, allows to pay attention to the correct execution modality and to the quality of movement. Reducing the velocity of muscle action allows a better breathing pattern and a correct body posture while performing resistance exercises [10]. Moreover, it is known that supervised resistance training is more effective than a non-supervised one for improving muscular strength [67].

Also, one of the main goals of exercise is to enhance self-awareness on the importance of being active, together with boosting the perception of well-being deriving from regular exercise. In this multidimensional perspective, individuals participating in a supervised resistance training program benefit from a correct execution modality and body posture, which serve for promoting adherence to a resistance exercise scheme in a non-supervised context (e.g. home, park).

We suggest low-intensity, low-velocity resistance training programs based on exercises that do not require special equipment and that can be easily performed individually without supervision. Non-instrumental resistance training with slow movements using body weight was found to be effective for improving body composition in healthy old individuals [68]. Moreover, a recent study provided evidences on the positive effects of resistance training on muscle strength in elderly individuals with either normal (1 s for each phase) and slow speed of movement (3 s for each phase) using body weight [52]. Based on these studies, the use of overloads (isotonic machines and/or free weights) in resistance training for health purposes does not appear mandatory. Given the didactic value of slow movement and the possibility to perform resistance training without supervision in a non-controlled environment, we recommend low-intensity, low-velocity resistance training programs for obese individuals using body weight and/or elastic bands. Some practical indications are the following:

1. At the beginning of the exercise period, an important focus should be given to self-awareness, postural control and breathing pattern. Strength training should be performed at low intensity and/or using body weight, so that individuals learn the proper exercise technique supervised by an expert trainer.
2. In low-intensity, low-velocity resistance training, we suggest a load of 50% of 1RM with slow speed of movement (3–5 s for each phase without rest) [8]. Blood flow restriction can be modulated by increasing the duration of the concentric and eccentric phases and reducing the relaxation time (the pause between repetitions), which induces a prolonged time under tension [55]. A load of 50% of 1RM performed at slow speed is adequate to generate a sufficient intramuscular pressure that reduces the muscle's blood flow and muscle oxygenation, mimicking the physiological, neuromuscular and hormonal adaptations that occur in blood flow restriction resistance training. Similarly, also for resistance training using body weight and/or elastic bands, velocity of muscle action should be reduced and controlled with a metronome.

   Perspectively, the effects of even slower contractions that increase the duration of each muscle action phase [69] should be studied, with the aim of reducing the exercise time to a still effective training regimen and possibly increase adherence to exercise prescription in obese patients.

3. For each muscle group, five progressive steps with slow movement should be suggested:
   (a) A single set without reaching muscular failure.
   (b) More sets without reaching muscular failure (e.g., two or three sets).
   (c) A single set reaching muscular failure.
   (d) More sets reaching muscular failure (e.g., two or three sets).
   (e) A single set with a gradual reduction of load until reaching muscular failure. This approach was previously proposed [70] and more recently used for obese individuals [9].
4. A whole-body kinetic chain approach is to be preferred: all major muscle groups are trained including upper body (pulling, pushing), torso (rotations) and lower body (squatting, lunging) movements. The choice of exercises should be based individually.
5. Global movements should be preferred, also performed with small tools (e.g. elastic bands, kettlebells), with the aim to ameliorate physical function in daily life activities.
6. Generally, emphasis should be devoted to the quality of movement. This approach intends to increase the self-awareness of the beneficial effects of resistance training and the feeling of well-being, thus providing the bases for continuing resistance training in a non-supervised environment.

References

1. Pescatello LS, MacDonald HV, Lamberti L, Johnson BT. Exercise for hypertension: a prescription update integrating existing recommendations with emerging research. Curr Hypertens Rep. 2015;17(11):87.
2. Pescatello LS, Franklin BA, Fagard R, Farquhar WB, Kelley GA, Ray CA, et al. American College of Sports Medicine position stand. Exercise and hypertension. Med Sci Sports Exerc. 2004;36(3):533–53.
3. Pollock ML, Franklin BA, Balady GJ, Chaitman BL, Fleg JL, Fletcher B, et al. Resistance exercise in individuals with and without cardiovascular disease. Circulation. 2000;101(7):828–33.
4. FitzGerald SJ, Barlow CE, Kampert JB, Morrow JR, Jackson AW, Blair SN. Muscular fitness and all-cause mortality: prospective observations. J Phys Act Health. 2004;1(1):7–18.
5. Jurca R, Lamonte MJ, Barlow CE, Kampert JB, Church TS, Blair SN. Association of muscular strength with incidence of metabolic syndrome in men. Med Sci Sports Exerc. 2005;37(11):1849–55.
6. Santilli V, Bernetti A, Mangone M, Paoloni M. Clinical definition of sarcopenia. Clin Cases Miner Bone Metab. 2014;11(3):177–80.
7. Rolland Y, Lauwers-Cances V, Cristini C, Abellan van Kan G, Janssen I, Morley JE, et al. Difficulties with physical function associated with obesity, sarcopenia, and sarcopenic-obesity in community-dwelling elderly women: the EPIDOS (EPIDemiologie de l'OSteoporose) Study. Am J Clin Nutr. 2009;89(6):1895–900.
8. Alberti G, Cavaggioni L, Silvaggi N, Caumo A, Garufi M. Resistance training with blood flow restriction using the modulation of the muscle's contraction velocity. Strength Cond J. 2013;35(1):42–7.
9. Scarin S, Aspesi V, Malchiodi Albedi G, Cimolin V, Cau N, Galli S, et al. Slow versus traditional strength training in obese female participants: preliminary results. Int J Rehabil Res. 2019;42(2):120–5.

10. Skjaerven LH, Kristoffersen K, Gard G. An eye for movement quality: a phenomenological study of movement quality reflecting a group of physiotherapists' understanding of the phenomenon. Physiother Theory Pract. 2008;24(1):13–27.
11. Fabris de Souza SA, Faintuch J, Valezi AC, Sant'Anna AF, Gama-Rodrigues JJ, de Batista Fonseca IC, et al. Postural changes in morbidly obese patients. Obes Surg. 2005;15(7):1013–6.
12. American College of Sports Medicine, Riebe D, Ehrman JK, Liguori G, Magal M. ACSM's guidelines for exercise testing and prescription. 10th ed. Philadelphia: Wolters Kluwer; 2018.
13. Sarsan A, Ardiç F, Ozgen M, Topuz O, Sermez Y. The effects of aerobic and resistance exercises in obese women. Clin Rehabil. 2006;20(9):773–82.
14. Cauza E, Hanusch-Enserer U, Strasser B, Ludvik B, Metz-Schimmerl S, Pacini G, et al. The relative benefits of endurance and strength training on the metabolic factors and muscle function of people with type 2 diabetes mellitus. Arch Phys Med Rehabil. 2005;86(8):1527–33.
15. Dunstan DW, Daly RM, Owen N, Jolley D, De Courten M, Shaw J, et al. High-intensity resistance training improves glycemic control in older patients with type 2 diabetes. Diabetes Care. 2002;25(10):1729–36.
16. Geliebter A, Maher MM, Gerace L, Gutin B, Heymsfield SB, Hashim SA. Effects of strength or aerobic training on body composition, resting metabolic rate, and peak oxygen consumption in obese dieting subjects. Am J Clin Nutr. 1997;66(3):557–63.
17. Welle S, Nair KS. Relationship of resting metabolic rate to body composition and protein turnover. Am J Phys. 1990;258(6 Pt 1):E990–8.
18. Kraemer W, Volek J, Clark K, Gordon S, Puhl S, Koziris L, et al. Influence of exercise training on physiological and performance changes with weight loss in men. Med Sci Sports Exerc. 1999;31(9):1320–9.
19. Schmitz KH, Jensen MD, Kugler KC, Jeffery RW, Leon AS. Strength training for obesity prevention in midlife women. Int J Obes. 2003;27(3):326–33.
20. Shaw I, Shaw BS. Consequence of resistance training on body composition and coronary artery disease risk. Cardiovasc J South Afr. 2006;17(3):111–6.
21. Fenkci S, Sarsan A, Rota S, Ardic F. Effects of resistance or aerobic exercises on metabolic parameters in obese women who are not on a diet. Adv Ther. 2006;23(3):404–13.
22. Hunter G, Kekes-Szabo T, Snyder S, Nicholson C, Nyikos I, Berland L. Fat distribution, physical activity, and cardiovascular risk factors. Med Sci Sports Exerc. 1997;29(3):362–9.
23. Hunter GR, Bryan DR, Wetzstein CJ, Zuckerman PA, Bamman MM. Resistance training and intra-abdominal adipose tissue in older men and women. Med Sci Sports Exerc. 2002;34(6):1023–8.
24. Ross R, Rissanen J, Pedwell H, Clifford J, Shragge P. Influence of diet and exercise on skeletal muscle and visceral adipose tissue in men. J Appl Physiol. 1996;81(6):2445–55.
25. Ross R, Rissanen J. Mobilization of visceral and subcutaneous adipose tissue in response to energy restriction and exercise. Am J Clin Nutr. 1994;60(5):695–703.
26. Treuth MS, Ryan AS, Pratley RE, Rubin MA, Miller JP, Nicklas BJ, et al. Effects of strength training on total and regional body composition in older men. J Appl Physiol. 1994;77(2):614–20.
27. Wilson PWF, D'Agostino RB, Sullivan L, Parise H, Kannel WB. Overweight and obesity as determinants of cardiovascular risk: the Framingham experience. Arch Intern Med. 2002;162(16):1867–72.
28. Maggio CA, Pi-Sunyer FX. Obesity and type 2 diabetes. Endocrinol Metab Clin N Am. 2003;32(4):805–22.
29. Pi-Sunyer FX. The obesity epidemic: pathophysiology and consequences of obesity. Obes Res. 2002;10(Suppl 2):97S–104S.
30. Sigal RJ, Kenny GP, Wasserman DH, Castaneda-Sceppa C, White RD. Physical activity/exercise and Type 2 Diabetes: a consensus statement from the American Diabetes Association. Diabetes Care. 2006;29(6):1433–8.
31. Dunstan DW, Daly RM, Owen N, Jolley D, Vulikh E, Shaw J, et al. Home-based resistance training is not sufficient to maintain improved glycemic control following supervised training in older individuals with Type 2 Diabetes. Diabetes Care. 2005;28(1):3–9.

32. Bompa TO, Buzzichelli C. Periodization training for sports. 3rd ed. Champaign: Human Kinetics; 2015.
33. Haff G, Triplett NT, National Strength & Conditioning Association (U.S.). Essentials of strength training and conditioning. 4th ed. Champaign, IL: Human Kinetics; 2016.
34. Niewiadomski W, Laskowska D, Gąsiorowska A, Cybulski G, Strasz A, Langfort J. Determination and prediction of one repetition maximum (1RM): safety considerations. J Hum Kinet. 2008;19(1):109–20.
35. American College of Sports Medicine. American College of Sports Medicine position stand. Progression models in resistance training for healthy adults. Med Sci Sports Exerc. 2009;41(3):687–708.
36. Schoenfeld BJ, Ogborn DI, Krieger JW. Effect of repetition duration during resistance training on muscle hypertrophy: a systematic review and meta-analysis. Sports Med. 2015;45(4):577–85.
37. Lacerda LT, Martins-Costa HC, Diniz RCR, Lima FV, Andrade AGP, Tourino FD, et al. Variations in repetition duration and repetition numbers influence muscular activation and blood lactate response in protocols equalized by time under tension. J Strength Cond Res. 2016;30(1):251–8.
38. Lieber RL. Skeletal muscle structure, function, and plasticity. Philadelphia: Lippincott Williams & Wilkins; 2002.
39. Kraemer WJ, Ratamess NA. Fundamentals of resistance training: progression and exercise prescription. Med Sci Sports Exerc. 2004;36(4):674–88.
40. Maiorana A, O'Driscoll G, Goodman C, Taylor R, Green D. Combined aerobic and resistance exercise improves glycemic control and fitness in type 2 diabetes. Diabetes Res Clin Pract. 2002;56(2):115–23.
41. Castaneda F, Layne JE, Castaneda C. Skeletal muscle sodium glucose co-transporters in older adults with type 2 diabetes undergoing resistance training. Int J Med Sci. 2006;3(3):84–91.
42. Loimaala A, Huikuri HV, Kööbi T, Rinne M, Nenonen A, Vuori I. Exercise training improves baroreflex sensitivity in type 2 diabetes. Diabetes. 2003;52(7):1837–42.
43. Rice B, Janssen I, Hudson R, Ross R. Effects of aerobic or resistance exercise and/or diet on glucose tolerance and plasma insulin levels in obese men. Diabetes Care. 1999;22(5):684–91.
44. Manning JM, Dooly-Manning CR, White K, Kampa I, Silas S, Kesselhaut M, et al. Effects of a resistive training program on lipoprotein—lipid levels in obese women. Med Sci Sports Exerc. 1991;23(11):1222–6.
45. Vincent HK, Bourguignon C, Vincent KR. Resistance training lowers exercise-induced oxidative stress and homocysteine levels in overweight and obese older adults. Obes Silver Spring Md. 2006;14(11):1921–30.
46. Lambers S, Van Laethem C, Van Acker K, Calders P. Influence of combined exercise training on indices of obesity, diabetes and cardiovascular risk in type 2 diabetes patients. Clin Rehabil. 2008;22(6):483–92.
47. Comstock BA, Thomas GA, Dunn-Lewis C, Volek JS, Szivak TK, Hooper DR, et al. Effects of acute resistance exercise on muscle damage and perceptual measures between men who are lean and obese. J Strength Cond Res. 2013;27(12):3488–94.
48. Ajisaka R. Cardiovascular safety of exercise in the elderly. Jpn J Phys Fitness Sports Med. 2003;52(Supplement):55–63.
49. Borst SE. Interventions for sarcopenia and muscle weakness in older people. Age Ageing. 2004;33(6):548–55.
50. Tanimoto M, Sanada K, Yamamoto K, Kawano H, Gando Y, Tabata I, et al. Effects of whole-body low-intensity resistance training with slow movement and tonic force generation on muscular size and strength in young men. J Strength Cond Res. 2008;22(6):1926–38.
51. Tanimoto M, Ishii N. Effects of low-intensity resistance exercise with slow movement and tonic force generation on muscular function in young men. J Appl Physiol. 2006;100(4):1150–7.
52. Watanabe Y, Madarame H, Ogasawara R, Nakazato K, Ishii N. Effect of very low-intensity resistance training with slow movement on muscle size and strength in healthy older adults. Clin Physiol Funct Imaging. 2014;34(6):463–70.

53. Watanabe Y, Tanimoto M, Ohgane A, Sanada K, Miyachi M, Ishii N. Increased muscle size and strength from slow-movement, low-intensity resistance exercise and tonic force generation. J Aging Phys Act. 2013;21(1):71–84.
54. Tamaki T, Uchiyama S, Tamura T, Nakano S. Changes in muscle oxygenation during weight-lifting exercise. Eur J Appl Physiol. 1994;68(6):465–9.
55. Formenti D, Perpetuini D, Iodice P, Cardone D, Michielon G, Scurati R, et al. Effects of knee extension with different speeds of movement on muscle and cerebral oxygenation. PeerJ. 2018;6:e5704.
56. Pearson SJ, Hussain SR. A review on the mechanisms of blood-flow restriction resistance training-induced muscle hypertrophy. Sports Med. 2015;45(2):187–200.
57. Schoenfeld BJ. The mechanisms of muscle hypertrophy and their application to resistance training. J Strength Cond Res Natl Strength Cond Assoc. 2010;24(10):2857–72.
58. Slysz J, Stultz J, Burr JF. The efficacy of blood flow restricted exercise: a systematic review & meta-analysis. J Sci Med Sport. 2016;19(8):669–75.
59. Loenneke JP, Wilson JM, Wilson GJ, Pujol TJ, Bemben MG. Potential safety issues with blood flow restriction training. Scand J Med Sci Sports. 2011;21(4):510–8.
60. Caballero AE. Endothelial dysfunction in obesity and insulin resistance: a road to diabetes and heart disease. Obes Res. 2003;11(11):1278–89.
61. Credeur DP, Hollis BC, Welsch MA. Effects of handgrip training with venous restriction on brachial artery vasodilation. Med Sci Sports Exerc. 2010;42(7):1296–302.
62. Bond V, Curry BH, Kumar K, Pemminati S, Gorantla VR, Kadur K, et al. Restricted blood flow exercise in sedentary, overweight African-American females may increase muscle strength and decrease endothelial function and vascular autoregulation. Aust J Pharm. 2017;20(1):23–8.
63. Nascimento D d C, Petriz B, da Cunha Oliveira S, Leite Vieira DC, Schwerz Funghetto S, Silva AO, et al. Effects of blood flow restriction exercise on hemostasis: a systematic review of randomized and non-randomized trials. Int J Gen Med. 2019;12:91–100.
64. Mertens I, Van Gaal LF. Obesity, haemostasis and the fibrinolytic system. Obes Rev. 2002;3(2):85–101.
65. Mueller KG, Hurt RT, Abu-Lebdeh HS, Mueller PS. Self-perceived vs actual and desired weight and body mass index in adult ambulatory general internal medicine patients: a cross sectional study. BMC Obes. 2014;1:26.
66. Sartorio A, Lafortuna CL, Conte G, Faglia G, Narici MV. Changes in motor control and muscle performance after a short-term body mass reduction program in obese subjects. J Endocrinol Investig. 2001;24(6):393–8.
67. Rustaden AM, Haakstad LAH, Paulsen G, Bø K. Effects of BodyPump and resistance training with and without a personal trainer on muscle strength and body composition in overweight and obese women—a randomised controlled trial. Obes Res Clin Pract. 2017;11(6):728–39.
68. Tsuzuku S, Kajioka T, Endo H, Abbott RD, Curb JD, Yano K. Favorable effects of non-instrumental resistance training on fat distribution and metabolic profiles in healthy elderly people. Eur J Appl Physiol. 2007;99(5):549–55.
69. Wilk M, Golas A, Stastny P, Nawrocka M, Krzysztofik M, Zajac A. Does tempo of resistance exercise impact training volume? J Hum Kinet. 2018;62:241–50.
70. Alberti G, Garufi M, Silvaggi N. Allenamento della forza a bassa velocità. Il metodo della serie lenta a scalare. Mariucci: Calzetti; 2012.

Aquatic Exercise

3

Michele Gobbi, Andrea Aquiri, Cecilia Monoli, Nicola Cau, and Paolo Capodaglio

Key Points

- Aquatic exercise yields protective effects against joint loading.
- The Osteoarthritis Research Society International, the American College of Rheumatology and the European League Against Rheumatism include aquatic exercise as an important treatment for pain.
- The immersed subject can exercise vigorously and is capable of increasing VO_2max over relatively short periods.
- Land-based high-intensity interval training is difficult to perform in obese subjects, but aquatic short-term low-volume HIIT is a feasible, time-efficient strategy to improve body composition, muscle oxidative capacity, fasting glucose, triglycerides level, blood pressure and fitness in obese subjects

Electronic Supplementary Material The online version of this chapter (https://doi.org/10.1007/978-3-030-32274-8_3) contains supplementary material, which is available to authorized users.

M. Gobbi (✉) · N. Cau · P. Capodaglio
Istituto Auxologico Italiano IRCCS, Piancavallo, Italy
e-mail: m.gobbi@auxologico.it

A. Aquiri
Athletic Trainer C.C. Aniene, Rome, Italy

C. Monoli
Milan Politechnic, Milan, Italy

P. Capodaglio (ed.), *Rehabilitation Interventions in the Patient with Obesity*,
https://doi.org/10.1007/978-3-030-32274-8_3

Excessive body weight increases mechanical stress to the joints and tissues and induces physical limitations and pain [1], leading to reduction of physical activity that contributes to the loss of muscle mass and strength. The combination of the above components contributes to higher BMI, decline in physical function, musculoskeletal pain and reduced quality of life [1–3]. In obese populations, traditional modes of aerobic exercise, such as walking and/or running, are often associated with increased risk of musculoskeletal injuries [4], thus reducing adherence to exercise prescription. Pain is one of the major determinants of ceasing physical activity in patients with obesity. The combination of obesity and knee osteoarthritis, most typically, creates a vicious cycle of pain, loss of functionality and disease progression. To interrupt this cycle, physical activity and weight loss can make an important contribution. Pain relief using analgesics and anti-inflammatory medications may have only a modest functional benefit while causing cardiovascular and gastrointestinal side effects. The recommendations of the Osteoarthritis Research Society International, the American College of Rheumatology and the European League Against Rheumatism also include aerobic, aquatic and resistance training as important treatment components [5, 6]. The American College of Sports Medicine generally recommends 30 min of moderate aerobic activity on land 5 days per week or 3 days of vigorous or combined aerobic activity and 1–4 sets (8–12 repetitions) of 8–10 resistance exercises to train the major muscle groups 2–3 days per week in non-consecutive days [7, 8]. Non-weight-bearing including aquatic exercises (AQE) are also recommended for the obese population to reduce stress on the lower extremities and spine [9, 10].

AQE is an exercise modality which can be defined as a group of exercises performed in water, mainly in the vertical position, with or without music or equipment, in shallow or deep water [5, 11]. It describes an environment for structured physical activity rather than a type of exercise. This confusion facilitates poor reporting and unclear definitions of the exact type of exercises used in clinical aquatic programs. The immersion of the body in water in a vertical position causes per se various modifications in the main apparatuses [12–16]:

Cardiovascular

- Redistribution of blood flow (thoracic "blood shift")
- Best venous return
- Increased central venous pressure
- Greater atrial filling
- Central hypervolaemia with increased systolic and cardiac output

Respiratory

- Decreased static lung volumes
- Increased respiratory rate in increased metabolic demand situations

Musculoskeletal

- Unloading of the joints
- Lower speed of movement due to fluid resistance
- Lower activation and recruitment of muscle groups

Renal

- Increase in diuresis and natriuresis

AQE is commonly used in Sports Medicine to improve athletes' skills, muscular tone and for strengthening and endurance training, but also to relieve pain and spams, relax and improve circulation [17]. In rehabilitation, AQE is recommended mainly for pre- and post-traumatic or post-surgical conditions [18] and in various chronic conditions such as fibromyalgia [19], osteoarthritis and rheumatological conditions [20], Parkinson [21], multiple sclerosis, muscular dystrophy, asthma [22], haemophilia [23], chronic obstructive pulmonary disease [24] and chronic heart diseases [25], balance disorders [26] and obesity [27]. Growing research evidence supports the value of AQE in improving function, quality of life or pain in arthritis [2, 3, 28, 29], low back pain [1], fibromyalgia [5, 17, 30] and after orthopaedic surgery [31, 32]. AQE can counteract kinesiophobia, a maladaptive strategy leading to the avoidance of physical activity because of pain-related fears [1]. It has been shown to improve 6-min walking test distance, hand grip strength and muscle mass, reduce body weight and fat mass and improve function and pain control [5, 33]. Walking/running on water treadmill increases energy expenditure, VO_2 and perceived exertion more than on land [34].

The main beneficiary of AQE are subjects with limitation during the execution of land-based exercises, due to aging, fear of falling and the aforementioned comorbidities. Its versatility and controlled conditions make it possible to define individualized protocols, allowing to combine different elements creating a cost-efficient environment [11, 35].

AQE seems to positively affect exercise compliance more than land-based programs and facilitate independent commitment after finishing supervised rehabilitation [36]. Contraindications for AQE are severe cardiovascular or cardiopulmonary disease, tracheotomy, diabetes, seizures, incontinence, mycosis, infections, open wounds or non-healing ulcers, chlorine allergy and contagious diseases. Surprisingly, to date, only two short-term (12–13 weeks) studies have compared the effectiveness of AQE and land-based training on aerobic fitness and body composition in obese people, demonstrating a similar improvement with the two exercise modes. However, the effectiveness on other cardio-metabolic risk factors (blood pressure, glycaemia, blood lipid levels) were not documented, and only one study used a nutritional intervention.

3.1 Physical Properties of Water

The physical features of water can be exploited to overcome the limitations to exercise on land. Most biological effects of immersion are related to the fundamental principles of hydrodynamics. The essential physical properties of water of interest are the following [28]:

Density: according to the Archimedes' principle, an obese patient has a greater vertical thrust than a normal-weight person [28]. The body's density is slightly less than that of water and averages a specific gravity of 0.974, with men higher than women. Lean body mass, which includes bone, muscle, connective tissue and organs, has a typical density of 1.1, whereas fat mass has a density of about 0.9.

Hydrostatic pressure: directly proportional to liquid density and immersion depth. Water exerts a pressure of 1 mm Hg/1.36 cm of water depth. An individual immersed in a depth of 120 cm is subjected to a force of 88.9 mm Hg, slightly greater than the normal diastolic blood pressure. Hydrostatic pressure reduces oedema in an injured body part and increases the venous return and the stroke volume with a reduction in total peripheral resistance [28]. Hormonal effects include alteration of renin-angiotensin aldosterone leading to diuresis, kaliuresis and natriuresis. Also, insulin sensibility can be improved because angiotensin II can downregulate the insulin resistance in skeletal muscle [30].

Buoyancy: an individual reaches floating equilibrium when 97% of his total body volume is submerged. Immersion to the waist provides a 40% offload of body weight, which becomes 60% at xiphoid level.

Viscosity: the magnitude of internal friction specific to a fluid during motion. A limb moving in water is subjected to the resistive effects of the fluid. Under turbulent flow conditions, this resistance increases as a log function of velocity. Resistance increases as more force is exerted, then dropping to 0 almost immediately after cessation of force. Thus, when a person ceases the movement because of pain, force suddenly drops as water viscosity damps the movement almost instantaneously. This allows enhanced control of strengthening activities within the patient's comfort range [28].

Thermodynamics: the therapeutic utility of water depends greatly on both its ability to retain and transfer heat or cold. Water is an efficient conductor, transferring heat 25 times faster than air. This makes the use of water in rehabilitation very versatile because water retains heat or cold while delivering it easily to the immersed body part. Water may be used therapeutically over a wide range of temperatures. Cold is often used in athletic training at temperatures of 10–15 °C to produce a decrease in muscle pain and speed recovery from overuse injury [5, 30]. Heat transfer begins immediately on immersion, and as the heat capacity of the human body is less than that of water (0.83 vs. 1.00), the body equilibrates faster than water does [28].

Body weight support (BWS): water offers a protective environment for obese individuals because of the buoyancy effects of immersion, which minimizes the risk of joint injury and creates a weight-assistant environment [17, 28], recommended by the Osteoarthritis Research Society International (OARSI), the American College of Rheumatology (ACR) and the European League Against Rheumatism (EULAR) as a principal non-pharmacological treatment of osteoarthritis and musculoskeletal disorder [5]. With body weight reduced, the individual can exercise vigorously and is capable of producing increases in VO_2max over relatively short periods. On land, aerobic exercise performed for long enough to produce conditioning is sometimes difficult to achieve. A training program that progresses from water to land as strength, endurance and tolerance build up may represent a more effective method of achieving conditioning and weight loss [28]. Unloading conditions alternative to water, like body weight support treadmills [32] or robot-assisted equipment [37], are also effective but present with very high costs.

In summary, the aquatic environment is different from land because of higher resistance to movement, "isokinetic" muscle contractions (maximal strength exerted throughout the range of movement, muscle contraction at consistent velocity), balance variations, due to a reduced plantar support, which stimulate control on the body centre of mass, and altered motor schema. As for the latter, the main factor, opposite to land-based exercise, is represented by Archimedes' force: in a subject running on the spot underwater, the main action is pushing the foot downwards rather than flexing the knees. Once the motor schema adapts to the water environment, work intensities higher than on land can be reached [38].

3.2 Pool Characteristics

According to the guidelines of the Aquatic Exercise Association (AEA), fitness goals should be pursued in water at 28–30 °C. Temperatures above 32 °C are recommended for passive work, relaxation techniques or for individuals with low movement levels, but not for aerobic or strength exercises. In cases of patients with low aquatic abilities, the Arthritis Foundation Guidelines suggest a superior limit range of water temperature of 31 °C [5]. Air temperature should not exceed 85° Fahrenheit (USA Swimming 2017). Indoor pool air humidity is in the range of 50–60% [11]. A section of the pool with a depth of 3.5–4.5 ft. (1–1.4 m) is considered ideal for most shallow-water programs [11]. The weight support is 90% of the body weight if the water reaches the neck and 50% if water reaches the hip [11]. Most public and competitive pools operate in the range of 27–29 °C, which is often too cool for general rehabilitative populations, because these populations are usually less active in water. Therapy pools operate in the range of 33.5–35.5 °C, which allows lengthy immersions and exercise activities sufficient to produce therapeutic effects without chilling or overheating. Hot tubs are usually maintained at 37.5–41 °C, although the latter temperature is rarely comfortable for more than a few minutes and even the lower typical temperature does not allow for active exercise.

3.3 Prescribing AQE

AQE has broad rehabilitative potential, ranging from the treatment of acute to chronic conditions. Because of this clinical adaptability, AQE represents a useful means in the rehabilitative toolbox [28]. It has beneficial applications in cardiovascular, cardiopulmonary, respiratory, musculoskeletal, neurological, metabolic, geriatric and psychiatric rehabilitation as well as in specific conditions like pregnancy, pain and osteoporosis [28]. Also, it does not negatively affect the respiratory system [39] and it appears a first choice treatment for lymphedema of the lower limbs [39], osteoarthritis and musculoskeletal pain [5], frailty and sarcopenia [33]. An AQE program should encompass cardiorespiratory endurance, resistance training and flexibility components. Specifically, the program should include the warm-up component (thermal warm-up, optional pre-stretch and cardiorespiratory warm-up, 5–15 min), the conditioning phase (depending on participant ability and experience, fitness status, needs and goals, water temperature, 20–120 min) and the cool-down component (5–15 min) [11]. Significant effects on cardiorespiratory adaptations of healthy individuals have been shown to occur after 8–12 weeks, three sessions per week and an average session duration of 60 min [40, 41].

Weight loss and fat mass loss follow a dose-response activity [7]. To maximize weight loss, ACSM suggests more than 250 min of moderate activity/weekly and up to 60 min moderate exercise/daily on land [4]. AQE allows to increase work load minimizing risk of musculoskeletal injuries. Subjects should be first familiarized with water, its viscosity, buoyancy and proprioception in water [42]. Only after this phase, underwater equipment can be added to increase exercise intensity. Then, frequency, duration and intensity of the exercise should be defined. Progression is a key factor: a 1 MET increase (1 MET = 3.5 mL O_2 × kg of body weight) correlates to a reduction of −7 cm in waist circumference, −5 mm Hg in systolic pressure, −88 mg/dL in triglyceridaemia, +7.72 mg/dL in HDL and −18 mg/dL in glycaemia [43].

3.4 Resistance/Circuit Training

On land, ACSM recommends 2–3 sets of resistance training per exercise, 8–10 repetitions at 60–75% of 1RM. ACSM suggests also for AQE to train from a minimum of 2 days/week with combined resistance and endurance training to improve muscle mass and reduce fat mass [7]. Resistance training in aquatic circuit training mode has been shown a valid strategy to improve fitness [5, 33], resting metabolic rate, metabolic responses and mitochondrial genesis [7, 8].

Resistance in water (or "drag") is expressed by the formula: Resistance (Newton) = $1/2\rho t CX V2At$, where ρt = density of the fluid (kg/m^3), CX = coefficient of friction, V = velocity (m/s) and At = projection of the frontal surface (m^2) combined of the limbs (and mobile parts of the bike) [38]. AQE professionals can increase or decrease intensity using inertia, acceleration, action/reaction, drag forces, buoyancy, levers and frontal resistance [11]. They can also use commercially available water equipment (see below), where the following parameters can be varied: movement velocity, size of water equipment, limb's lever arm, hydrodynamic position of the moving segment and equipment.

Swimming gloves or rubber dumbbells and ankle cuffs are particularly suited for patients who suffer from hand osteoarthritis and are unable to hold other accessories such as dumbbells or barbells. Made of neoprene, the handheld gloves enhance the support surface of the hands and allow the upper body to work more effectively.

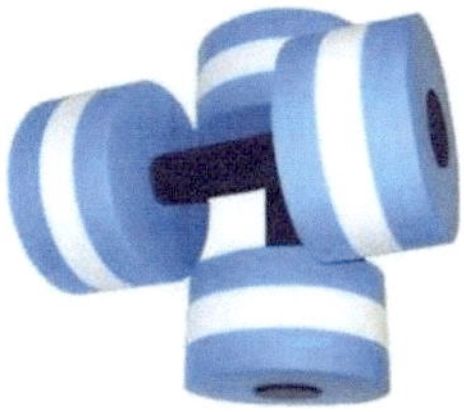
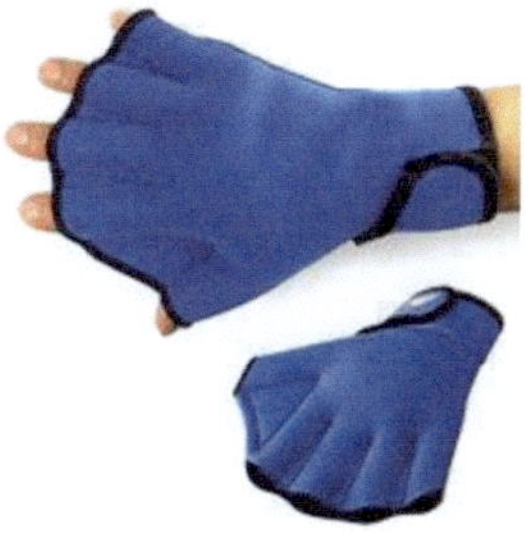
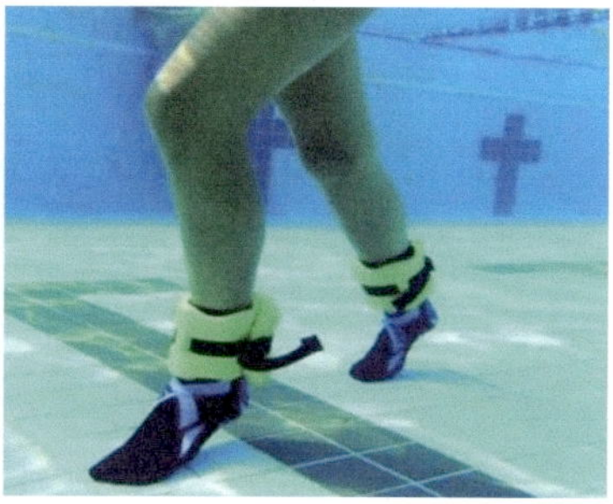

Swimming training fins are useful for backstroke swimming and core exercise with backstroke legs from semi-seated position.

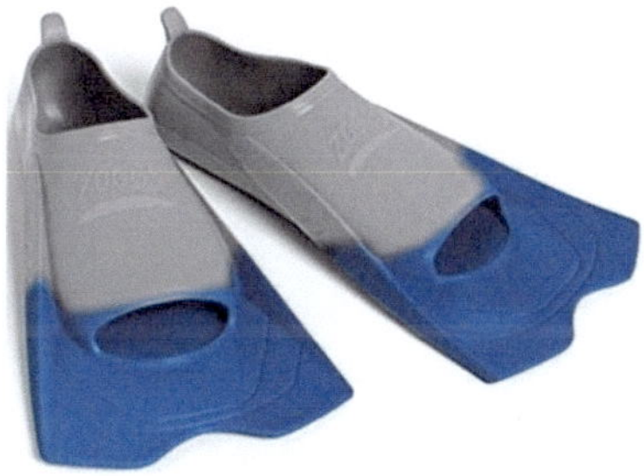

Superior belt favours floating during the execution of exercises which do not require plantar loading.

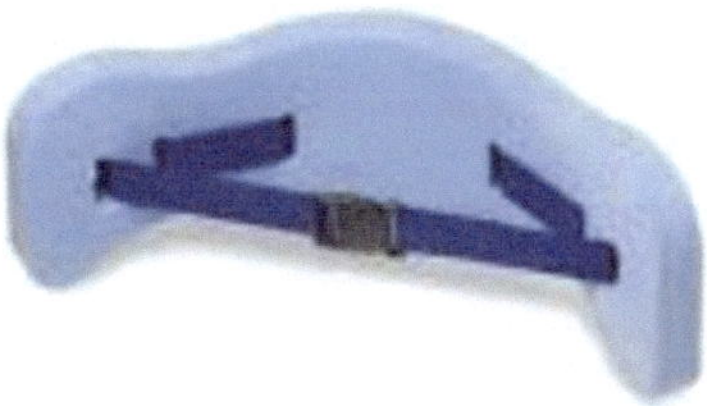

Aquatic trampoline trains balance and proprioceptive capacity, strengthens the lower limbs and has a draining effect on lower limb oedema. Compared to its land-based equivalent, it provides resistance during the downward push and a rebound effect with an accelerated upward phase. It can be used to treat patients with lymphedema [39].

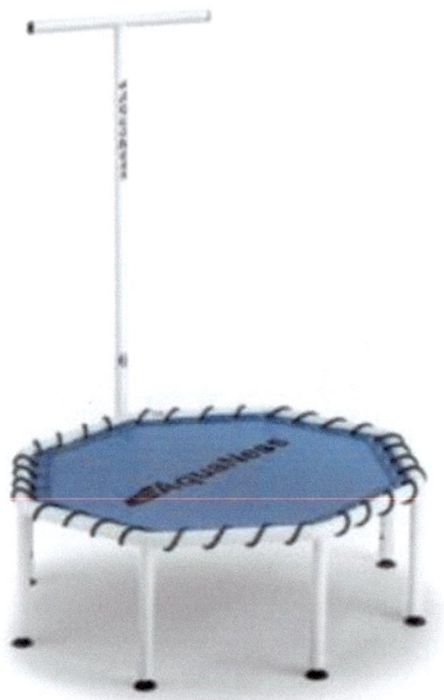

Acquapole is a versatile resistance training equipment. It allows progression of loading, depending on the distance from the upper end to the water surface. The deeper the immersion in water, the less the fatigue in exertions in the sagittal plane (i.e. traction) perceived.

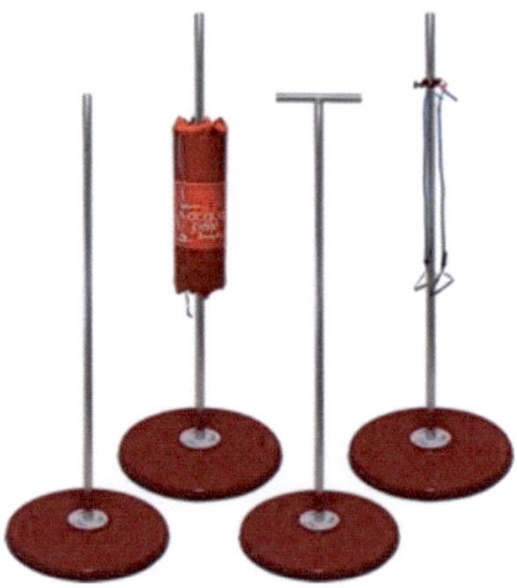

Handrail is a very adaptable water handrail.

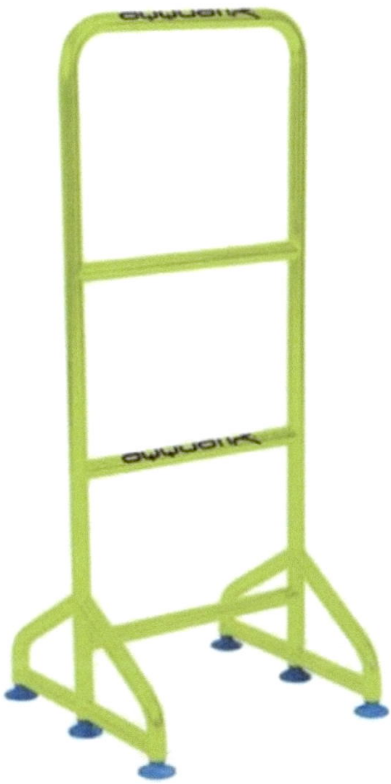

3.5 Aerobic Training

Different models of underwater bikes are available. Some have flaps on the pedals or other mechanical systems to increase resistance. Seats adapted for overweight patients are available.

Water treadmills are usually mechanical with a set of inclination. Some models have a belt and others independent bushings on cylindrical axes forming the inclined plane. Belt treadmills can be made of rubber or tracks (Fig. 3.1). Water shoes are recommended, especially in the latter types of treadmills. For high BMI values, treadmills with rubber belt may not be adequate. All of the aforementioned equipment cannot measure the mechanical load imposed.

Patients with sedentary habits and no familiarity with physical exercise may feel that AQE affect motor schema. Hence, in those cases, a sensible approach to AQE could be with bike and treadmill first.

Examples of all water exercises are described in the **video material** accompanying this chapter as Electronic Supplementary Material (Courtesy of www.vat-academy.it).

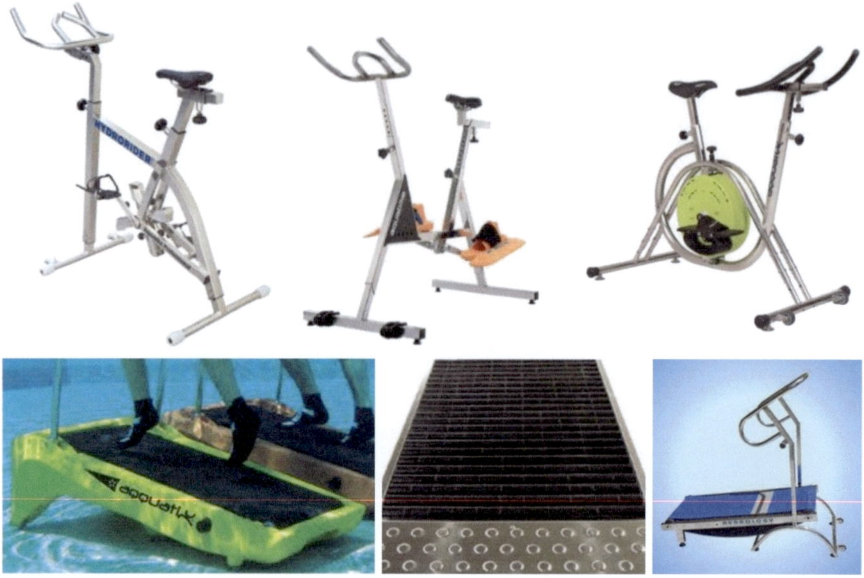

Fig. 3.1 Different belt types: rubber, independent rollers, tracks

3.6 High-Intensity Interval Training (HIIT)

HIIT is characterized by explosive, intermittent bouts of vigorous activity with rest or lower-intensity activity in between. The variables in a HIIT protocol are duration, intensity, rest, workout modality, number of repetitions, number of sets and rest between sets. HIIT has been shown to provide larger improvements in performance capacity than traditional training [44–46]. Burgomaster et al. [47] and Gibala et al. [48, 49] demonstrated that a 2-week HIIT can increase oxidative capacity of the skeletal muscle, glycogen content at rest, systemic lipid oxidation capacity, vascular function, performance as measured by a "time-to-exhaustion" test and maximal oxygen uptake and reduce lactate production during exercise [47, 48, 50, 51]. A 12-week HIIT significantly reduced abdominal subcutaneous and visceral fat tissue and increased fat-free mass in obese subjects [52]. Growth hormone, which yields a distinct lipolytic capacity, was found markedly increased after only 1 HIIT session, with marked reduction in long-term plasmatic cortisol [53].

Most of the adult population fails to adhere to the physical activity guidelines due to lack of time [54]. Timewise, HIIT could be a valid solution compared to prolonged moderate-intensity steady-state exercise [54]. In patients with obesity, the cardiac output (Q (L/m)) is reduced, leading to reduced oxygenation [55]. In AQE, the increase in blood flow to the central regions can reach 700 mL/min. This shift in blood flow increases the final diastolic volume and, consequently, the systolic volume. Thus, during AQE, both maximal and exercise heart rates are lower than the rates reached on land [56]. The increase in cardiac output is also secondary to the increase in stroke volume, meaning less cardiac stress and lower oxygen demand [57].

The short-term low-volume HIIT is a time-efficient strategy to improve body composition, muscle oxidative capacity, fasting glucose, triglyceride levels, blood pressure and fitness in obese subjects on land [58] and in water [9]. Longer intervals (i.e. 120 s) do not seem to provide advantages over continuous exercise for obese adults who do not exercise regularly [59].

VO2max and HR values are affected by water. For this reason, when using a water bike or treadmill it is more practical and accurate to use the external power output (Watt or METs) for planning a correct HIIT. The maximum workload determined with an incremental test or theoretical HRmax calculated with the aquatic formula [9] should be used. Short HIIT protocols based on 15-, 30- or 60-s bouts are recommended in obese subjects [9, 49].

Gibala [49] proposed a low-volume protocol for subjects with metabolic disorders consisting of 10 × 60 s work bouts at constant intensity of 90% HRmax with 60-s recovery, while other HIIT protocols require greater intensities. However, the minimal intensity and training volume needed to potentiate the effect of the stimulus adaptation on outcomes such as mitochondrial biogenesis and relevant health markers is still unclear. For AQE in patient with obesity, HIIT represents the latest novelty: with this modality, patients exploit fully the aquatic properties to safely achieve high HR ranges, otherwise not reachable on land, with little contraindications.

3.7 AQE Protocols

To define an aquatic protocol for patients with obesity we should take into consideration the following factors: age, gender, degree of obesity and comorbid conditions, nutritional state, anthropometrics, attitude to exercise and fitness, aquatic ability, training duration, short- and long-term goals and characteristics of the pool. The recommended water exercise modalities are summarized in Table 3.1.

3.8 Progression of AQE: An Example

- Week 1: the first week is explorative with respect to the new environment. The exercises should be carried out, through free exploration and guided discovery of the physical laws of water. It is very important for the patient to adapt his motor and body patterns to the aquatic environment.
- Weeks 2–4: aerobic exercise (30-minute exercise with HR monitoring).
- Weeks 5–6: implement resistance exercises two sessions per week, 4–6 exercises involving large muscle groups per session, 1–2 sets of 8–15 repetitions per exercise. Patients should be monitored with HR and OMNI scale.
- Weeks 7–9: add up to six exercises of resistance training and up to three sets of 8–15 repetitions per exercise.
- Weeks 10–14: mix of resistance and aerobic in circuit training (see Table 3.1).
- Week 15+: introduce the low-volume HIIT with bouts of 15, 30 and 60 s (see Table 3.1) with a progression during the week starting with 5 × 60 s, adding one set every week to reach ten sets.

Table 3.1 The recommended water exercise modalities for resistance, aerobic and high-intensity interval training

	Frequency	Duration	Type	Equipment	Volume/rest/ intensity
Resistance training	≥2–3 sessions/ week	15–45 min	8–12 exercises/ session involving large muscle groups (also in circuit[a])		Volume: 2–5 sets of 8–15 repetitions for each exercise Rest time: from 20 to 120 s, depending on volume and intensity Intensity: prescription of effort by using OMNI scale (score 5–9)
Aerobic training	≥2–3 sessions/ week	Up to 60 min	Low-intensity steady state	Bike, treadmill or bodyweight	Volume: >250 min/week Intensity: 60–70% AHRD
HIIT	2–3 sessions/ week	4–20 min depending on protocol	Bike, treadmill, resistance training	Bike, treadmill, water equipment	Volume and intensity: 10 sets × 60 s at 90% AHRD

[a]Circuit training performed on land [60] and adapted to water [35]: 2–4 sets of 8–12 exercises at 60–80% HR_{max} or 20–40 s of each exercise with 0–30 s rest between exercises performed at maximum velocity, 3-min rest between sets

3.9 Monitoring

The aquatic fitness community has long been aware that HR is lower in water than on land while exercising. For this reason, it is important to determine the Aquatic Heart Rate Deduction (AHRD) when calculating a target HR for water exercise. Environmental condition, medication, caffeine and excessive movement when entering the pool can affect rate responses. To determine target HR, 1-min HR while standing out of the pool for 3 min and a 1-min HR after being in water for 3 min should be measured. The AHRD is calculated by subtracting HR in water from HR on land. It is also possible to use a standard deduction (−17 beat/min), but it can over- or underestimate HR_{max}.

(220 − age − aquatic deduction) × desired intensity percentage

To determine the desired intensity percentage, we suggest the following HR equations:

1. Peak HR formula by applying AHRD to the traditional peak HR equation (% HR_{max}):
   (220 − age − AHRD) × desired intensity percentage

Table 3.2 The use of HR to estimate exercise intensities that coincide with $\%VO_2$ max (land based)

$\%VO_2$ max	% HRR	% HR_{max}
40	40	64
50	50	71
60	60	77
70	70	84
80	80	91
85	85	94

Based on Karvonen method ($HR = (HR_{max} - HR_{min}) \times$ (intended fraction) + HR_{rest}) [61, 62]

2. Peak HR formula by applying AHRD to the Karvonen formula:
   [(220 − age − RHR(reserved heart rate) − AHRD) × desired intensity percentage] + basal heart rate

HR can be used to estimate exercise intensities that coincide with the land-based $\%VO_2$ max (Table 3.2).

Most literature focuses on assessing the subject's state before and after the water training, using different types of questionnaires, the evaluation of heart rate with chest strap [6, 27, 57, 63] or the level of oxygen in the blood with pulse oximetry (SaO_2) [64]. Measurements pre- and post-activity are used to get generic idea of the patient's condition. This limitation is mainly due the humid environment and to the scarce availability of waterproof tools or monitoring equipment leading to risk of contamination and electrical accidents [64]. To date, the literature fails to propose a continuous monitoring system with wearable sensors applicable to the water environment. However, there are some basic systems to monitor activity underwater: swim trackers able to monitor the swim activity in terms of laps, meters, times, heart rate and calories burned (i.e. Swimmo©). There are commercially available aquatic heart rate monitors, also without thoracic belt, like Polar M430 or Vantage M. Unfortunately, these systems do not provide information about the kinematic of the movements. Technologies based on wearables (*Inertial Measurement Unit, IMU*) or video based (i.e. Kinovea) can add kinematic data. At present, however, limitations in data reliability, due to their use underwater, still exist.

Continuous monitoring of physical activity in terms of quality and quantity of movements would help assess the objective value of water-based exercises, allowing feedback and monitoring of the patient's conditions, thus limiting the subjective component.

Due to the difficulty in estimating the 1 RM for determining workload in water, the Omni-Perceived Exertion Scale for Resistance Exercise [5] can be adopted using a score range of 5–7 [7].

References

1. Vincent H, Zdziarski L, Wasser J. Chronic pain management in the obese patient: a focused review of key challenges and potential exercise solutions. J Pain Res. 2015;8:63. https://doi.org/10.2147/jpr.s55360.

2. MacLellan G, et al. Impact of a multidisciplinary weight management service on musculoskeletal pain in obese individuals. Obes Facts. 2017;10:182.
3. Bliddal H, Leeds AR, Christensen R. Osteoarthritis, obesity and weight loss: evidence, hypotheses and horizons—a scoping review. Obes Rev. 2014;15:578–86.
4. Donnelly JE, et al. Appropriate physical activity intervention strategies for weight loss and prevention of weight regain for adults. Med Sci Sports Exerc. 2009;41:459–71.
5. Yázigi F, et al. The PICO project: aquatic exercise for knee osteoarthritis in overweight and obese individuals. BMC Musculoskelet Disord. 2013;14:320.
6. Rewald S, et al. Effect of aqua-cycling on pain and physical functioning compared with usual care in patients with knee osteoarthritis: study protocol of a randomised controlled trial rehabilitation, physical therapy and occupational health. BMC Musculoskelet Disord. 2016;17:1–14.
7. Westcott WL, Winett RA, Annesi JJ, Wojcik JR, Anderson ES, Madden PJ. Prescribing physical activity: applying the ACSM protocols for exercise. Phys Sportsmed. 2009;37:51–8.
8. Westcott WL. Resistance training is medicine. Curr Sports Med Rep. 2012;11:209–16.
9. Boidin M, et al. Effect of aquatic interval training with Mediterranean diet counseling in obese patients: results of a preliminary study. Ann Phys Rehabil Med. 2015;58:269–75.
10. Greene NP, et al. Comparative efficacy of water and land treadmill training for overweight or obese adults. Med Sci Sports Exerc. 2009;41:1808–15.
11. Association, A. E. Aquatic fitness professional manual 7th edition. (Human Kinetics Champaign, IL, 2018).
12. Arborelius M, Ballidin UI, Lilja B, Lundgren CE. Hemodynamic changes in man during immersion with the head above water. Aerosp Med. 1972;43:592–8.
13. Avellini BA, Shapiro Y, Pandolf KB. Cardio-respiratory physical training in water and on land. Eur J Appl Physiol Occup Physiol. 1983;50:255–63.
14. Convertino VA, Tatro DL, Rogan RB. Renal and cardiovascular responses to water immersion in trained runners and swimmers. Eur J Appl Physiol Occup Physiol. 1993;67:507–12.
15. Nakamitsu S, et al. Effect of water temperature on diuresis-natriuresis: AVP, ANP, and urodilatin during immersion in men. J Appl Physiol. 1994;77:1919–25.
16. Perini R, Milesi S, Biancardi L, Pendergast DR, Veicsteinas A. Heart rate variability in exercising humans: effect of water immersion. Eur J Appl Physiol Occup Physiol. 1998;77:326–32.
17. Lim JY, Tchai E, Jang SN. Effectiveness of aquatic exercise for obese patients with knee osteoarthritis: a randomized controlled trial. PM R. 2010;2:723–31.
18. Asimenia G, et al. Aquatic training for ankle instability. Foot Ankle Spec. 2013;6:346–51.
19. McVeigh JG, McGaughey H, Hall M, Kane P. The effectiveness of hydrotherapy in the management of fibromyalgia syndrome: a systematic review. Rheumatol Int. 2008;29:119–30.
20. Rewald S, et al. Aquatic circuit training including aqua-cycling in patients with knee osteoarthritis: a feasibility study. J Rehabil Med. 2015;47:376–81.
21. Mooventhan A, Nivethitha L. Scientific evidence-based effects of hydrotherapy on various systems of the body. N Am J Med Sci. 2014;6:199–209.
22. Grande AJ, et al. Water-based exercise for adults with asthma. Cochrane Database Syst Rev. 2014;(7):CD010456.
23. Von Mackensen S, et al. The impact of a specific aqua-training for adult haemophilic patients—results of the WATERCISE study (WAT-QoL). Haemophilia. 2012;18:714–21.
24. McNamara RJ, McKeough ZJ, McKenzie DK, Alison JA. Water-based exercise in COPD with physical comorbidities: a randomised controlled trial. Eur Respir J. 2013;41:1284–91.
25. Teffaha D, et al. Relevance of water gymnastics in rehabilitation programs in patients with chronic heart failure or coronary artery disease with normal left ventricular function. J Card Fail. 2011;17:676–83.
26. Booth CE. Water exercise and its effect on balance and gait to reduce the risk of falling in older adults. Act Adapt Aging. 2004;28:45–57.
27. Wadell K. Water-based exercise is more effective than land-based exercise for people with COPD and physical comorbidities. J Physiother. 2014;60:57.
28. Becker BE. Aquatic therapy: scientific foundations and clinical rehabilitation applications. PM R. 2009;1:859–72.

29. King LK, March L, Anandacoomarasamy A. Obesity & osteoarthritis. Indian J Med Res. 2013;63:185–93.
30. Delevatti R, Marson E, Kruel LF. Effect of aquatic exercise training on lipids profile and glycaemia: a systematic review. Rev Andal Med Deporte. 2015;8:163–70.
31. LaRoche DP, Marques NR, Cook SB, Masley EA, Morcelli MH. Augmenting strength-to-weight ratio by body weight unloading affects walking performance equally in obese and nonobese older adults. Age (Omaha). 2016;38:21.
32. Mao YR, et al. The effect of body weight support treadmill training on gait recovery, proximal lower limb motor pattern, and balance in patients with subacute stroke. Biomed Res Int. 2015;2015:175719.
33. de Souza Vasconcelos KS, et al. Land-based versus aquatic resistance therapeutic exercises for older women with sarcopenic obesity: study protocol for a randomised controlled trial. Trials. 2013;14:1–7.
34. Dolbow DR, Farley RS, Kim JK, Caputo JL. Oxygen consumption, heart rate, rating of perceived exertion, and systolic blood pressure with water treadmill walking. J Aging Phys Act. 2008;16:14–23.
35. Borreani S, et al. Aquatic resistance training: acute and chronic effects. Strength Cond J. 2014;36:48–61.
36. Vincent HK, Heywood K, Connelley J, Hurley RW. Weight loss and obesity in the treatment and prevention of osteoarthritis. PM R. 2013;4:1–15.
37. Ammann-Reiffer C, Bastiaenen CHG, Meyer-Heim AD, van Hedel HJA. Effectiveness of robot-assisted gait training in children with cerebral palsy: a bicenter, pragmatic, randomized, cross-over trial (PeLoGAIT). BMC Pediatr. 2017;17:1–9.
38. Frangolias DD, Rhodes EC. Metabolic responses and mechanisms during water immersion running and exercise. Sport Med. 1996;22:38–53.
39. Dionne A, Goulet S, Leone M, Comtois A-S. Aquatic exercise training outcomes on functional capacity, quality of life, and lower limb lymphedema: pilot study. J Altern Complement Med. 2018;24:1007–9.
40. Sanders ME, Takeshima N, Rogers ME, Colado JC, Borreani S. Impact of the S.W.E.A.T.™ water-exercise method on activities of daily living for older women. J Sports Sci Med. 2013;12:707–15.
41. Takeshima N, et al. Water-based exercise improves health- related aspects of fitness in older women. Med Sci Sport Exerc. 2002;34:544–51.
42. Han SK, Kim MC, An CS. Comparison of effects of a proprioceptive exercise program in water and on land the balance of chronic stroke patients. J Phys Ther Sci. 2013;25:1219–22.
43. Schwingshackl L, Dias S, Strasser B, Hoffmann G. Impact of different training modalities on anthropometric and metabolic characteristics in overweight/obese subjects: a systematic review and network meta-analysis. PLoS One. 2013;8:e82853.
44. Wisløff U, et al. Superior cardiovascular effect of aerobic interval training versus moderate continuous training in heart failure patients: a randomized study. Circulation. 2007;115:3086–94.
45. Tjønna AE, et al. Aerobic interval training vs continuous moderate exercise as a treatment for the metabolic syndrome: "A Pilot Study". Circulation. 2008;118:170–6.
46. Hwang C-L, Wu Y-T, Chou C-H. Effect of aerobic interval training on exercise capacity and metabolic risk factors in people with cardiometabolic disorders. J Cardiopulm Rehabil Prev. 2011;31:378–85.
47. Burgomaster KA, et al. Similar metabolic adaptations during exercise after low volume sprint interval and traditional endurance training in humans. J Physiol. 2008;586:151–60.
48. Gibala MJ, et al. Short-term sprint interval versus traditional endurance training: similar initial adaptations in human skeletal muscle and exercise performance. J Physiol. 2006;575:901–11.
49. Gibala MJ, Little JP, Macdonald MJ, Hawley JA. Physiological adaptations to low-volume, high-intensity interval training in health and disease. J Physiol. 2012;590:1077–84.
50. Burgomaster KA. Six sessions of sprint interval training increases muscle oxidative potential and cycle endurance capacity in humans. J Appl Physiol. 2005;98:1985–90.

51. Rakobowchuk M, et al. Sprint interval and traditional endurance training induce similar improvements in peripheral arterial stiffness and flow-mediated dilation in healthy humans. Am J Physiol Integr Comp Physiol. 2008;295:R236–42.
52. Heydari M, Freund J, Boutcher SH. The effect of high-intensity intermittent exercise on body composition of overweight young males. J Obes. 2012;2012:480467.
53. Peake JM, et al. Metabolic and hormonal responses to isoenergetic high-intensity interval exercise and continuous moderate-intensity exercise. Am J Physiol Metab. 2014;307:E539–52.
54. Keating SE, Johnson NA, Mielke GI, Coombes JS. A systematic review and meta-analysis of interval training versus moderate-intensity continuous training on body adiposity. Obes Rev. 2017;18:943–64.
55. Salvadori A, et al. Oxygen uptake and cardiac performance in obese and normal. Respiration. 1999;66:25–33.
56. Rebold MJ, Kobak MS, Otterstetter R. Influence of a tabata interval training program on performance variables. J Strength Cond Res. 2013;27:3419–25.
57. Michaud TJ, Brennan DK, Wilder RP, Sherman NW. Aquarunning and gains in cardiorespiratory fitness. J Strength Cond Res. 1995;9:78–84.
58. Gillen JB, Percival ME, Ludzki A, Tarnopolsky MA, Gibala MJ. Interval training in the fed or fasted state improves body composition and muscle oxidative capacity in overweight women. Obesity. 2013;21:2249–55.
59. Martinez N, Kilpatrick MW, Salomon K, Jung ME, Little JP. Affective and enjoyment responses to high-intensity interval training in overweight-to-obese and insufficiently active adults. J Sport Exerc Psychol. 2015;37:138–49.
60. Seo Y, Noh H, Kim SY. Weight loss effects of circuit training interventions: a systematic review and meta-analysis. Obes Rev. 2019;20:1642–50. https://doi.org/10.1111/obr.12911.
61. Chewning BJM, Krist PS, Figueiredo PAP De. Monitoring your aquatic heart rate: increasing accuracy with the Kruel aquatic adaptation by June M. Chewning, Paula S. Krist and Paulo A. Poli de Figueiredo Aquatic exercise Association Research Committee Project, May 2008–July 2009. (2010).
62. Robergs RA, Landwehr R. The surprising history of the "HRmax=220-age" equation. J Exerc Physiol Online. 2002;5:1–10.
63. Fedor A, Garcia S, Gunstad J. The effects of a brief, water-based exercise intervention on cognitive function in older adults. Arch Clin Neuropsychol. 2015;30:139–47.
64. Perk J, Perk L, Bodén C. Cardiorespiratory adaptation of COPD patients to physical training on land and in water. Eur Respir J. 1996;9:248–52.

4 Nutrition and Exercise

Raffaella Cancello, Elisa Lucchetti, Michele Gobbi, and Amelia Brunani

Key Points

- A balanced diet (carbohydrates, proteins, lipids) together with proper hydration is important in exercise.
- A very-high-protein intake does not necessarily improve muscle mass and may have adverse effects on calcium homeostasis and some metabolic functions.
- Leucine is the amino acid residue with major evidence of efficacy in fat-free mass maintenance.
- Fat-free mass decrease during weight loss is affected by multiple factors (including level of energy intake, diet composition, duration of dieting, sex, age, baseline adiposity, prolonged inactivity).

R. Cancello (✉)
Obesity Unit and Laboratory of Nutrition and Obesity Research, Department of Endocrine and Metabolic Diseases, IRCCS Istituto Auxologico Italiano, Milan, Italy
e-mail: r.cancello@auxologico.it

E. Lucchetti
Experimental Laboratory for Auxo-Endocrinological Research, IRCCS Istituto Auxologico Italiano, Piancavallo-Verbania, Italy
e-mail: e.lucchetti@auxologico.it

M. Gobbi
Rehabilitation Unit and Research Laboratory in Biomechanics and Rehabilitation, IRCCS Istituto Auxologico Italiano, Piancavallo-Verbania, Italy
e-mail: gobbi@auxologico.it

A. Brunani
Division of Rehabilitation Medicine, IRCCS Istituto Auxologico Italiano, San Giuseppe Hospital, Piancavallo-Verbania, Italy
e-mail: brunani@auxologico.it

P. Capodaglio (ed.), *Rehabilitation Interventions in the Patient with Obesity*,
https://doi.org/10.1007/978-3-030-32274-8_4

- Nutrition and exercise should be carefully planned in morbidly obese patients complicated by diabetes, nonalcoholic fatty liver disease, chronic kidney diseases, obstructive sleep apnea, heart failure, and osteoarthrosis because in these critical conditions the fat-free mass maintenance is crucial to prevent malnutrition and to avoid the worsening of disability.
- Sarcopenic obesity is an underestimated problem and should be carefully considered in weight loss plans.

4.1 Carbohydrates, Proteins, Lipids, and Exercise

A nutrition program should guarantee an adequate energy supply (especially before exercise) with an adequate intake of nutrients such as carbohydrates, proteins, and lipids (balanced meal) for the maintenance of muscular activity and with a proper hydration (water and mineral salts).

In order to perform healthy exercise, it is important to know the energy sources to which the muscle draws to be able to contract and then generate strength but also the activity of different nutrients. The main substrate oxidized during moderate activity (50–70% VO_2max) is represented by carbohydrates, at least in the first 30 min of activity [1, 2]. Numerous evidences indicate that a high-carbohydrate intake is essential for maintaining a good nutritional status during exercise. The total content in carbohydrates of an organism is around 350–500 g, almost all distributed in the form of glycogen: 70–79% muscle glycogen (250–400 g), 20% hepatic glycogen (80–100 g), and less than 1% (2–5 g) circulating glucose [3]. In theory, the stocks of carbohydrates in the human body would allow moderate exercise for a maximum of 3 h. Muscular fatigue, which prevents the effective continuation of exercise, is due to the exhaustion of glycogen stocks in the body. Carbohydrate timing can influence postexercise rates of glycogen resynthesis [4, 5]. Depletion of muscle glycogen induces a strong drive for its own resynthesis. Even in the absence of postexercise carbohydrate intake, glycogen synthesis occurs at rates of 1–2 mM/kg of wet muscle weight/h, through gluconeogenesis or lactate [6, 7]. Recommended daily intakes of carbohydrates are commonly reported to be 5–12 g/kg/day, with the upper limit of this range reserved for athletes trained at moderate-high intensities (≥70% VO_2max) for more than 12 h/week [8]. A "glycogen storage threshold" with an average intake of 7–10 g/kg body mass of carbohydrates has been established with dose-response studies [9]. The timing and the frequency of carbohydrates intake (large meal vs. small snacks) does not affect glycogen storage in longer-term recovery, despite differences in blood glucose and insulin response to be carefully considered in diabetic patients [10]. The exact timing of a meal rich in carbohydrates is still a matter of debate and under investigation [8].

It was observed that the co-ingestion of less carbohydrates (0.8 g/kg/h) together with a little protein amount (0.2–0.4 g/kg/h) in the postexercise can assist glycogen repletion and storage and, at the same time, stimulate muscle protein synthesis [11].

This is particularly important in sarcopenic subjects or in patients affected by obesity during weight loss to counteract the loss of lean/muscular mass. During an exercise at 60% of the VO_2 max for 1 h, the protein oxidation contributes only for the 5% of the total energy expenditure. However, when the stocks of muscle glycogen are reduced, oxidation of proteins can increase to cover 10–15% of total energy expenditure with protein consumption and negative effects on performance (especially in athletes). This protein consumption can be antagonized by adding resistance exercises to the aerobic session. Essentially, dietary protein requirement is described as the minimum level of protein necessary to maintain short-term nitrogen balance under conditions of controlled energy intake. Physiological protein requirements are conventionally defined by studies on nitrogen balance [12]. Anabolism can be the cause of additional protein requirements (such as during growth and pregnancy or in critically ill patients). Protein requirements or recommendations are usually expressed either in relative terms (g/kg of body weight/day) or as a percentage of energy (% of total daily energy). The first estimate of protein requirements dates back to the latter half of the nineteenth century with several revisions based on the first nitrogen balance studies [13–15]. Before the Second World War, the recommended amount of protein requirements was 1.0 g/kg of body weight/day. This value was higher than that recommended later for almost four decades, *i.e.*, 0.8 g/kg body weight/day. All of these recommendations are general and make no distinction between genders and age groups, which is due to a lack of adequate scientific data for each subgroup. Since 1970s the Food and Agriculture Organization (FAO) and the World Health Organization (WHO) have determined the reference requirements for proteins and essential amino acids in humans as operational data for assessing the quality of dietary intake as protein sources and in order to prevent and control human malnutrition [16]. Significant progress has been made on this issue during recent decades. On one side, consensus on the level of protein intake based on the nitrogen balance has been reached, but, on the other, reference methods for measuring the need for each essential amino acid remain a matter of debate, due to large individual variability. A precise and complete definition of the nature of the need for nitrogen and amino acids remains difficult to formulate, because of the complexity of the metabolic pathways and the multiple roles of amino acids. These compounds are indeed precursors of protein synthesis and of many nitrogenous substrate molecules, substrates for energy metabolism and for certain amino acids with "signalling" function. Thus, the evaluation of the protein requirement and the quality of the protein intake to satisfy this need depends on physiological conditions, individual criteria, and criteria chosen to assess the need. Finally, the quality of protein intake is mainly assimilated to the facility of absorption and composition in essential amino acids (EAA), such as leucine, isoleucine, valine, lysine, threonine, tryptophan, methionine, phenylalanine, and histidine. There is no information on the variability of requirements for individual single amino acid residue. Therefore, approximate values have been calculated on the assumption that the interindividual coefficient of variation of the requirements for amino acids is the same as that for total protein, *i.e.*, 12% [17]. Under certain circumstances, specific amino acid supplements, such as branched-chain amino acids (BCAAs, *i.e.*, leucine, isoleucine, and valine), may improve exercise performance and recovery from exercise as well as the rates of protein synthesis, decreasing the rate of protein degradation. BCAA ingestion has been shown to be beneficial during aerobic exercise, decreasing the net rate of protein degradation [18] and also during exhaustive aerobic exercise, delaying the muscle glycogen depletion [19]. Food-derived proteins contain approximately 25% of BCAAs. Consuming whey protein during the exercise session may represent a natural strategy to avoid BCAA deficiency; however, an attempt should be made to obtain all recommended BCAAs from whole food protein sources. Out of the three BCAAs, the amino acid leucine appears to play the most significant role in stimulating protein synthesis [20] through activation of the mammalian target of rapamycin (mTOR) signaling pathway in skeletal muscle cells and other cell types and acting also via two key metabolites: α-ketoisocaproate (α-KIC) and β-hydroxy-β-methylbutyrate (HMB) [21]. The recommended dose of 55 mg leucine/kg/day is optimal in young adults, but this recommendation remains to be confirmed in larger cohorts. At present, the optimal leucine intake for older individuals is still undetermined. Based on studies on healthy men, leucine doses >500 mg/kg/die may be considered potentially unsafe, due to a transient increase in plasma ammonia concentrations [22]. Little data exist on the comprehensive metabolic effects of large amounts of dietary protein (in the order of 300–400 g/day). Intakes of this magnitude would result in some degree of prolonged hyper-aminoacidemia, hyper-ammonemia, hyper-insulinemia, and hyper-glucagonemia and some conversion to fat. However, the metabolic and physiological consequences of such states are currently unknown. The upper limit of protein intake is debated, with many experts advocating levels up to 2.0 g/kg/day to be safe without concerns about kidney function [17].

Lipids, especially non-esterified free fatty acids (NEFAs) and triglycerides, are oxidized during exercise [23]. During low-intensity aerobic exercises (40–50% VO_2max), NEFAs contribute to 40% of the supply of energy during the first hour of exercise and up to 70% in the following 3–4 h. A more intense muscular exercise tends to consume preferentially glucose and to spare NEFAs. The preferential use of NEFA with respect to glucose also depends from the level of training: the greater the training, the higher the use of NEFAs instead of sugars [24]. For this reason, low-intensity aerobic exercises are indicated in insulin-dependent diabetic patients because they allow a slow and gradual glucose use, thus resulting in a lower risk of hypoglycemia and taking advantage of the positive effects of complete NEFA oxidation under aerobic conditions. The regulation of the active muscle NEFA uptake can be summarized with a four-step process, consisting of (1) increased energy demand by the contracting muscle, (2) delivery of NEFA to the muscle, (3) transport of NEFA into the muscle by fatty acid transporters, and (4) activation of the fatty acids and either oxidation or re-esterification into intracellular lipids then stored into the intramuscular triacylglycerol droplets located next to the mitochondria [25]. Endurance training increases the capacity of the muscle to uptake NEFAs. The way to elevate the plasma NEFA concentration, which is an important determinant of the active muscle NEFA uptake and subsequent oxidation, is still under investigation. Currently, much research is focusing on how to induce an increase in fat/NEFA oxidation to improve performance, sparing carbohydrates for high-intensity (endurance) exercise.

4.2 Water, Micronutrients and Exercise

From a nutritional point of view, water replenishment is essential during exercise and must precede the sense of thirst. Even slight dehydration increases the sense of psychophysical fatigue and can trigger dangerous effects [26, 27]. High-intensity exercise in athletes and regularly active individuals typically results in dehydration that progressively hinders physical performance and mental capacity [28]. A water loss of 1–5% of body weight can reduce physical performance, while greater water loss can be particularly dangerous (heat stroke, hyperthermia up to convulsions, and coma). These effects must be taken into account when replenishing the water under high-temperature and high-humidity environmental conditions, in which sweating also causes a considerable loss of electrolytes (sodium, potassium, magnesium) [28]. It is recommended to drink 300 ml of water (and/or hypo-isotonic saline solutions) 2 h before the exercise session and 250 ml every 20–30 min of exercise to constantly hydrate the body when the exercise is prolonged over time. Different water amount may depend on type and duration of exercise [29]. Recent evidence suggests that the consumption of postexercise deep ocean mineral water may improve muscle function and recovery after exercise [30–32].

Establishing a precise daily requirement for micronutrients during exercise is difficult, as there is considerable individual variation depending on age, gender, body weight, physical activity levels, type of activity, and individual food habits. Recommendations for micronutrient intake in the normal diet have been formulated from observational studies on healthy populations, along with some detailed nutrient balanced studies associated with particular levels of intake. A balanced and various diet rich in raw fruits, vegetables, and cereals guarantees the right intake of almost all vitamins, mineral salts, and fibers needed. Interestingly, fruits and vegetables rich in antioxidant polyphenols have demonstrated important antagonistic effects on oxidative stress and exercise-induced lipid peroxidation [30]. Out of all vitamins, vitamins C and E seem to positively influence perception of general fatigue and heart rate in adults with obesity performing moderate exercise and following a low-calorie diet [33]. However, there is no clinical work demonstrating a clear therapeutic efficacy of vitamin supplementation in humans, as opposed to experimental data on rats [34, 35].

4.3 Role of Protein and Amino Acids in Fat-Free Mass (FFM) Preservation During Weight Loss

The aim of weight loss in obese subjects should be the loss of fat mass (FM) excess in the body. However during this process, inevitably and unintentionally, a variable proportion of weight loss is fat-free mass (FFM), which includes water and muscular mass. The assessments of FFM loss, as a proportion of total weight loss, could provide an important measure of the safety of individual weight loss methods when treating obesity. However, the point at which the proportional loss of FFM is excessive and potentially hazardous is still unclear. FFM loss decrease during weight loss depends on several factors including the induced caloric deficit, its duration, physical activity levels, eventually the type of bariatric surgical procedure used, and the magnitude of weight loss over time. The mechanisms responsible for the induced decrease in FFM (reduced muscle protein synthesis, increased breakdown, or both) have not been extensively clarified [36]. Two studies evaluating the effect of short-term caloric restriction (~30–40% energy deficit-day) on the rate of muscle protein synthesis in young and middle-aged men and women who were overweight and obese found that calorie restriction decreases the postprandial rate of muscle protein synthesis and decreases or does not change the basal rate of muscle protein synthesis [37, 38]. On the contrary, moderate calorie restriction is able to induce 5–10% weight loss in 4–6 months and increased the rate of muscle protein synthesis [39, 40]. The occurring loss of FFM during prolonged moderate caloric restriction is therefore mediated by increased muscle proteolysis rather than suppressed muscle protein synthesis. Adults require a minimum of protein intake of at least 0.66 g/kg/die to maintain nitrogen balance [41]. Nitrogen balance depends on nitrogen needed for both the maintenance and, in the case of growth, additional protein deposition in newly formed tissues. An average value of 70% can be considered for the efficiency of dietary protein utilization, whereas this value can vary with factors such as protein quality. Age-related changes in protein metabolism, such as the decrease in whole body protein synthesis from 17.4 g/kg/day in newborns to 6.9 g/kg/day in infants and 3.0 g/kg/day in adults to 1.9 g/kg/day in the elderly, result in different protein requirements. Age-dependent protein requirements imply differing roles of dietary protein in different age groups: it appears that in specific age groups higher protein intakes mainly affect body composition rather than body weight. In the elderly, a sustained protein intake may attenuate the physiological loss of FFM. Despite a reduction in energy requirements, protein requirements are unaltered in the elderly. This results from a decreased protein synthesis and a lower protein absorption, coinciding with larger protein catabolism. Age-related loss of FFM could be viewed as an effect of aging itself, rather than the result of insufficient protein intake. However, maintaining protein intake could stimulate muscle protein synthesis which may slow down the loss of FFM also during aging. Compared with adults, this means that the relative proportion of protein in the diet should increase in order to counteract the unfavorable effects of aging on protein metabolism. Information gained from recent reviews strengthens the scientific foundation for older overweight and obese adults to consume protein intakes at least at 1.0 g/kg/day to preserve lean mass as part of a successful weight loss intervention [42]. During positive energy balance (or dietary energy excess), inadequate protein intake (less than the RDA of 0.8 g/kg/die) results in loss of total body fat-free and muscle mass (~0.2–0.5% per week) [36]. The inadequate protein intake during energy deficit (such as during low calory diet) may accelerate the decrease in lean body mass, including FFM.

The questions is “How much protein is required to elicit improvements in body weight management?” Meta-analyses focused on this topic, including short-term energy restriction as well as long-term weight maintenance studies, indicate that the amount of protein necessary to promote weight management improving cardio-metabolic risks lies somewhere in between 1.2 and 1.6 g of protein/kg/day (which is an average of 89–119 g protein/day for adult women or 104–138 g protein/day for adult men) [43, 44]. However, other evidence suggests that also a lower protein amount (0.8 g protein/kg/day) during energy restriction might be sufficient for body weight and fat mass losses, whereas higher protein amounts (1.2 g protein/kg/day) are required for the preservation of lean mass [45]. To further support a specific protein quantity that is required to elicit improvements in weight management, Bosse J.D. and Dixon B.M. [45] categorized 25 higher-protein weight loss studies, on the basis of those who show successful weight loss, compared with those who did not. The change in protein intake (from habitual intake) was compared between groups. An average increase in protein consumption of 28.6% beyond habitual protein intake was needed to elicit significant weight loss [46]. Thus, if habitual protein intake in US adults (age range 19–70 years) is, on average, 88 g/day (1.07 g protein/kg/day), then the addition of only ~25–30 g protein/day (up to 113–118 g/day or 1.38 g protein/kg/day) would potentially be sufficient to elicit long-term improvements in weight management during weight loss [46].

On the other hand, a very-high-protein intake does not necessarily improve muscle mass amount and could have adverse effects on calcium homeostasis and metabolic functions, especially on glucose metabolism. There are some evidences that suggest that high-protein intake is involved in the pathogenesis of insulin resistance and type 2 diabetes, such as increasing the acid load [36]. As important as total daily protein intake is the distribution of dietary protein intake over day time, because of the appearance of a refractory period during which muscle protein synthesis, once stimulated by amino acids, cannot be stimulated again (also called "muscle-full" phenomenon). Some evidences suggest that a more even distribution of protein intake across meals is associated with more appendicular lean body mass than is a skewed protein intake (least for breakfast, most at dinner) in free living older adults [36]. A moderate, meal-driven approach to daily protein consumption, aware of the interplay of protein anabolism, costs, and daily energy consumption, should then be considered. High-protein (1.2–1.6 g/kg body weight/die) diet plans used after bariatric surgery are commonly used in order to prevent protein malnutrition, a common postoperative observed phenomenon [41]. In bariatric patients, adherence to an energy-restricted, relatively high-protein diet is associated with improvement in nutritional status; improvements in the feelings of satiety, with body loss; and improvement in body composition. Regarding the protein source, the amino acid leucine appears to be relevant for maintaining muscle mass [47]. Besides sufficient intake of high-quality protein, the strategies to reduce the loss of skeletal muscle mass during weight loss must include resistance exercise. Resistance exercise stimulates muscle protein synthesis, which in turn supports muscle mass preservation and muscle function. The number of weight loss trials in overweight or obese adults is limited, and trials combining resistance exercise with a high-protein diet or daily protein redistribution provide scanty and contradictory results. At present, the recommended dietary allowance (RDA) for protein is 0.8 g/kg/day and is age independent, while protein requirements of older adults (>65 year) is higher, and recommended protein intake ranges from 1.0 to 1.2 g/kg/day. Specific evidence-based recommendations for obese older adults during weight loss do not exist at present.

Exercise induces a mechanical load of skeletal muscles and bone, the magnitude of which varies with the chosen activity and is often viewed as a way to reduce FFM loss when dieting. Activities vary in type, amount, and duration, making exact estimates of FFM effects difficult. Reported reductions in body fat mass with no or small increases in lean tissues (i.e., FFM and skeletal muscle mass) without measuring muscle strength or function. The proportion of weight loss as lean tissue varies over time and is determined by multiple factors including level of energy intake, diet composition, time of dieting, gender, baseline adiposity, inactivity, type and level of added activity, and the subject's metabolic state or the hormonal response. In conclusion, higher-protein diets provide improvements in satiety, body weight management, and/or cardio-metabolic risk factors compared with lower-protein diets in obese patients, especially in elderly obese patients [47]. Although greater satiety, weight loss, fat mass loss, and/or the preservation of lean mass is often observed with increased protein consumption, the lack of dietary compliance with prescribed diets in free-living adults makes it challenging to confirm a sustained protein effect in the long term.

4.4 Nutrition and Exercise in Morbidly Obese Patients

In the context of critical illness, evidence suggests that exogenous protein/amino acid supplementation has the potential to favorably impact whole body protein balance. Whether this translates into the retention of muscle, greater muscle strength, and improved survival and physical recovery of critically ill patients remains uncertain. Obesity-related diseases are different kinds of severe diseases associated with obesity [48]. The sham etiopathogenetic mechanisms that cause obesity produce the development of several clinical conditions. For instance, insulin resistance is involved in type 2 diabetes, present in 20.1% of obese patients and lipid metabolism alteration in the nonalcoholic fatty liver disease (NADH) in 25–45% of patients. A combination of mechanisms (endocrine such as adipokines from adipose tissue, metabolic such as increased oxidative stress for elevation in free radicals, and a state of chronic low-grade inflammation) concur to induce hypertension, cardiac and vascular dysfunctions, and heart failure, which increase by 41% every 5 kg/m^2. Hypertension, type 2 diabetes per se or with diabetic nephropathy, protein overload, and adipokine and ectopic lipid accumulation produce kidney dysfunction (obesity-related glomerulopathy) in 13–33% of obese patients [49], reduced respiratory function, a decline in FFM resulting in reduced exercise tolerance and peripheral muscle weakness, responsible for chronic obstructive pulmonary disease (COPD) and obstructive sleep apnea syndrome (OSAS) (incidence of 30–60% in severe obesity). Inflammation and mechanical overload due to large fat mass induces joint complications such as osteoarthritis (OS): arthrosis of the knee is increased by approximately 15% for each additional point of BMI > 27 kg/m^2.

Nutritional and exercise interventions must consider patients with obesity with more attention, because, especially when obesity-related diseases are present, maintaining FFM during weight loss prevents the development of malnutrition or worsening of disability. For this reason, we reported the data available in the literature on diet and exercise specifically for those patients.

The Diabetes Prevention Program, which involved 3234 participants with obesity and prediabetes, demonstrated that body mass reduction by 7% accompanied by regular physical activity (NICE 2012) led to a 58% reduction in type 2 diabetes morbidity [50]. The aim of the intervention was a lowering of blood glucose or glycated hemoglobin (HbA1c) levels. Nutritional and lifestyle indications are favorable to a moderate weight loss (3–7% of initial body weight) with lower fat intake (20–50 g/day or <30% total intake and <15% saturated fat), increased fibers, limiting intake of carbohydrate (<30%), and physical activity (30–40 min/day or 150 min/week). It has also been observed that typical consumption of 3 meals/day (notwithstanding additional snacking or carbohydrate-containing drinks) means that people can spend more than half the day in a postprandial or post-absorptive state [51]. Low-carbohydrate diets could protect the beta cell by reducing insulin demand. On the contrary, beta cell exhaustion might be due to frequent and prolonged episodes of hyperglycemia [52]. Exercise training, whether aerobic or resistance training or a combination of the two, improves glucose regulation because it enhances skeletal muscle glucose uptake using both insulin-dependent and insulin-independent mechanisms, and regular exercise results in sustained improvements in insulin sensitivity. The aerobic training has been shown to increase skeletal muscle mitochondrial content and oxidative enzymes, resulting in dramatic improvements in glucose and fatty acid oxidation and increased expression of proteins involved in insulin signaling. Exercise intensity, volume, and frequency are associated with reductions in HbA1c; however, a consensus has not been reached on whether one type of exercise is a better determinant than the other [53]. For patients in insulin treatment, dose adjustments are often required in preparation to exercise [54] because hypoglycemia is the most common adverse event, and it is the greatest barrier to exercise for many patients. A number of factors can affect the insulin strategies used for exercise including intensity, duration, and type of activity. In general, the bolus insulin dose should be reduced by 25–75%, depending on the duration and intensity of exercise, for activities that occur in the postprandial. To reduce the risk of hypoglycemia for prolonged aerobic exercise well after meal absorption (*i.e.*, 3 or more hours after a meal), basal insulin dose reductions are recommended well before (60–90 min) the start of exercise, when possible. In the case of hypoglycaemia, the integration of carbohydrates (for example 30–60 g for > 1 h of exercise at ~ 60% of the maximum heart rate = 120–240 kcal), still remains the simplest management. For anaerobic exercise, adjustments in insulin are often not required during the activity, but small bolus insulin corrections may be required after exercise if hyperglycemia ensues.

NAFLD is divided into the histological categories of (1) isolated hepatic steatosis and (2) presence of hepatocellular injury with or without fibrosis [55]. Diet and exercise are the mainstay treatment: using a variety of interventions, either by diet alone or in combination with different exercise prescriptions, a 40% (ranging from

20% to 81%) reduction in liver fat was reported. The degree of hepatic fat reduction was proportional to the intensity of the lifestyle intervention, and generally a loss of at least 3–5% of body weight improves steatosis, but a greater weight loss (up to 10%) may be needed to improve necro-inflammation [56]. The ideal diet for patients with NAFLD has yet to be determined. The Mediterranean diet was compared with an isocaloric low-fat, high-carbohydrate diet during a 6-week crossover study and was associated with reduced liver fat and improved insulin sensitivity without differences in weight loss. A 2-week carbohydrate-restricted diet (<20 g/day of carbohydrates) compared with a reduced calorie diet (range, 1200–1500 kcal/day) resulted in similar weight loss between the groups; however, the carbohydrate-restricted group had a higher percentage reduction in hepatic fat (mean of 55 ± 14%) compared with the reduced calorie diet group (mean of 28 ± 23%) ($P < 0.001$). Limited data suggest that aerobic exercise results in greater reduction in hepatic fat than does resistance training, and it is suggested that this effect may be independent of weight loss. The intensity and duration of exercise appear related to the results because it is demonstrated that the highest intensity exercise (>250 min/week −1) improved metabolic parameters and significant hepatic fat reduction.

Few guidelines for overweight or obese patients with early chronic kidney diseases (CKDs) suggest caloric restriction under medical control to achieve weight loss. Recently, the Australian and New Zealand Nephrology Society [57] recommended a dietary intervention included a calorie-restricted diet (deficit of 500 calories from the usual diet or a set calorie intake of 740–1410 calories/day) with some physical activity. The result was weight reduction and improved outcomes in albuminuria and proteinuria in mild to moderate CKDs. It is reported that a reduction of 3.6 kg/m^2 of BMI is associated with a reduction of 1.3 g/day in proteinuria. A low-protein diet (LPD) of 0.6–0.8 g/kg/day is recommended for the management of CKD [58], but there are variability in protein intake depending on CKD stages, and average protein intake was 1.04 g/kg·ideal body weight (IBW)/day or 0.81 g/kg·actual body weight (ABW)/day in those with advanced stages of CKD. Implementation of LPD as proper dietary regimen is recommended to retard decline of GFR and initiation of dialysis. Guidelines recommend much higher protein intake (1.2–1.4 g/kg IBW/day) in end-stage renal failure patients treated with dialysis. During LPD, close monitoring is necessary for nutritional status to avoid malnutrition or protein energy wasting. Given the adequate calorie intake (30–35 kcal/kg·ABW/day), it is needed to avoid protein catabolism and malnutrition under protein restriction ≤0.6 g/kg·ABW/day. In extreme obesity, nutritional requirements is difficult to calculate; for practical use, we provide a nutritional body weight in patients who are more than 20% of their ideal body weight with this equation: $\text{nutritional}_{BW} = \text{ideal}_{BW} + (0.25*(\text{actual}_{BW} - \text{ideal}_{BW}))$ also if it lacks of a scientific basis. In relation to CKD stage, protein management is not enough; a striking reduction of either phosphate load and/or absorption (vegetal proteins) or salt intake is needed (no more than 2 g/day of than 5 g/day of salt unless contraindicated because of volume depletion). In a study with Dietary Approaches to Stop Hypertension (DASH) diet model (salt intake <5 g/daily and 22% protein intake) in conjunction with a 40-min bike ride every other day for 12 weeks, a statistically significant reduction was obtained for body weight of 8% with diet alone and 11%

with diet and aerobic exercise with a reduction in albuminuria and an improvement in eGFR which is augmented by exercise co-intervention [59].

Lifestyle modifications to induce weight loss with diet program, changes in sedentary and/or physical activities/exercise along with behavioral procedures (such as keeping food and activity logs, goal setting, stimulus control, and managing emotional eating and food cravings) are effective treatments for obese patients with OSAS. More recently, several larger randomized controlled trials, with LCD or VLCD, produced an average weight loss with a range from 3% to 18% with improvements in AHI ranging from 3 to 62% [60]. The conventional hypocaloric diet of 1200–1800 kcal daily leads to modest weight loss; most dramatic weight loss in 6 months was registered with very-low-calorie diets (VLCDs), which provide fewer than 800 kcal/day [61]. The benefits of Mediterranean diet also seem to extend to OSAS, with greater improvement in AHI during rapid eye movement sleep at 6 months probably with a mechanism independent of weight loss but related to fat redistribution. Furthermore, losing ≥5% of initial weight may be associated with improvements in sleep duration and quality. Guidelines recommend also a moderate-intensity physical activity of at least 150 min a week or vigorous-intensity physical activity for at least 60 min a week as part of a healthy lifestyle.

Although COPD has traditionally been associated with involuntary weight loss, malnutrition, and muscle mass depletion, the prevalence in obesity has been reported to be between 18 and 54%. Previously systematic meta-analysis showed that nutritional support, mainly in the form of oral nutritional supplements, showed significantly greater increases in mean total protein (14.8 g daily) and energy intakes (236 kcal daily) that improves anthropometric measures, and grip strength in COPD [62]. A low-calorie, high-protein diet coupled with a replacement meal plan and dietetic consultations has been reported to improve the dietary quality and eating behaviors and muscle mass maintenance [63]. Exercise and high-intensity physical activity can support healthy weight loss and improve the frequent coexisted components of the metabolic syndrome [64]. Studies have focused on aerobic exercise interventions for weight loss using a range of modalities, including walking, stationary cycling, and elliptical cross trainers, and the evidence seems to support this approach. There may be additional gains and other benefits, for example, on body composition, muscle strength, and cardiovascular fitness, through the addition of high-intensity or resistance exercise.

The role of intensive lifestyle interventions, such as intentional weight loss with hypocaloric/low-fat diet and exercise training, in patients with established chronic HF has been more studied [65], but specific recommendations for weight management did not exist. Advice regarding weight management is difficult because of the lack of evidence-based guidelines. Other than restricting sodium intake to <2 g daily, there are no specific dietary HF guidelines. Intentional weight loss in a patient with coexistent obesity and HF may improve exercise capacity, NYHA classification, and quality of life. Body composition may be more important; lean muscle mass is a major determinant of cardiorespiratory fitness in HF. A recent study reported that loss of lean mass or sarcopenia was associated with lower muscle strength, exercise capacity, and quality of life in patients with HF. Weight loss leads to reduction in LV mass and diastolic dysfunction but the mechanism remains unclear [66]. Moderate continuous training is efficient, safe, and well tolerated by HF patients, and it is recommended by the Heart Failure Association Guidelines [67]. Improvement in exercise capacity of HF patients undergoing continuous aerobic exercise training is primarily determined by the total energy expenditure, such as the product of training intensity, session duration, session frequency, and program duration of the training program. In addition to continuous moderate-intensity aerobic training, and also high-intensity and low-intensity interval training models, respiratory training and strength training demonstrated efficacy in this setting. It became progressively clear that different organ systems, such as the heart, skeletal muscle, vascular function, respiratory function, and neurohormonal systems are involved in HF disease progression and modulation by exercise training [68]. In observational cohort studies, improvements in fitness levels and weight loss on longitudinal follow-up have been associated with better LV diastolic function and favorable LV remodeling phenotypes, as well as lower risk of overall HF.

Clinical guidelines for osteoarthritis (OA) strongly encourage the use of diet, a caloric restriction to induce a 10% weight loss, combined with exercise to relieve pain and improve function [69]. Although definitions of Mediterranean diet (MD) vary, all of them include high consumption of fruit, vegetables, legumes, nuts, seeds, and cereals; greater intakes of fish and seafood; moderate consumption of dairy products, poultry, and eggs; and frequent, but moderate, intake of red wine and olive oil as the main sources of dietary lipids [70]. This diet was associated with better quality of life and decreased pain, disability, and depressive symptoms and with a significant improvement in knee cartilage as assessed by MRI [71]. MD is rich in polyphenols which prevent inflammation and cartilage destruction, resulting in a prevention of osteoarthritis-related musculoskeletal inflammation. MD also produces a lower *n*-6 to *n*-3 fatty acid (FA) ratio. Compounds derived from *n*-3 FA decrease gene expression of proteinase cartilage lesions and inflammatory cytokines. Rehabilitation for osteoarthritis (OA) widely includes land- and water-based exercise therapy, strength training, self-management and education, biomechanical interventions, and participation in regular physical activities. Aerobic physical activity and muscle-strengthening exercise may help reduce symptoms and improve joint function for hip or knee OA. The delivery of exercise programs varies by amount and magnitude of work (level of resistance, frequency, duration, and progression), supervision (type, mode of delivery), and setting (home, community/gym, healthcare setting) [72]. The prescribed exercise program consists of aerobic (15 min), resistance-training (20 min), a second aerobic (15 min), and cool-down (10 min) phases. Strength training is particularly relevant to offset any loss of muscle and bone mass resulting from weight loss.

4.5 Nutrition and Exercise in Obese Patients with Sarcopenia

The term "*sarcopenia*" (composed of the two Greek words "*sarco*, meat," and "*penia*, loss") was first used in 1989 by Rosemberg [73, 74] to describe the loss of muscle mass correlated with aging. Actually the clinical staging of sarcopenia is

Table 4.1 Clinical staging of sarcopenia (EWGSOP2 criteria)

Staging	Muscle mass	Muscle strength		Muscle function
Pre-sarcopenia	↓	–		–
Sarcopenia	↓	↓	or	↓
Severe sarcopenia	↓	↓	and	↓

based on criteria developed by The Working Group on Sarcopenia in Older People (EWGSOP2) that represent an update of the original definition and suggests the criteria for diagnosis of sarcopenia: (1) low muscle quantity, (2) low muscle strength, and (3) low physical performance. When all these conditions are present, the sarcopenia is severe (Table 4.1) [75].

Sarcopenic obesity (SO) is defined as the coexistence of sarcopenia and obesity [76], where sarcopenia is a progressive and generalized skeletal muscle disorder that is associated with deterioration in quality of life (QoL), a higher risk of frailty, activities of daily living (ADL) disability, instrumental ADL disability, and all-cause mortality. Sarcopenic obesity is commonly, not exclusively, related to aging. In fact, aging is accompanied by a gradual loss of muscle mass (or fat-free mass (FFM)) and a parallel increase in fat mass also in normal-weight subjects. In obesity a relative increase of fat mass in relation to muscle mass (or FFM) is due to the depot of adipose tissue, most importantly in the muscles. Since individuals with obesity have a greater quantity of both fat mass and lean mass, they could have a "normal" absolute amount of muscle mass and may not appear to be sarcopenic, even if their muscle mass is inadequate for their size. Therefore, a greater BMI could mask the presence of sarcopenia, and the classic definition of sarcopenia could underestimate the real sarcopenic state in overweight and obese subjects. Actually, there are no commonly accepted criteria for diagnosis of SO. Muscle mass could be measured by different validated techniques, but the diagnosis is not always easily available. In clinical practice, more precise nutritional intervention studies with protein and amino acid supplementation/redistribution in daily meals when dieting, will help to induce a proper weight (mainly fat) loss, with improvement of muscle mass in terms of increased lean mass and, more importantly, muscle strength and function. There are few validated techniques for measuring muscle strength. The handgrip strength measured under standard conditions with a handheld dynamometer is closely related to the muscle power of the lower extremity and the area of the calf cross-sectional area. Knee flexion/extension torque can be measured with isometric/isokinetic dynamometers suitable for research studies, but their use in clinical practice is limited [77]. Muscle function of the lower extremities can be assessed also by measuring gait speed or with the timed up-and-go test. Practical diagnostic cutoffs for gait speed are considered to be <0.8 m/s [2] or <1.0 m/s. Suggested cutoff points for reduced muscle strength measured by handgrip strength are <20 kg for women and <30 kg for men [78]. Recent studies identifying the coexistence of impaired bone health (osteopenia/osteoporosis), reduced muscle mass or strength (sarcopenia), and increased obesity in middle-aged and older women have led to the proposal of "osteo-sarcopenic obesity," but there is insufficient evidence to support this clinical condition as a distinct entity [79]. Lifestyle interventions, including calorie restriction and physical activity, are hallmarks of SO treatment [80]. Weight loss in younger adults (age 45–65 years) led to a not negligible loss of lean mass after calorie restriction (average of 4% reduction), which was partially compensated by increasing aerobic activity (2% reduction in lean mass in participants who had augmented weight loss from aerobic activity, $P = 0.05$). Unopposed diet therapy without exercise in older frail adults ≥65 years with obesity led to a marked loss of lean mass at 6 months and 1 year (−3.5 kg and −3.2 kg, respectively), compared to the diet and exercise group, where the loss of lean mass was partially mitigated (−1.7 kg and −1.8 kg, respectively). Energy deficits created by acute calorie restriction could downregulate muscle protein synthesis and increase proteolysis, which contributes to reduced muscle mass. Increased dietary protein stimulates muscle protein synthesis, and the association of aerobic exercise, resistance training, and their combination increase muscle protein synthesis in older adults despite age-related decreases in anabolic signaling. The source of protein, timing of intake, and specific amino acid constituents (e.g., leucine) can also be determinants for the increasing muscle mass and strength. In particular, leucine supplementation enhances myofibrillar protein synthesis in older men consuming lower- and higher-protein diets with and without exercise. Whey protein, a milk-derived protein, has been shown to be very effective in stimulating postprandial muscle protein accretion in older men, which has been ascribed to its fast digestion and absorption kinetics and the high leucine content [81]. The PROT-Age group recommends 1.0–1.1 g/kg protein/day in divided doses. Dietary protein that is derived from animal source products, rather than from plant-based sources, seems most effective eliciting muscle protein synthesis. The distribution of protein intake throughout the day or pulse feeding at main meals could be beneficial for the stimulation of muscle protein synthesis in patients with SO. Interestingly, a more evenly distribution of dietary protein intake, that is, every 3–4 h (the "spread diet"), led to a higher protein synthesis rates (25%, $p = 0.003$) and is associated with higher muscle strength, physical performance, and skeletal muscle mass in older adults. A trial of older adults with obesity consisted of a hypocaloric diet with an energy deficit of 500–750 kcal/day on average, 1 g high-quality protein, plus either 60 min of progressive aerobic exercise and resistance training or 75–90 min of both aerobic exercise and resistance training, 3 times a week. We need further evidence to support the effect of supplemental protein on functional outcomes in patients with SO. High-protein diets consisting of 1.0–1.2 g/kg/day should be prescribed with caution to prevent renal dysfunction as evidenced by observational data, as higher doses have recently demonstrated no changes in lean mass. Nutritional interventions to prevent and/or alleviate osteo-sarcopenic obesity components include adequate intake of protein (>0.8 g/kg/day), calcium (1200 mg/day), magnesium (320 mg/day), and vitamin D (800 IU/day), and increasing consumption of foods containing omega-3 PUFAs (1 g/day) and fiber (25 g/day for women). Moderate-intensity physical activity programs significantly improve physical functioning, attenuate intermuscular fat accumulation, and improve muscle quality. Exercise prescription should take into account the intensity, volume, frequency, and progression of training [81]. Aerobic exercise has the potential to improve aerobic capacity by initiating mitochondrial adaptation, enhancing cardiovascular function (e.g., increased stroke volume capacity) and increasing the capillary density of the muscle tissue. Resistance exercise is currently seen as the most effective exercise strategy in order to elicit muscle hypertrophy and to improve muscle function and strength in older adults. In an 8-week randomized controlled trial that included 60 sarcopenic obese older adults (aged 65–75), it was demonstrated that aerobic exercise significantly led to improvements in body fat mass (−0.7 kg, $p < 0.05$) and visceral fat (−6 cm^2, $p < 0.05$), maintaining the skeletal muscle mass (+0.1 kg, $p < 0.05$), as compared to the control group. In the same study, resistance exercise resulted in the maintenance of skeletal muscle mass (+0.1 kg, $p < 0.05$), decreased fat mass (−1.0 kg, $p < 0.05$), and increased grip strength (3.5 N/kg, $p < 0.05$), as compared to the non-exercise group. There was only one study available on the effects of combined exercise in 139 sarcopenic obese women undergoing 3 months of biweekly, 60-min combined exercise showing a 17.8% increase (SE: 4.2, $p = 0.119$) in knee extension strength, a significant increase in arm (1.8%, SE: 0.6, $p < 0.05$) and leg muscle mass (2.2, SE: 0.7, $p < 0.05$), and a decrease in the total body fat mass (−5.5%, SE: 0.9, $p < 0.05$), compared to the control group. A study of the effects of a 12-week program of resistance training in older women ($N = 62$, mean age 68 years; mean BMI 27 kg/m^2) found that performing three sets of exercise three times a week has beneficial effects on the risk factors for osteo-sarcopenic obesity including skeletal muscle mass and strength. Sarcopenia should no longer be considered as a purely geriatric clinical condition as it occurs also in young adults especially when suffering from severe obesity. Therefore it is important to pay attention also to the younger age groups with severe obesity in order to prevent complications due to the coexistence of obesity and sarcopenia, such as risk of fracture, physical disability, and cardiovascular complications. Further research on nutritional aspects and their role in the prevention of muscle mass loss when dieting are needed. In particular more precise nutritional intervention studies with protein and amino acid supplementation/redistribution in daily meals when dieting will help to induce a proper weight (mainly fat) loss, with improvement of muscle mass in terms of increased lean mass and, more importantly, muscle strength and function.

References

1. Spriet LL. New insights into the interaction of carbohydrate and fat metabolism during exercise. Sports Med. 2014;44(Suppl 1):S87–96.
2. Maughan RJ, Greenhaff PL, Leiper JB, Ball D, Lambert CP, Gleeson M. Diet composition and the performance of high-intensity exercise. J Sports Sci. 1997;15(3):265–75.
3. Adeva-Andany MM, González-Lucán M, Donapetry-García C, Fernández-Fernández C, Ameneiros-Rodríguez E. Glycogen metabolism in humans. BBA Clin. 2016;5:85–100. https://doi.org/10.1016/j.bbacli.2016.02.001. eCollection 2016 Jun
4. Coyle EF, Coggan AR, Hemmert MK, Ivy JL. Muscle glycogen utilization during prolonged strenuous exercise when fed carbohydrate. J Appl Physiol. 1986;61(1):165–72.
5. Coyle EF, Coggan AR, Hemmert MK, Lowe RC, Walters TJ. Substrate usage during prolonged exercise following a preexercise meal. J Appl Physiol. 1985;59(2):429–33.

6. Maehlum S, Hermansen L. Muscle glycogen concentration during recovery after prolonged severe exercise in fasting subjects. Scand J Clin Lab Invest. 1978;38(6):557–60.
7. Hermansen L, Vaage O. Lactate disappearance and glycogen synthesis in human muscle after maximal exercise. Am J Phys. 1977;233(5):E422–9.
8. Kerksick CM, Arent S, Schoenfeld BJ, Stout JR, et al. International society of sports nutrition position stand: nutrient timing. J Int Soc Sports Nutr. 2017;14:33. https://doi.org/10.1186/s12970-017-0189-4. eCollection 2017
9. Burke LM, Kiens B, Ivy JL. Carbohydrates and fat for training and recovery. J Sports Sci. 2004;22(1):15–30.
10. Costill DL. Carbohydrate nutrition before, during, and after exercise. Fed Proc. 1985;44(2):364–8.
11. Beelen M, Burke LM, Gibala MJ, van Loon LJC. Nutritional strategies to promote postexercise recovery. Int J Sport Nutr Exerc Metab. 2010;20(6):515–32.
12. Hoffer LJ, et al. Human protein and amino acid requirements. JPEN J Parenter Enteral Nutr. 2016;40(4):460–74. https://doi.org/10.1177/0148607115624084.
13. Carpenter KJ. Protein and energy. A study of changing ideas in nutrition. Med Hist. 1995;39(3):389–90.
14. McCay D. The protein element in nutrition. Edward Arnold, London, 1912, and Longmans. New York: Green & Co.; 1912. p. 172–8.
15. FAO/WHO/UNU. Energy and protein requirements. Report of a Joint Expert Consultation. World Health Organ Tech Rep Ser. 1985;724:1–206.
16. FAO/WHO/UNU. Expert consultation on protein and amino acid requirements in human nutrition. (2002: Geneva, Switzerland) Protein and amino acid requirements in human nutrition: report of a joint FAO/WHO/UNU expert consultation. (WHO technical report series; no. 935) 1. Proteins. 2. Amino acids. 3. Nutritional requirements. I. World Health Organization. II. Food and Agriculture Organization of the United Nations. III. United Nations University. IV. Title. V. Series. ISBN 92 4 120935 6 (NLM classification: QU 145) ISSN 0512-3054.
17. Blomstrand E, Newsholme EA. Effect of branched-chain amino acid supplementation on the exercise-induced change in aromatic amino acid concentration in human muscle. Acta Physiol Scand. 1992;146(3):293–8.
18. Blomstrand E, Ek S, Newsholme EA. Influence of ingesting a solution of branched-chain amino acids on plasma and muscle concentrations of amino acids during prolonged submaximal exercise. Nutrition. 1996;12(7–8):485–90. https://doi.org/10.1016/S0899-9007(96)91723-2.
19. Kimball SR, Jefferson LS. Signaling pathways and molecular mechanisms through which branched-chain amino acids mediate translational control of protein synthesis. J Nutr. 2006;136(1 Suppl):227S–31S.
20. Wang X, Proud C. The mTOR pathway in the control of protein synthesis. Physiology (Bethesda). 2006;21:362–9.
21. Pencharz PB, Elango R, Ball RO. Determination of the tolerable upper intake level of leucine in adult men. J Nutr. 2012;142(Suppl):2220S–4S.
22. Frayn KN. Fat as a fuel: emerging understanding of the adipose tissue-skeletal muscle axis. Acta Physiol (Oxford). 2010;199(4):509–18. https://doi.org/10.1111/j.1748-1716.2010.02128.
23. van Hall G. The physiological regulation of skeletal muscle fatty acid supply and oxidation during moderate-intensity exercise. Sports Med. 2015;45(Suppl 1):S23–32. https://doi.org/10.1007/s40279-015-0394-8.
24. Hoppeler H, Weibel ER. Limits for oxygen and substrate transport in mammals. J Exp Biol. 1998;201:1051–64.
25. Stearns RL, Casa DJ, Lopez RM, McDermott BP, Ganio MS, Decher NR, Scruggs IC, West AE, Armstrong LE, Maresh CM. Influence of hydration status on pacing during trail running in the heat. J Strength Cond Res. 2009;23:2533–41.
26. Barr SI. Effects of dehydration on exercise performance. Can J Appl Physiol. 1999;24:164–72.
27. Maughan RJ, Shirreffs SM. Dehydration and rehydration in competitive sport. Scand J Med Sci Sports. 2010;20(Suppl 3):40–7.

28. Hamer M, Ingle L, Carroll S, Stamatakis E. Physical activity and cardiovascular mortality risk: possible protective mechanisms? Med Sci Sports Exerc. 2012;44(1):84–8.
29. Harty PS, Cottet ML, Malloy JK, Kerksick CM. Nutritional and supplementation strategies to prevent and attenuate exercise-induced muscle damage: a brief review. Sports Med Open. 2019;5:1. https://doi.org/10.1186/s40798-018-0176-6.
30. Keen DA, Constantopoulos E, Konhilas JP. The impact of post-exercise hydration with deep-ocean mineral water on rehydration and exercise performance. J Int Soc Sports Nutr. 2016;13(1):17. https://doi.org/10.1186/s12970-016-0129-8.
31. Hou C-W, Tsai Y-S, Jean W-H, Chen C-Y, Ivy JL, Huang C-Y, et al. Deep ocean mineral water accelerates recovery from physical fatigue. J Int Soc Sports Nutr. 2013;10:7. https://doi.org/10.1186/1550-2783-10-7.
32. Franz MJ, Van Wormer JJ, Crain AL, et al. Weight-loss outcomes: a systematic review and meta-analysis of weight-loss clinical trials with a minimum 1-year follow-up. J Am Diet Assoc. 2007;107:1755–67.
33. Naziroğlu M, Butterworth PJ. Protective effects of moderate exercise with dietary vitamin C and E on blood antioxidative defense mechanism in rats with streptozotocin-induced diabetes. Can J Appl Physiol. 2005;30(2):172–85.
34. Kutlu M, Naziroğlu M, Simsek H, Yilmaz T, Sahap Kükner A. Moderate exercise combined with dietary vitamins C and E counteracts oxidative stress in the kidney and lens of streptozotocin-induced diabetic-rat. Int J Vitam Nutr Res Gen. 2005;75(1):71–80.
35. Cava E, Yeat NC, Mittendorfer B. Preserving healthy muscle during weight loss. Adv Nutr. 2017;8(3):511–9.
36. Pasiakos SM, Cao JJ, Margolis LM, Sauter ER, Whigham LD, McClung JP, Rood JC, Carbone JW, Combs GF Jr, Young AJ. Effects of high-protein diets on fat-free mass and muscle protein synthesis following weight loss: a randomized controlled trial. FASEB J. 2013;27: 3837–47.
37. Murphy CH, Churchward-Venne TA, Mitchell CJ, Kolar NM, Kassis A, Karagounis LG, Burke LM, Hawley JA, Philips SM. Hypoenergetic diet-induced reductions in myofibrillar protein synthesis are restored with resistance training and balanced daily protein ingestion in older men. Am J Physiol Endocrinol Metab. 2015;308:E734–43.
38. Campbell WW, Haub MD, Wolfe RR, Ferrando AA, Sullivan DH, Apolzan JW, Igay HB. Resistance training preserves fat-free mass without impacting changes in protein metabolism after weight loss in older women. Obesity (Silver Spring). 2009;17:1332–9.
39. Villareal DT, Smith GI, Shah K, Mittendorfer B. Effect of weight loss on the rate of muscle protein synthesis during fasted and fed conditions in obese older adults. Obesity (Silver Spring). 2012;20:1780–6.
40. Martens EA, Westerterp-Plantenga MS. Protein diets, body weight loss and weight maintenance. Curr Opin Clin Nutr Metab Care. 2014;17(1):75–9.
41. Kim JE, O'Connor LE, Sands LP, Slebodnik MB, Campbell WW. Effects of dietary protein intake on body composition changes after weight loss in older adults: a systematic review and meta-analysis. Nutr Rev. 2016;74(3):210–24.
42. Leyd HJ, Carnell NS, Mattes RD, Campbell WW. Higher protein intake preservers lean mass and satiety with weight loss in pre-obese and obese woman. Obesity. 2017;15:421–9.
43. Layman DK, Evans E, Browm JI, Seyler J, Erickson DJ, Boileau RA. Dietary protein and exercise have additive effects on body composition during weight loss in adult woman. J Nutr. 2005;135:1903–10.
44. Soenen S, Martens EA, Hochstenbach-Waelen A, Lemmens SG, Westerterp-Plantenga MS. Normal protein intake is require for body weight loss and weight maintenance, and elevated protein intake for additional preservation of resting energy expenditure and fat free mass. J Nutr. 2013;143:591–6.
45. Bosse JD, Dixon BM. Dietary protein in weight management: a review proposing protein spread and change theories. Nutr Metab. 2012;9:81.
46. Faria SL, Faria OP, Buffington C, et al. Dietary protein intake and bariatric surgery patients: a review. Obes Surg. 2011;21:1798–805.

47. Leidy HJ, Clifton PM, Astrup A, Wycherley TP, Westerterp-Plantenga MS, Luscombe-Marsh ND, Woods SC, Mattes RD. The role of protein in weight loss and maintenance. Am J Clin Nutr. 2015;101(6):1320S–9S.
48. Kinlen D, Cody D, O'Shea D. Complications of obesity. QJM. 2018;111(7):437–43.
49. D'Agati VT, Chagnac A, De Vries APJ, Levi M, Porrini E, Herman-Edelstein M, Praga M. Obesity-related glomerulopathy: clinical and pathologic characteristics and pathogenesis. Nat Rev Nephrol. 2016;12(8):453–71. National Institute for Health and Clinical Excellence. Preventing Type 2 Diabetes: Risk Identification and Interventions for Individuals at High Risk; NICE Guidelines (PH38); Updated: September 2017; National Institute for Health and Clinical Excellence: London, UK, 2012.
50. Knowler WC, Barrett-Connor E, Fowler SE, Hamman RF, Lachin JM, Walker EA, Nathan DM, Diabetes Prevention Program Research Group. Reduction in the incidence of type-2 diabetes with lifestyle intervention or metformin. N Engl J Med. 2002;346(6):393–403.
51. Monnier L, Colette C. Target for glycemic control: concentrating on glucose. Diabetes Care. 2009;32:S199–204.
52. Eizirik DL, Korbutt GS, Hellerström C. Prolonged exposure of human pancreatic islets to high glucose concentrations in vitro impairs the beta-cell function. J Clin Investig. 1992;90(4):1263–8.
53. Kirwan JP, Sacks J, Nieuwoudt S. The essential role of exercise in the management of type 2 diabetes. Cleve Clin J Med. 2017;84(7 Suppl 1):S15–21.
54. Zaharieva DP, Riddell MC. Insulin management strategies for exercise in diabetes. Can J Diabetes. 2017;41(5):507–16.
55. Rinella ME. Nonalcoholic fatty liver disease a systematic review. JAMA. 2015; 313(22):2263–73.
56. Chalasani N, Younossi Z, Lavine JE, et al. American Gastroenterological Association; American Association for the Study of Liver Diseases; American College of Gastroenterology. The diagnosis and management of non-alcoholic fatty liver disease: practice guideline by the American Gastroenterological Association, American Association for the Study of Liver Diseases, and American College of Gastroenterology. Gastroenterology. 2012;142(7):1592–609.
57. Lambert K, Beer J, Dumont R, Hewitt K, Manley K, Meade A, Salamon K, Campbell K. Weight management strategies for those with chronic kidney disease: a consensus report from the Asia Pacific Society of Nephrology and Australia and New Zealand Society of Nephrology 2016 renal dietitians meeting. Nephrology. 2018;23(10):912–20.
58. Ko GJ, Obi Y, Tortoricci AR, Kalantar-Zadeh K. Dietary protein intake and chronic kidney disease. Curr Opin Clin Nutr Metab Care. 2017;20(1):77–85.
59. Straznicky NE, Grima MT, Lambert EA, Eikelis N, Dawood T, Lambert GW, Nestel PJ, Masuo K, Sari CI, Chopra R, Mariani JA, Schlaich MP. Exercise augments weight loss induced improvement in renal function in obese metabolic syndrome individuals. J Hypertens. 2011;29(3):553–64.
60. Xanthopoulos MS, Berkowitz RI, Tapia IE. Effects of obesity therapies on sleep disorders. Metab Clin Exp. 2018;84(7):109–17.
61. Tham KW, Lee PC, Lim CH. Weight management in obstructive sleep apnea medical and surgical options. Sleep Med Clin. 2019;14(1):143–53.
62. Collins PF, Stratton RJ, Elia M. Nutritional support in chronic obstructive pulmonary disease: a systematic review and meta-analysis. Am J Clin Nutr. 2012;95(6):1385–95.
63. McLoughlin RF, McDonald VM, Gibson PG, Scott HA, Hensley MJ, MacDonald-Wicks L, Wood LG. The impact of a weight loss intervention on diet quality and eating behaviours in people with obesity and COPD. Nutrients. 2017;9(10):pii:E1147.
64. James BD, Jones AV, Trethewey RE, Evans RA. Obesity and metabolic syndrome in COPD: is exercise the answer? Chron Respir Dis. 2018;15(2):173–81.
65. Pandey A, Patel KV, Vaduganathan M, Sarma S, Haykowsky MJ, Berry JD, Lavie CJ. Physical activity, fitness, and obesity in heart failure with preserved ejection fraction. J Am Coll Cardiol HF. 2018;6(12):975–82.

66. McDowell K, Petrie MC, Raihan NA, Logue J. Effects of intentional weight loss in patients with obesity and heart failure: a systematic review. Obes Rev. 2018;19(9):1189–204.
67. Ponikowski P, Anker SD, Bueno H, et al. 2016 ESC Guidelines for the diagnosis and treatment of acute and chronic heart failure: the task force for the diagnosis and treatment of acute and chronic heart failure of the European Society of Cardiology (ESC) developed with the special contribution of the Heart Failure Association (HFA) of the ESC. Eur Heart J. 2016;37(27):2129–200.
68. Cattadori G, Segurini C, Picozzi A, Padeletti L, Anzà C. Exercise and heart failure: an update. ESC Heart Fail. 2018;5(2):222–32.
69. Messier SP, Callahan LF, Beavers DP, Queen K, Mihalko SL, Miller GD, Losina E, Katz JN, Loeser RF, Quandt SA, DeVita P, Hunter DJ, Lyles MF, Newman J, Hackney B, Jordan JM. Weight-loss and exercise for communities with arthritis in North Carolina (we-can): design and rationale of a pragmatic, assessor-blinded, randomized controlled trial. BMC Musculoskelet Disord. 2017;18(1):91.
70. Morales-Ivorra I, Romera-Baures M, Roman-Viñas B, Serra-Majem L. Osteoarthritis and the mediterranean diet: a systematic review. Nutrients. 2018;10(8):pii:E1030.
71. Bortoluzzi A, Furini F, Scirè CA. Osteoarthritis and its management—epidemiology, nutritional aspects and environmental factors. Autoimmun Rev. 2018;17(11):1097–104.
72. Nguyen C, Lefevre-Colau MM, Poiraudeau S, Rannou F. Rehabilitation (exercise and strength training) and osteoarthritis: a critical narrative review. Ann Phys Rehabil Med. 2016;59(3):190–5.
73. Rosenberg I. Summary comments: epidemiological and methodological problems in determining nutritional status of older persons. Am J Clin Nutr. 1989;50:1231–3.
74. Cruz-Jentoft AJ, Sayer AA. Sarcopenia. Lancet. 2019;393(10191):2636–46.
75. Dávalos-Yerovi V, Marco E, Sánchez-Rodríguez D, Guillen-Solà A, Duran X, Pascual EM, Muniesa JM, Escalada F, Duarte E. Sarcopenia according to the revised european consensus on definition and diagnosis (EWGSOP2) criteria predicts hospitalizations and long-term mortality in rehabilitation patients with stable chronic obstructive pulmonary disease. J Am Med Dir Assoc. 2019;20(8):1047–9. https://doi.org/10.1016/j.jamda.2019.03.019.
76. Polyzos SA, Margioris AN. Sarcopenic obesity. Hormones. 2018;17:321–31.
77. Cruz-Jentoft AJ, Baeyens JP, Bauer JM, Boirie Y, Cederholm T, Landi F, Martin FC, Michel JP, Rolland Y, Schneider SM, Topinková E, Vandewoude M, Zamboni M. Sarcopenia. European consensus on definition and diagnosis: report of the European Working Group on Sarcopenia in Older People. Age Ageing. 2010;39(4):412–23.
78. Bischoff SC, Boirie Y, Cederholm T, Chourdakis M, Cuerda C, Delzenne N, Deutz NE, Fouque D, Genton L, Gil C, Koletzko B, Leon-Sanz M, Shamir R, Singer J, Singer P, Stroebele-Benschop N, Thorell A, Weimann A, Barazzoni C. Towards a multidisciplinary approach to understand and manage obesity and related diseases. Clin Nutr. 2017;36:917e938.
79. Bauer JM, Cruz Jentoft AJ, Fielding RA, Kanis JA, Reginster JV, Bruyère O, Cesari M, Chapurlat R, Al Daghri N, Dennison E, Kaufman JM, Landi F, Laslop A, Locquet M, Maggi S, McCloskey E, Perna S, Rizzoli R, Rolland Y, Rondanelli M, Szulc P, Vellas B, Vlaskovska M, Cooper C. Is there enough evidence for osteosarcopenic obesity as a distinct entity? A critical literature review. Calcif Tissue Int. 2019;105(2):109–24.
80. Batsis JA, Villareal DT. Sarcopenic obesity in older adults: aetiology, epidemiology and treatment strategies. Nat Rev Endocrinol. 2018;14(9):513–37.
81. Trouwborst I, Verreijen A, Memelink R, Massanet P, Boirie Y, Weijs P, Tieland M. Exercise and nutrition strategies to counteract sarcopenic obesity. Nutrients. 2018;10:605.

The Role of Specific Motor Control Exercises

5

Dianne E. Andreotti, Sean G. T. Gibbons, and Francesco Cantarelli

Key Points

- Motor control is necessary for efficiently controlled movement.
- Numerous comorbidities associated with obesity can negatively influence motor control.
- Specific motor control exercises address the different characteristics of motor control and can be beneficial for obese patients.
- A comprehensive subclassification model and clinical reasoning process is essential for correct application of specific motor control exercises.

5.1 Motor Control, Pain and Specific Exercises

5.1.1 Motor Control

Motor control can be defined as the processing of information by the central nervous system (CNS) to organize the musculoskeletal system for postural control, coordinated movements, and actions [1, 2] together with the execution of the

D. E. Andreotti (✉)
SMARTERehab, St. John's, NL, Canada

S. G. T. Gibbons
SMARTERehab, St. John's, NL, Canada

Memorial University of Newfoundland, St. John's, NL, Canada

McMaster University of Hamilton, Hamilton, ON, Canada

F. Cantarelli
SMARTERehab, St. John's, NL, Canada

University of Brescia, Brescia, Italy

P. Capodaglio (ed.), *Rehabilitation Interventions in the Patient with Obesity*,
https://doi.org/10.1007/978-3-030-32274-8_5

movement itself. This complex process relies on the integration of sensory information, perception, motor planning, and movement execution. All these processes take place at the same time, with many brain areas working in parallel.

Motor control depends on a sensory motor system able to integrate many physiological mechanisms such as vision, vestibular function, tactility, and proprioception with muscle activity and neurocognitive functions and processing [3, 4]. For this integration the CNS is required to constantly manage the continuous bidirectional flow of data between the body and the external environment [5].

We believe that efficient motor control leads to efficiently controlled movement that could be seen as the correct amount of muscle activity for the requested task with the least amount of conscious effort [6]. In other words, without forgetting that there is variability in motor control, a subject demonstrates efficient motor control not just when the movement appears correct but also when his/her posture and movements are maintained and performed in an easy and automatic way, with a low sensation of effort and a high sensation of accuracy and precision. From a clinical point of view, motor control is strictly related to the quality with which posture and movement are performed. It is assessed through observation of the patient's specific muscle activation and movement strategies that then allow us to interpret how the central nervous system is elaborating sensory input and motor output. When observing and assessing a patient, the following questions are all related to the patient's motor control efficiency: is the alignment of the body regions correct, is the trajectory of the movement ideal, is the movement pattern appropriate for the task, is the muscle activity well distributed. When attempting to answer, we are trying to evaluate if the patient has sufficient motor control for the required task or if rehabilitation is necessary.

For example, when looking at a person's trunk in free sitting, we should concentrate on the spinal position and the activity of the abdominals and back extensor muscles. If the subject's motor control in this position is efficient for the back, ideally we will see a gentle physiological curve of the thoracic spine towards flexion and of the lumbar spine towards extension (avoiding any end of range passive positions) with the transition point between one curve and the other located at the thoraco-lumbar junction. The shoulders and hips will be aligned on the sagittal plane and the line of gravity will fall between the ischial tuberosities. The abdominals and back extensors should be active, to sustain this position, but the muscle tone should be homogeneously distributed without a prevalent contraction of the abdominals, of the paraspinals, or of the more lateral, longer trunk muscles.

Pain may or may not be present in people demonstrating poor motor control. Pain in a body region can provoke alterations in muscle activity [7] and in the way a person moves. However, in many situations, especially when considering chronic pain of an insidious onset, movement pattern alterations occur first, causing an overload of the tissues in that body region that then become symptomatic [8]. For this reason we need clinical strategies and indicators to not only assess pain but also movement patterns and to assist in evaluating when and if the motor control rehabilitation process is effective in modifying provocative postures and/or functional movements such as gait, sit to stand, reaching or bending forward.

5.1.2 Specific Motor Control Exercises (SMCE)

Some authors suggest that changing the manner in which a person controls his/her body is the main goal in active exercises called motor control exercises [2]. SMCE can be considered motor skill training if we consider that motor skill training, also known as procedural learning, takes place when the person is asked to practice a motor skill (or is asked to contract specific muscles) with the aim to improve or acquire a combination of motor functions such as muscle contraction, speed, accuracy, and consistency of a movement or movement sequence [9, 10]. When considering active exercise, important changes in cortical map reorganization has been documented at the brain level only with skill training. The nature of changes seen with strength and endurance training is different [11, 12]. For example, in our clinical experience, strength training modifies some features of movement but not the movement quality nor does it resolve an imbalance between muscle synergists. Motor skill training has the potential to change the way a person moves, influencing posture, functional movements, and specific muscle activation. In other words, motor skill training has the potential to change the person's motor control through sensory motor and cortical changes.

Three categories of SMCE are needed to address the different characteristics of motor control, and each category requires specific facilitation strategies to guide the patient during the motor control training.

Category 1: Specific motor control stability exercises (*SMCSE*) are highly specific isometric contractions of the deep muscles called *local stabilizers* [13] that have been shown to be more specific for translation control [14–16]. The exercises aim to bias segmental control and are generally performed using slow, isometric contractions controlled through palpation or scanning. The patient is asked to hold the contraction for ten seconds and to repeat ten times while breathing normally.

Category 2: Specific movement pattern control exercises (*SMPCE*) are exercises where one joint or region is consciously and easily maintained in a neutral position and an adjacent joint or region is independently moved while maintaining normal breathing. The exercises are generally performed with slow, low force repetitive movements [17, 18] requiring coordination of the muscle activation to avoid co-contraction rigidity.

Category 3: Specific global muscle imbalance retraining (*SGMIR*) are exercises that specifically bias the more one joint superficial muscles called *global stabilizers* [13] that produce and control movement and are responsible for global stability. The patient is asked to maintain an inner range contraction of a specific muscle for ten seconds and to repeat the contraction ten times maintaining normal breathing and without fatigue. The exercises can also address the multi-joint superficial muscles called *global mobilisers* [13] if the patient is requested to lengthen the muscle in question.

5.1.3 Motor Skill Training

The nature of motor skill training requires a voluntary and therefore cortical control of the contraction and/or movement performed. The execution of every exercise is monitored using observation, palpation and, when needed, instrumental support (e.g., technologies such as ultrasound). This is to guarantee the quality of the movement or contraction requested since it must be precise to be effective. When the patient experiences a low sensation of effort when performing a correct exercise, usually a progression in the training can be made by reducing the facilitation and/or changing elements within the exercise. Progression of the exercise could be an element that facilitates neuroplasticity [19], but it must be made within the correct timeframe. In fact, as seen in our clinical practice, an increase in the difficulty of a requested task can lead to failure of the rehabilitation if the change is made too early and the patient is not ready for it. Success in the rehabilitation is therefore dependent on the ability of the physiotherapist to guide the patient with the specific movement or specific muscle activation pattern and progression.

During the rehabilitation training, the performance is monitored and corrected using verbal cues, motor imagery, sensory motor feedback, and manual facilitation. For example, to achieve the correct neutral position of the lumbar spine, often the patient is facilitated if asked to think of lifting his/her sacrum from below. Clinically we frequently see that this leads to a multifidus contraction and the correct execution of the task. If the patient is asked to simply tilt his pelvis anteriorly, the execution more often involves a high activation of longissimus and/or iliocostalis leading to a global extension of both the lumbar and thoracic spines.

5.1.4 Exercise Prescription

The exercises are prescribed based on a comprehensive subclassification model (see Table 5.1) and clinical reasoning process. To benefit from SMCE, the patient must have mechanical pain, adequate motor skill learning ability, low behavioral issues, and low comorbid medical symptoms. To aid the clinical reasoning, the Motor Control Abilities Questionnaire (MCAQ) may be used. This is a self-report tool which was developed to identify the ability to learn SMCE [21]. The Neuro-Immune-Cardiometabolic-Endocrine screening tool may be used to identify comorbid medical symptoms [22].

The clinical reasoning process has four key aspects. (1) The therapist should match a MPC test to the functional activity that aggravates the patient's symptoms. For example, if sit to stand is the aggravating activity for the lumbar spine, the test seen in Fig. 5.1 would be used. This tests the patient's ability to control a neutral lumbar spine position during a sit to stand activity. (2) If a patho-anatomical diagnosis is available, the anatomical location of this should be within the region of the MPC test and the aim of treatment. Control of a referred pain region is less likely to be beneficial. (3) If there is a translation control deficit present, specific exercises would be prescribed to control this. Although SMCPE have the potential to help translation control and related symptoms, the only known way to fully rehabilitate a translation deficit is with targeted SMCSE. (4) The underlying cause of the poor motor control must also be addressed. Table 5.2 illustrates the most common causes of poor movement patterns using leaning forward in standing as an example. These should be addressed concurrently or as suitable during the progression of the rehabilitation.

A sample of SMCE, which can be useful for obese patients, is provided below.

Table 5.1 Overview of subclassification model

NICE syndrome*	Behavioral factors	Pain mechanisms	Neurological factors	Movement and motor function	Patho-anatomical
Subclassification and mechanisms					
• Comorbid medical symptoms • Comorbid medical conditions • Chronic low-grade systemic inflammation	• Clinical disorders • Maladaptive cognitions • Social factors	• Nociceptive • Neuropathic • Central sensitization • Central body image pain	• Motor skill learning abilities • Sensory motor function • Neurocognitive function • Body image spectrum • Low and high muscle tone	• Movement pattern control • Functional movement • Translation control • Motor fitness • Directional preference	• Articular • Myofascial • Neurodynamic • Connective tissue
Functional causes					
• Nutritional compromise • Environmental exposures • Behavioral factors • Infection	• NICE syndrome • Neurological factors • Adverse childhood exposures • Adverse adult exposures • Social factors	• NICE syndrome • Sensory motor gating • Behavioral factors • Ongoing tissue pathology	• Atypical birth history or early life • Neurodevelopmental disorders • NICE syndrome • Behavioral factors • Injury	• Sensory motor deficit • Restricted movement • Neurodevelopmental • Fatigue • Loading factors	• Trauma • Altered movement patterns • NICE syndrome

Ref. [20].
*neuro-immune, cardiometabolic and endocrine

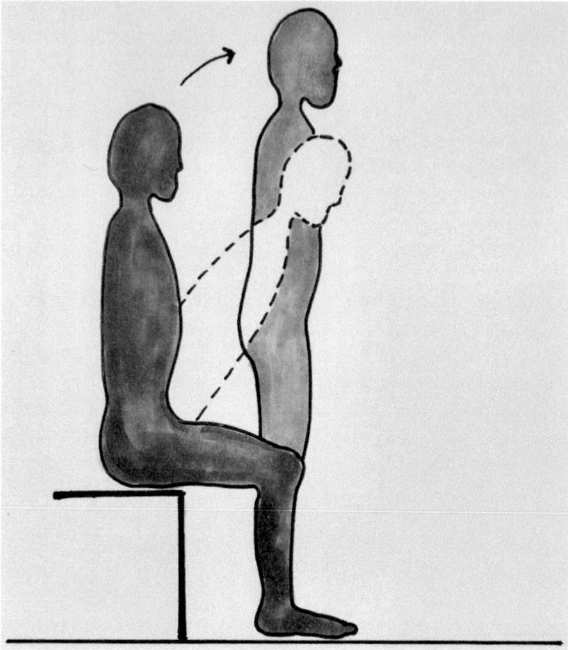

Fig. 5.1 A test of the patient's ability to control a neutral lumbar spine position and flex the hips during a sit to stand activity

Table 5.2 Examples of common causes of poor MPC: leaning forward in standing

Restrictions to movement	Hamstring tightness (and neurodynamic reactivity) OA of the hip Obesity
Sensorimotor function	Reduced proprioception (vibration) Neurodevelopmental disorders
Fatigue	May be due to reduced proprioception
Loading factors	Habitual activities at end-range postures Altering body position Longer lever during lifting
Other	Over 60 years of age Weakness Dual tasking Muscle tone changes with low-grade inflammation

Ref. [23]

5.2 Motor Control and Obesity: Literature and Subclassification

5.2.1 What Is Different About Adults with Obesity?

Obesity is a multifactorial and complex presentation. There are lifestyle, genetic, environmental, social, and cultural factors involved. Obesity is considered a chronic low-grade inflammatory disease [24]. It is associated with neuro-immune [25–27], cardiometabolic dysfunction [28–30], and endocrine dysregulation [31–35]. These neuro-immune, cardiometabolic, and endocrine (NICE) factors are directly and indirectly associated with numerous comorbidities and their associated symptoms. The central and peripheral nervous systems are influenced, which in turn influence the motor system. This, along with the morphological changes and associated challenges, create considerable changes in motor function.

Numerous comorbidities are associated with obesity. They include cardiovascular disease [36], hypertension, several types of cancer [37], stroke [38], diabetes and pre-diabetes [39], gastroesophageal reflux disease [40, 41], cholelithiasis [42], obstructive sleep apnea and reduced sleep health [43], and mental health problems [38]. Severe obesity has been associated with an increased rate of death from all causes and decreased life expectancy. This is regardless of age, smoking, educational level, geographic region, and physical activity levels [44].

Obesity is also an established risk factor for degenerative joint disease or osteoarthritis [37, 45–47], osteoporosis [37], and lower urinary tract symptoms and pelvic floor disorders including pelvic organ prolapse, stress urinary incontinence, overactive bladder, and fecal incontinence [48, 49].

5.2.2 Subclassification

Subclassification is currently recommended to help guide the rehabilitation of neuromuscular disorders such as low back pain [50]. This is based on the premise that certain therapies are more appropriate for subgroups based on their individual presentation. In brief, with this approach, patients are placed in groups based on clinical presentation criteria, physical assessment, questionnaires, or investigations. A targeted therapy is then created from this profile. A category may be considered a subgroup if it identifies a poor prognosis, provides a diagnosis or describes an underlying mechanism for the presentation, or predicts a response to therapy [51]. Common subclassification categories include *behavioral factors* (prognosis), *pain mechanisms* (mechanism), *movement patterns and spinal control* (mechanism), and *patho-anatomical* (diagnosis). Recently *neurological factors* (motor skill learning ability) [52] and *comorbid medical symptoms* [53] have been added for their ability to predict a response to therapy (Table 5.1).

Obesity represents a unique population of neuromusculoskeletal disorders. In order to identify if someone is suitable for SMCE, it is important to understand if they have the ability to learn the exercises [21] and can respond to the rehabilitation. SMCE require more sensory motor and neurocognitive function than general exercise; therefore, some people are unable to learn the exercises [54]. Preliminary work suggests that widespread subjective comorbid medical symptoms limit the ability to respond to the rehabilitation, despite having learnt the exercises. It is hypothesized that the mechanism responsible for this is low-grade inflammation that influences muscle tone and/or pain threshold [53].

5.2.3 Subclassification Categories Influencing SMCE

5.2.3.1 Behavioral Factors

There is often a stigma associated with obesity and people often have to deal with various forms of discrimination and prejudice [55–63]. Body image is one of the most common behavioral issues in obesity [64]. Body image may be defined as the degree of satisfaction about appearance [65]. It has three categories: cognitive (perception of physical appearance), subjective (satisfaction about appearance), and behavioral (avoidance of exposures, anxiety, and discomfort). There is a much higher incidence of anxiety and depression in obese subjects compared to normal-weight subjects [66]. Bipolar is also a common comorbid condition [44]. Behavioral factors can have unhelpful effects on motor function. Various behavioral factors have been shown to influence muscle tone [67, 68], change movement patterns [69], alter the timing of spinal muscles [70], and influence respiratory patterns [71, 72]. They are also associated with the presence of primitive reflexes [73] which can influence motor function [74].

5.2.3.2 Neurological Factors

Obesity is associated with altered brain structure and plasticity [75]. Reduced neurocognitive function has been found over the life span [76–78].

Numerous sensory motor functions are altered in obesity including the perception of the intensity of peripheral pain [79–81], vibratory sensation and temperature [82], sense of satiety [83], gastric motor functions [84], ability to discriminate between object weights [85], tactile acuity of the knees [86], and tactility-based body part representations [87]. Further, obesity may alter the sensory messages from the foot plantar mechanoreceptors [88]. The central processing and/or function of somatosensory afferents may be altered in obesity. Sensory and motor nerve impulses are lower in obesity [89] as well as motor unit activation [90] and muscle spindle input to alpha motor neurons. This, in turn, may decrease muscle tone [91]. Motor behavior is the output of the sensory integration process which involves the individual, the task being carried out, and the environment in which it takes place [92, 93]. Obese subjects have reduced postural control [94] and require greater attention for control [95]. Clumsiness is commonly reported by obese subjects [96] and there is an increased risk of falls [97, 98].

5.2.3.3 Motor Function

With the excess mass, the physical body shape is altered in obesity. This alters body geometry and the line of gravity which limits the variability of normal movement. Given this altered body image, sensory motor changes, and possible central processing influences on obesity, it would be expected that numerous alterations in motor behavior would be observed in these subjects. In general, there are limitations to overall range of movement, with variable compensations, and movements are performed more slowly [38], especially in antigravity actions [99].

The effect of obesity is variable across movement tasks [100]; however there are some general patterns. There are alterations during sit to stand, [99, 101, 102], trunk flexion [37, 94, 103, 104], lifting, reaching [105], and lateral flexion [104].

During gait, speed is slower with a reduced step length, step frequency, shorter swing, and longer single and double stance phase [37]. There is increased rearfoot motion, with forefoot abduction [106]. Gait characteristics in Class III obesity resemble changes in gait following a cerebrovascular accident [107].

There are considerable differences in respiratory function in obese subjects. They have a heightened demand for ventilation, an elevated breathing workload, respiratory muscle inefficiency, and diminished respiratory compliance [108] and capacity [109]. During normal breathing, they tend to have a rapid and shallow breathing pattern due to an elevated oxygen consumption [110, 111]. This may have widespread implications since the diaphragm has multiple functions. The diaphragm provides the largest influence on intra-abdominal pressure and has a role in spinal control [15, 112]. The diaphragm's respiratory function is superimposed on the spinal stabilization function as well as on micturition, defecation, and possibly parturition. The diaphragm also plays a crucial role in the vascular and lymphatic systems and is greatly involved in gastroesophageal functions such as in swallowing and emesis and as an anti-reflex barrier [113].

There is general agreement that obese subjects, compared to normal-weight persons, have lower maximal strength when relative body mass is considered although there is greater absolute maximum strength [114]. Obesity can affect isometric, concentric, and eccentric muscle force [114–116] and is not the same across body site and function [115, 116]. This effect is mostly seen in antigravity muscles where the greater size acts as a chronic overload stimulus [114].

The differences above were discussed with reference to adults. It should be noted that many of these changes have been observed in children and adolescent populations. There may also be gender differences and a worsening of certain characteristics based on the magnitude of obesity. However, taken together, these changes in motor behavior impact on activities of daily living and quality of life in obese subjects. This provides the opportunity for a SMCE intervention to assist obese subjects.

5.3 Posture, Movement and Obesity: The Clinical Analysis

In obese subjects excess weight imposes abnormal mechanics on body movements and provokes standing and sitting postures that are not always biomechanically ideal or well controlled. In standing the additional abdominal mass contributes to increased lumbar lordosis and anterior pelvic tilt and causes an anterior shift of the body center of gravity relative to the ankle joint [97, 117]. To compensate, obese subjects tend to lean the upper trunk backwards and flex the thoracic spine. This lumbar posture indicates long and inefficient lower abdominal and gluteal muscles that are unable to maintain the correct lumbar-pelvic alignment. The posture is sustained by the longer thoracic muscles going from the upper trunk to the pelvis such as iliocostalis, longissimus, and external obliques that attempt to maintain stability between the trunk and the pelvis. Unfortunately these muscles also limit ribcage mobility and segmental rotation and extension of the thoracic spine and don't provide deep muscle control and stability for the lumbar spine. As a result, trunk lateral flexion and rotation occurs mainly in the lumbar spine increasing the possibility of excessive translation and joint overload that may lead to chronic low back pain. This trunk rigidity will also have a negative effect on the fine automatic postural adjustments needed to maintain postural stability and will limit the posterolateral expansion of the lower ribcage rendering efficient diaphragmatic breathing difficult and the apical respiration pattern dominate.

Three common problems seen in obesity can be linked to motor control deficits and muscle imbalances due to obese posture: chronic low back pain [104, 118], reduction in respiratory capacity [109, 119, 120], and urinary incontinence [121]. Mechanisms of respiration, continence, and lumbar stability are intertwined. The pelvic floor muscles and the diaphragm not only play an important role in continence and breathing, but, together with the transversus abdominis, the deep fibers of lumbar multifidus and possibly the psoas major form the deep lumbar cylinder, responsible for providing lumbopelvic stability through correct intra-abdominal pressure [122–124]. These common symptom presentations seen in obese subjects would lead to believe that the deep lumbar cylinder is often insufficient and the longer and more superficial trunk muscles dominate in their attempt to compensate.

Also in standing, due to the thoracic flexion and the weight and circumference of the upper arms, we find the scapulae of obese subjects protracted and depressed and the upper limbs rolled anteriorly into medial rotation. The apical breathing pattern previously mentioned and the biomechanically disadvantaged position of the scapulae and upper limbs pulls the cervical spine into increased lordosis predisposing the patient to mid-cervical translation and shoulder impingement symptoms.

Obese subjects also stand with a wider than normal stance partly due to the circumference of the thighs and possibly to facilitate balance. In one leg stance, we see increased pelvic obliquity [125] indicating poor control of the lumbar pelvic region and insufficient gluteal activation. The hips often tend to be in medial rotation, the knees in valgus and hyperextension, and the ankles rotated outward in excessive plantar flexion and pronation with a collapse of the medial longitudinal arch. In gait, push-off at the ankle is inefficient [97] because the mid-foot is not in a stable close-packed supinated position facilitating the push-off and the plantar flexor muscles are unable to generate sufficient force in a lengthened, end-of-range position. Lack of stability at the hip and pelvis due to inefficient gluteal muscle activation not only promotes incorrect joint loading of the lower limbs and lumbar spine predisposing the patient to chronic musculoskeletal pain [126–128] and degenerative changes [129, 130] at the lumbar spine, hip, knee, and foot but also has the potential to negatively influence gait speed and postural stability thus increasing the risk of falls and injury common to this patient group.

Obese subjects tend to sit in thoracic and lumbar flexion, while the mid-cervical spine is often in anterior translation and/or excessive upper cervical extension.

The scapulae are again protracted and depressed further loading the cervical spine. The lower limbs are in abduction to allow space for the abdominal mass.

5.4 Musculoskeletal Rehabilitation in Obesity

The clinical analysis of the typical postures and movement patterns seen in obesity suggest some appropriate SMCE for musculoskeletal rehabilitation when the patient meets subclassification criteria.

5.4.1 Therapeutic Steps

The therapeutic steps required for SMCE are varied and individual for each patient. Therefore, the following proposals cannot be considered to be a treatment protocol but simply examples of possible exercises to correct common conditions. We would like to stress that precision, concentration, and neurocognitive and sensory motor requirements are required not only in the specific exercises requested but also during the integration into functional movements such as walking, stair climbing, reaching, bending, and going from sitting to standing.

Precision control of the exercises is ideally provided through palpation or technological support such as ultrasound or biofeedback; however, the excess adipose tissue in obese subjects makes both difficult, if not impossible, and therefore control is somewhat limited compared to what is possible in normal-weight subjects. Decreased proprioception and altered body image, if present, will slow rehabilitation progress. However, it is also true that any improvement in posture and in the breathing pattern of an obese patient has potential for significant positive change.

During the rehabilitation it is not only important to choose the correct exercises for the individual patient but, when necessary, the best facilitation strategy. Motor imagery is ideal and can be assisted by sensory motor strategies such as tactility, position changes to alter levers and loads, guided hands-on movement, and especially proprioception. As the rehabilitation progresses and the patient improves, the facilitation that was previously needed should be reduced and eventually eliminated.

The exercises should be continued until they can be performed with low effort, without facilitation, and can be integrated into functional activities that were previously difficult and/or provocative. The time required for this is varied depending on the underlying mechanisms present including motor skill learning ability determined by the MCAQ and NICE comorbidities previously diagnosed and, of course, the patient's compliance.

5.4.2 Where and How to Start?

A major problem for obese subjects is when the multi-joint superficial muscles become dominant to the more proximal segmental muscles altering the trajectory of joint movement, limiting freedom and variety of movement and possibly giving rise to joint and tissue overload. Therefore the analysis of the patient's posture and movement patterns and any symptoms present will guide us in our choice of where and how to begin.

Proximal stability is essential for correct distal movement and, as in all movement, is dependent on an efficient sensory motor system. It is important to appreciate that movement control is not always a question of strength but of the ability to rapidly perceive and adjust muscle activity to changes in load. The perception of which muscle is activating, as well as how strong is the activation, is an essential part of specific motor control rehabilitation. Strength training is then built on efficient motor control.

5.4.3 Lumbar-Pelvic Neutral

A useful starting point for the rehabilitation of obese subjects is the acquisition of the lumbar-pelvic neutral position in various positions; lying, sitting, and standing. Lumbar-pelvic neutral is the patient's midrange position between anterior and posterior pelvic tilt where the deep segmental muscles are solicited. As seen in Fig. 5.2, the patient, when seated, is asked to anteriorly tilt the pelvis initiating from the sacrum and not by extending the thoracic spine. In this way, the contraction of segmental lumbar multifidus is dominant over the long trunk muscles, thus facilitating lumbar segmental control and proximal stability. In sitting, obese patients tend to be in end-of-range posterior tilt and lumbar flexion, and so the activation of segmental lumbar multifidus, internal obliques, and psoas major together with iliacus is a priority for lumbar-pelvic control. In standing however, they are often in excessive anterior tilt, and therefore the internal obliques and gluteus maximus are essential to obtain proximal stability and control the neutral lumbar-pelvic position referred to as neutral. In standing the patient is asked to posteriorly tilt the pelvis by lifting from the pubic bone. The lower abdominal wall should lift and flatten without limiting lower ribcage expansion and thoracic mobility, and the patient should be aware of a bilateral gluteal contraction.

The pelvic floor muscles, very often insufficient in obese subjects, represent the floor of the deep lumbar cylinder and co-activate with the deep abdominal muscle, transversus abdominis, and the diaphragm [122]. Activation of the pelvic floor muscles can facilitate lower abdominal activation. Different commands can be used to facilitate the pelvic floor muscles. One example for men is to lift the testicles as if walking into a cold lake and women to gently close the anus and then the urethra lifting the pelvic floor (Fig. 5.3). The lower abdominal wall should tension.

The neutral lumbar-pelvic position should never be maintained with high load co-contraction rigidity and breath holding. Neutral assists postural correction and postural control and becomes the starting position for all SMPCE that challenge lumbar-pelvic control. The ability to perceive and control neutral should be slowly integrated into all daily activities.

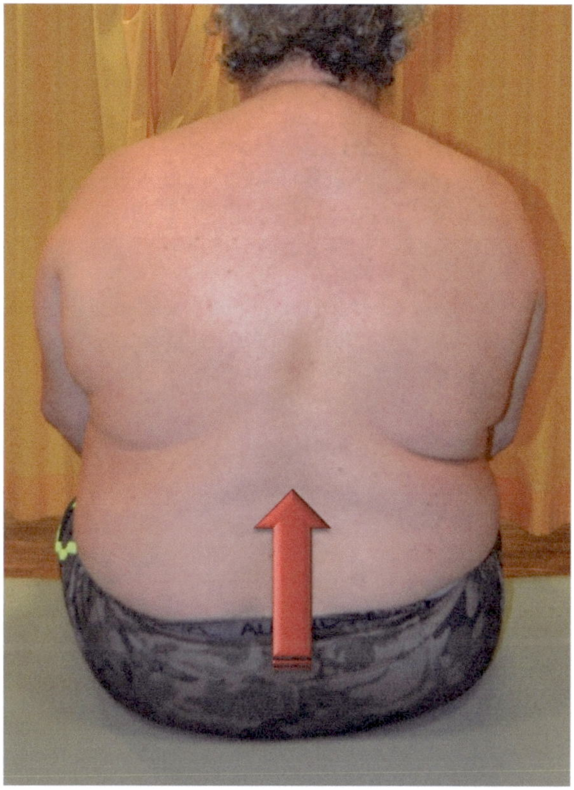

Fig. 5.2 The patient is asked to anteriorly tilt the pelvis initiating from the sacrum and not by extending the thoracic spine

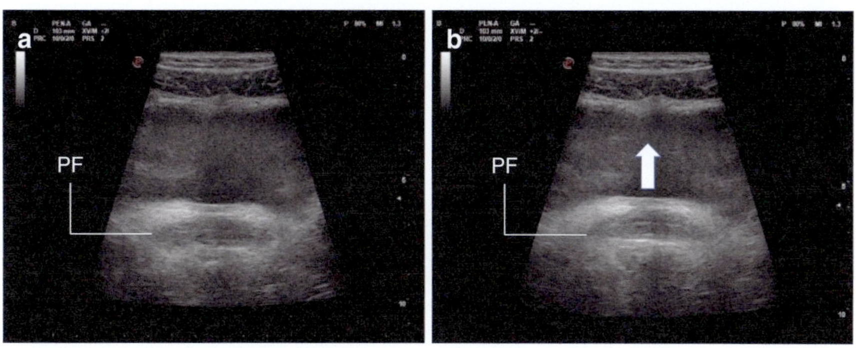

Fig. 5.3 Correct voluntary pelvic floor (PF) contraction in a normal-weight subject. (**a**) Resting position of the pelvic floor; (**b**) the pelvic floor elevates during the contraction

5.4.4 Examples of SMCE

Initially the SMCE can begin in positions that provide sensory information to facilitate postural control such as inclined sitting, sitting with a back support, or standing against a wall. As progress is made, the same exercise can again become challenging by eliminating the postural support and decreasing any sensory feedback given by hands, towels, or supports. The choice of which exercise to choose is dependent on the treatment priority of the patient and his/her ability for motor learning. All exercises must be carried out while maintaining lumbar-pelvic neutral and must not be provocative. Skin creases are often seen in the lumbar and cervical spines possibly indicating excessive anterior segmental translation. If the patient's symptoms correspond to this anatomical area, then SMCSE should be added to the treatment prescription.

Exercise 1: Diaphragmatic breathing	
Aim:	Improve respiratory function
	Reduce joint and muscle stress in the cervical region
Starting position:	Supine, side lying, or inclined sitting in lumbar-pelvic neutral
Exercise:	Breathe in nasally expanding and lifting the lower ribcage posterolaterally without lifting the sternum. Continue breathing diaphragmatically
Facilitation and/or feedback if necessary:	Elastic band, towel, or hands on the lower ribcage to provide light resistance increasing sensory input (Fig. 5.4)
	Hand on the sternum to control that the sternum does not lift
	Hand on the pelvis to control lumbar-pelvic neutral

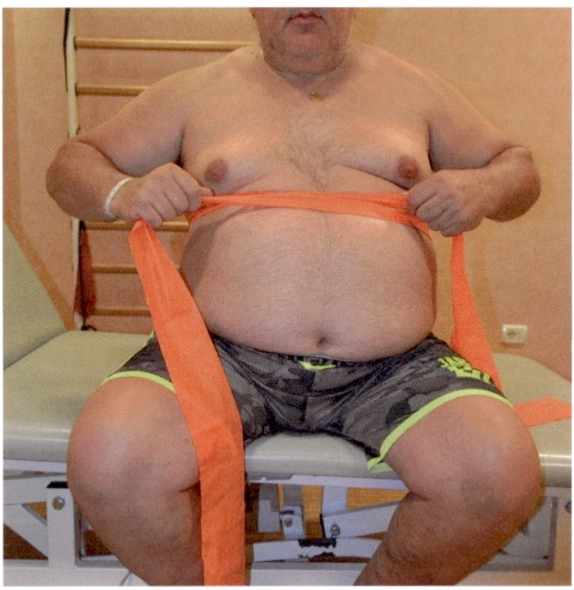

Fig. 5.4 During the diaphragmatic breathing exercise, an elastic band, towel, or hands are placed on the lower ribcage to facilitate by providing a light resistance to increase sensory input

Exercise 2: Thoracic posture and mobility	
Aim:	Decrease thoracic and ribcage rigidity
	Decrease dominance of long thoracic extensors and improve activation of thoracic multifidus
Starting position:	Standing or sitting in lumbar-pelvic neutral
Exercise:	Place one index finger at the sternal notch and the other at the xiphoid process
	Lift the sternum by extending the thoracic spine to mid-range without altering the lumbar spine or pelvis (Fig. 5.5) (10 repetitions 10 s) progression—in mid-range thoracic extension, rotate only the thoracic spine freely to the left and then to the right (10 repetitions) (Fig. 5.6)
Facilitation and/or feedback if necessary:	One hand controls the sternal lift while other hand controls lumbar-pelvic neutral

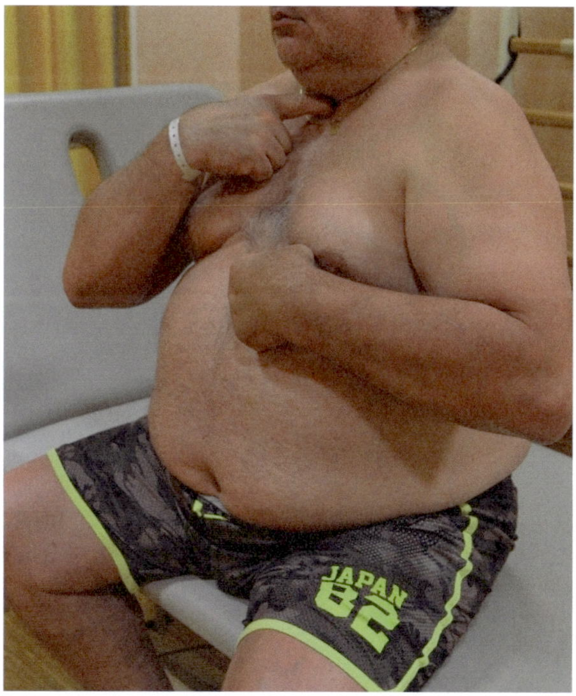

Fig. 5.5 Place one index finger at the sternal notch and the other at the xiphoid process and extend the thoracic spine segmentally by lifting the sternum without pelvic movement

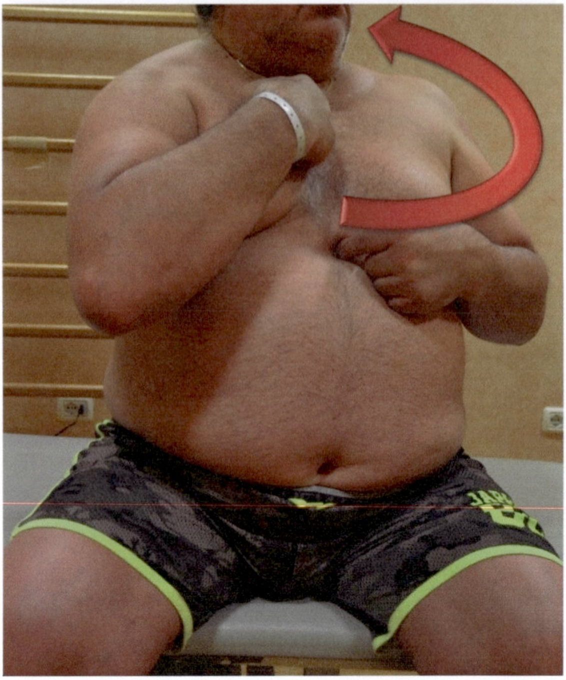

Fig. 5.6 Rotate the thoracic spine freely while maintaining thoracic extension, lumbar-pelvic neutral, and a diaphragmatic breathing pattern

Exercise 3: Lumbar-pelvic control in lying	
Aim:	Increase lumbar-pelvic control under load of the lower limb
	Ensure that hip flexion and rotation can occur independently to lumbar-pelvic movements
Starting position:	Supine in lumbar-pelvic neutral or inclined lying if supine is poorly tolerated
Exercise:	Do unilateral hip flexion by sliding one foot up the plinth to the level of the opposite knee without hiking or rotating the pelvis and return to the starting position (Fig. 5.7). Go only as far as lumbar-pelvic control can be maintained. Repeat with the opposite leg (10 repetitions each leg)
	Progression—in the flexed position, externally rotate the hip without rotating the pelvis (Fig. 5.8). Go only as far as control can be maintained. Repeat with the opposite leg (10 repetitions each leg)
Facilitation and/or feedback if necessary:	Facilitate the sliding movement by placing a firm, slippery surface under the legs and a towel under the moving foot
	Hands control lumbar-pelvic neutral

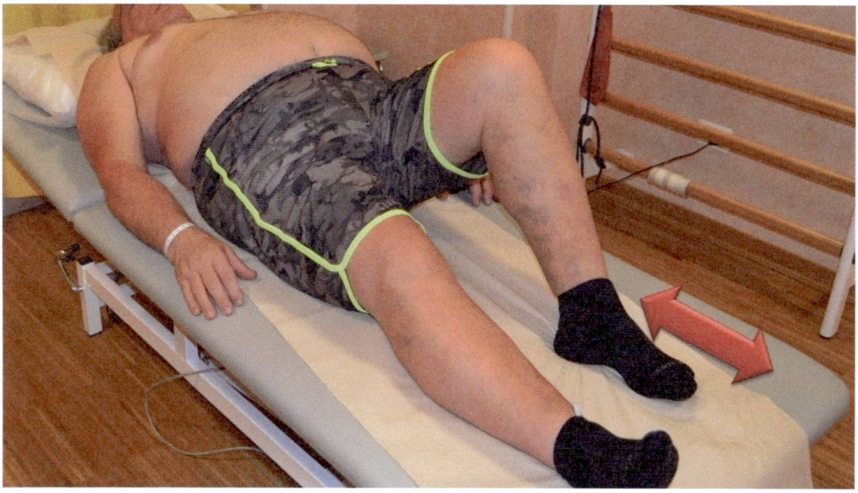

Fig. 5.7 Slide one foot up the plinth to the level of the opposite knee without hiking or rotating the pelvis. Go as far as the lumbar-pelvic control can be maintained

Fig. 5.8 Externally rotate the hip without rotating the pelvis as far as the lumbar-pelvic control can be maintained

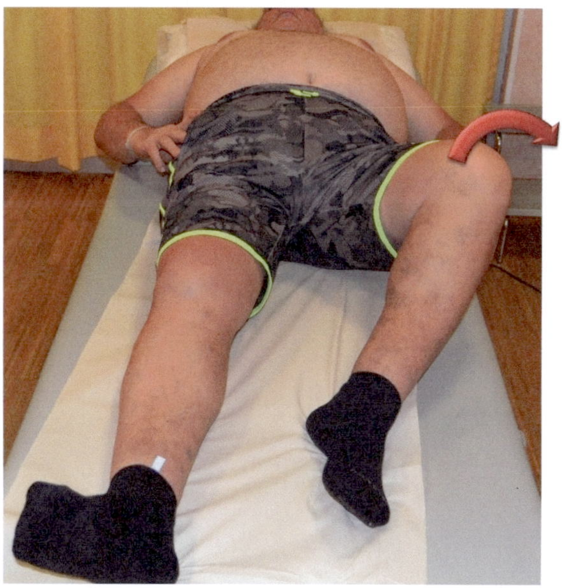

Exercise 4: Lumbar-pelvic control in standing	
Aim:	Correct pelvic obliquity in one leg stance to prepare for walking and stairs
Starting position:	Free standing in lumbar-pelvic neutral with the feet in correct alignment under the hip joints as much as possible
Exercise:	Shift the body weight over one foot without altering the alignment of the pelvis and then return to the mid position (Fig. 5.9). Go only as far as pelvic control allows. Repeat going to the opposite side (10 repetitions to each side)
	Progression—shift to one side and then lift the opposite heel (Fig. 5.10)
	Shift to one side, lift the opposite foot, and place it on a book
	Gradually progress to stair height
Facilitation and/or feedback if necessary:	In lumbar-pelvic neutral, stand against a wall for sensory input to assist postural stability
	Hands on pelvis to control lumbar-pelvic neutral

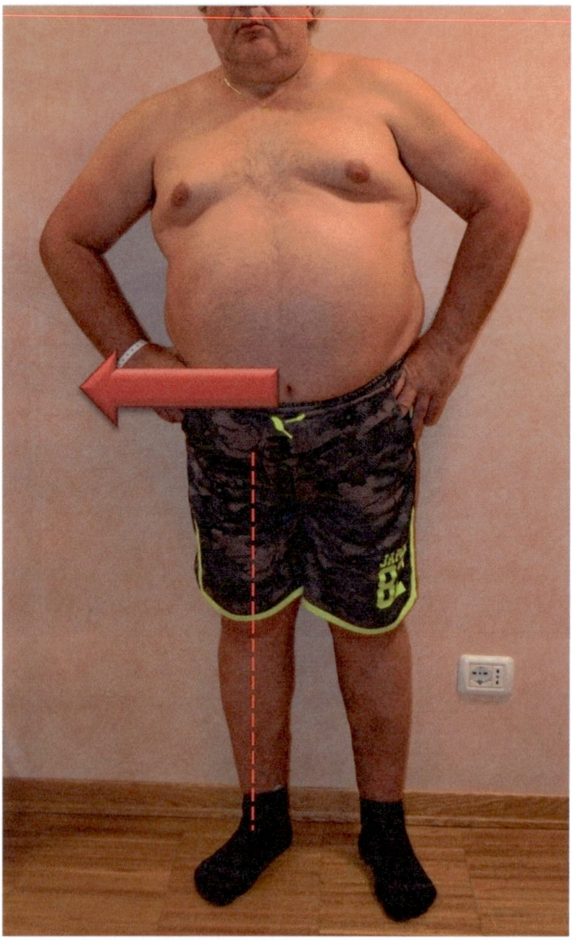

Fig. 5.9 In preparation for walking with lumbar-pelvic control, shift the body weight over one foot without altering the alignment of the pelvis

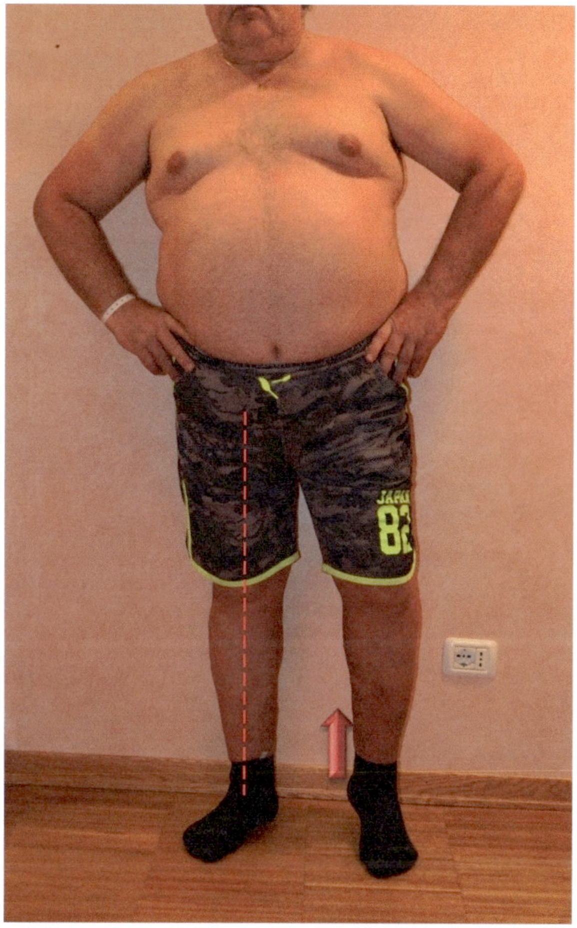

Fig. 5.10 In preparation for stair climbing with lumbar-pelvic control, shift the body weight over one foot and then lift the opposite heel. Progress to placing the foot onto a small step

Exercise 5: Bilateral lower limb flexion	
Aim:	Correct lower limb alignment to improve gait and stair climbing and facilitate eccentric and concentric activation of gluteus maximus
Starting position:	Free standing or standing against a wall for sensory input to assist postural stability with the feet under the hip joints as much as possible
Exercise:	Squat, flexing both hips and knees simultaneously while maintaining good alignment of the trunk and lower limbs (hip and knee joints in line with the second metatarsal) (Fig. 5.11). Return to the starting position. Gluteus maximus and medius should remain active during both the eccentric and concentric parts of the exercise. Go only as far the alignment remains correct and glutei remain active (10 repetitions)
	Progression—in one leg standing, without changing the lower limb alignment and the gluteus activation, rotate the pelvis in both directions on the flexed lower limb (10 repetitions to each side)

Facilitation and/or feedback if necessary:	Use a laser beam to control the alignment of the lower limb (Fig. 5.12)
	Hand on pelvis to control lumbar-pelvic neutral
	Hand on gluteus maximus just distal to the ischial tuberosity or gluteus medius just cranially and posteriorly to the greater trochanter to control activation (Fig. 5.13)
	During the progression exercise, an object can be placed just lateral to the knee to provide sensory input for the lower limb alignment control

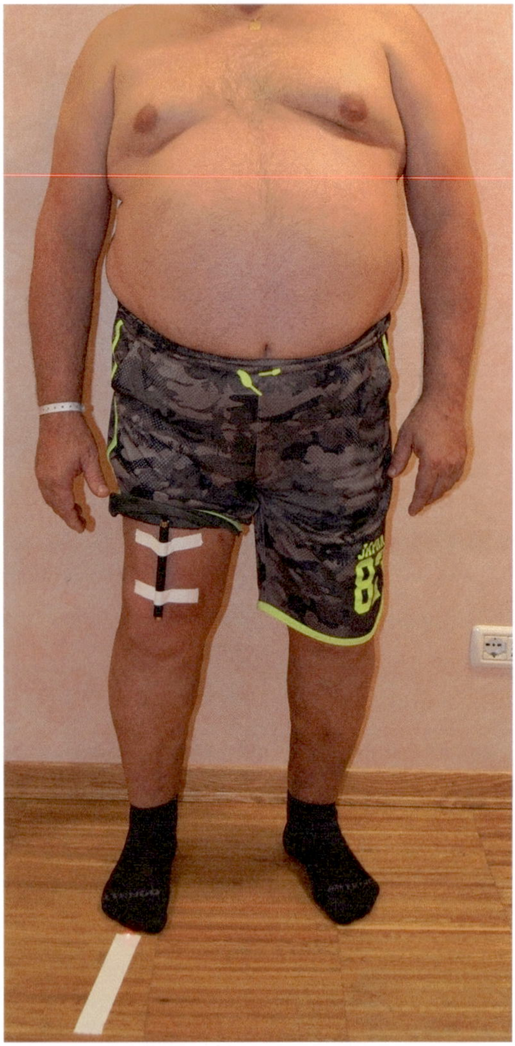

Fig. 5.11 Flex both hips and knees simultaneously while maintaining good alignment of the trunk and lower limbs (hip and knee joints should remain in line with the second metatarsal)

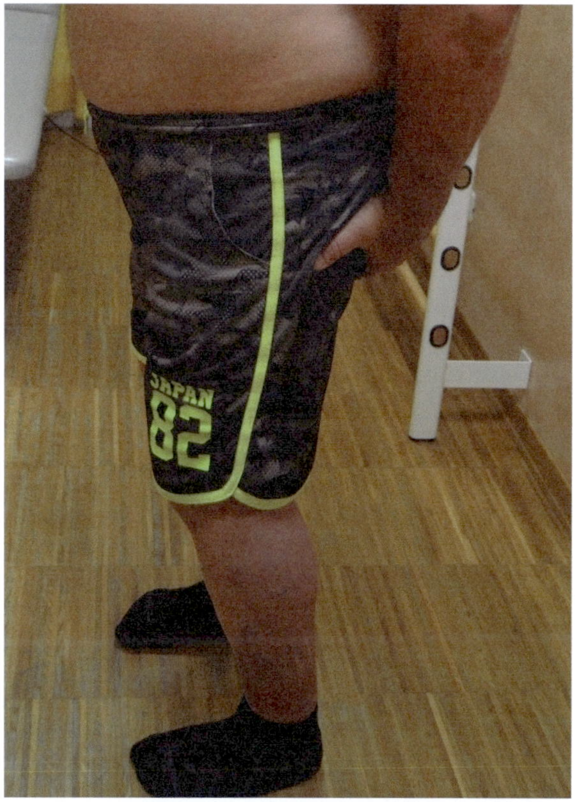

Fig. 5.12 Palpate gluteus maximus just distal to the ischial tuberosities

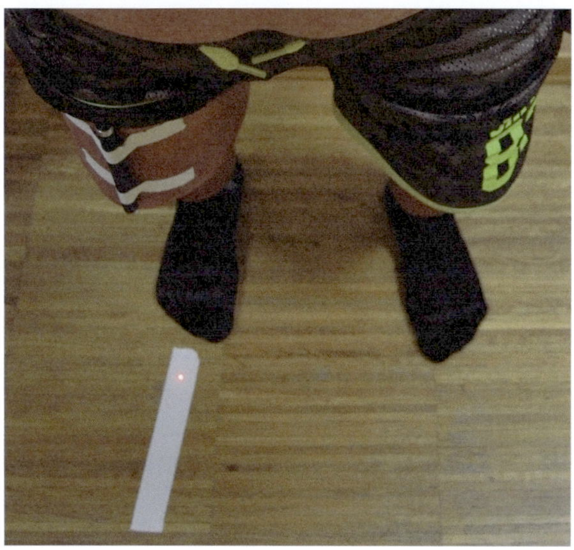

Fig. 5.13 A laser beam can be used to control the correct alignment of the lower limb during flexion in functional tasks such as stairs or squatting down

Exercise 6: Sit to stand	
Aim:	Facilitate a better gluteal contraction and trunk coordination to decrease torque at the knees when standing up or sitting down
Starting position:	Sitting in lumbar-pelvic neutral on a high stool with feet supported on the floor and in correct lower limb alignment. Progress to normal chair height
Exercise:	Flex the trunk forward at the hips bringing the weight over the feet and stand up using a gluteal contraction and not trunk extension. Slowly return to the starting position with eccentric gluteal control (10 repetitions)
Facilitation and/or feedback if necessary:	Hand on pelvis to control lumbar-pelvic neutral
	Palpate gluteus maximus bilaterally, just distal to the ischial tuberosities, to control activation throughout the exercise

Exercise 7: Lower limb external rotation	
Aim:	Facilitate a gluteus medius contraction in inner range to improve pelvic control and lower limb alignment
	Starting position: side lying in lumbar-pelvic neutral with hips and knees flexed
Exercise:	Maintain the feet together and lift the upper leg by externally rotating the hip to end range without pelvic movement. Slowly return to the starting position (10 repetitions 10 s with each leg)
Facilitation and/or feedback if necessary:	Hand on pelvis to control lumbar-pelvic neutral and pelvic rotation
	Palpate gluteus medius just cranially and posteriorly to the greater trochanter to ensure a contraction throughout the concentric and eccentric movement (Fig. 5.14)

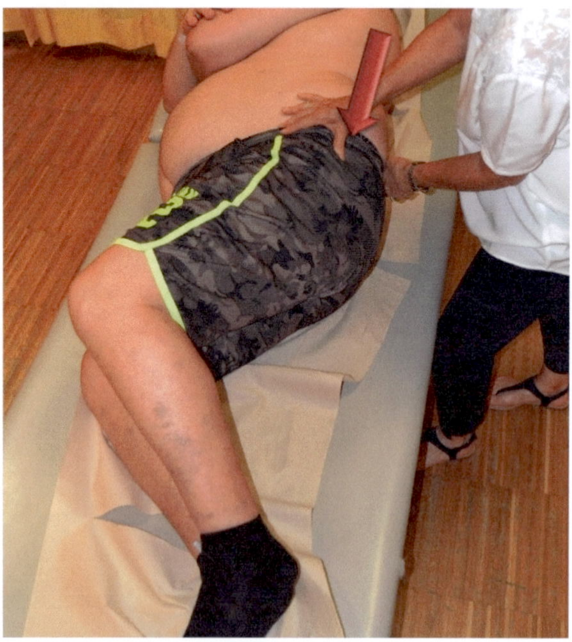

Fig. 5.14 Palpate gluteus medius just cranially and posteriorly to the greater trochanter

5.5 Conclusion

Obesity is a complex problem that benefits from multidisciplinary interventions. There is a role in obesity for SMCE for various motor function and motor behavior issues.

References

1. Shumway-Cook A, Woollacott M. Motor control: issues and theories. In: Motor control: translating research into clinical practice. 4th ed. Philadelphia: Lippincott Williams & Wilkins; 2011.
2. van Dieën JH, Reeves NP, Kawchuk G, et al. Analysis of motor control in patients with low back pain: a key to personalized care? J Orthop Sports Phys Ther. 2019;49(6):380–8.
3. Quatman-Yates CC, Quatman CE, Meszaros AJ, et al. A systematic review of sensorimotor function during adolescence: a developmental stage of increased motor awkwardness? Br J Sports Med. 2012;46(9):649–55.
4. Gibbons SGT. Problem solving in specific motor control exercise rehabilitation. Neuromusc Rehab Rev. 2011;1(1):7–13.
5. Hodges PW, Moseley GL. Pain and motor control of the lumbopelvic region: effect and possible mechanisms. J Electromyogr Kinesiol. 2003;13(4):361–70.
6. Strassl H, Andreotti Jackson D, Cantarelli F, et al. Spezifische Übungen zur Verbesserung der Bewegungskontrolle: ihre Rolle und Regeln in der Rehabilitation. Sportphysio. 2016;04:16–22.
7. Hodges PW, Danneels L. Changes in structure and function of the back muscles in low back pain: different time points, observations, and mechanisms. J Orthop Sports Ohys Ther. 2019;49(6):464–76.
8. Hides JA, Donelson R, Lee D, et al. Convergence and divergence of exercise-based approaches that incorporate motor control for the management of low back pain. J Orthop Sports Phys Ther. 2019;49(6):437–52.
9. Makino H, Hwang EJ, Hedrick NG, et al. Circuit mechanisms of sensorimotor learning. Neuron. 2016;92(4):705–21.
10. Marich AV, Hwang CT, Salsich GB, et al. Consistency of a lumbar movement pattern across functional activities in people with low back pain. Clin Biomech (Bristol, Avon). 2017;44:45–51.
11. Adkins DL, Bojchuk J, Remple MS, et al. Motor training induces experience-specific patterns of plasticity across motor cortex and spinal cord. J Appl Physiol. 2006;101(6):1776–82.
12. Jensen JL, Marstrand PC, Nielsen JB. Motor skill training and strength training are associated with different plastic changes in the central nervous system. J Appl Physiol. 2005;99(4):1558–68.
13. Gibbons SGT, Comerford MJ. Strength versus stability. Part 1: concept and terms. Orthop Div Rev. 2001;
14. Richardson C, Jull G, Hodges P, et al. Therapeutic exercise for spinal segmental stabilization in low back pain. Edinburgh: Churchill Livingstone; 1999.
15. Hodges P, Kaigle HA, Holm S, et al. Intervertebral stiffness of the spine is increased by evoked contraction of transversus abdominis and the diaphragm: in vivo porcine studies. Spine. 2003;28(23):2594–601.
16. Richardson CA, Hides JA. The rationale for a motor control programme for the treatment of spinal muscle dysfunction. In: Boyling JD, Jull GA, editors. Grieve's modern manual therapy. 3rd ed. Edinburgh: Churchill Livingstone; 2005.

17. Gibbons SGT Sub-classification of core stability exercise for the purpose of a systematic review. Proceedings of: The 6th Interdisciplinary World Congress on Low Back Pain. November 7–11; Barcelona, Spain, 2007.
18. Lehtola V, Luomajoki H, Leinonen V, et al. Efficacy of movement control exercises versus general exercises on recurrent sub-acute nonspecific low back pain in a sub-group of patients with movement control dysfunction. Protocol of a randomized controlled trial. BMC Musculoskelet Disord. 2012;13:55.
19. Christiansen L, Madsen MJ, Bojsen-Møller E, et al. Progressive practice promotes motor learning and repeated transient increases in corticospinal excitability across multiple days. Brain Stimul. 2018;11(2):346–57.
20. Gibbons SGT. Can manual therapists diagnose instability of the sacro-iliac joint? Manuelletherapie (German). 2015;19(5):211–6. https://doi.org/10.1055/s-0035-1570013.
21. Gibbons SGT. The development, initial reliability and construct validity of the motor control abilities questionnaire. Man Ther. 2009;14(S1):S22.
22. Gibbons SGT. Preliminary development of items to identify a neuro-immune-autonomic-endocrine involvement in complex pain presentations. Man Ther. 2016;25:e109–10.
23. Gibbons SGT. What are the functional mechanisms of altered movement patterns during trunk flexion tasks? The need for further sub-classification: a systematic review. Proceedings of "Expanding Horizons": The 11th International Conference of IFOMT. July 4–8; Glasgow, Scotland. 2016.
24. Castro AM, Macedo-de la Concha LE, Pantoja-Meléndez CA. Low-grade inflammation and its relation to obesity and chronic degenerative diseases. Rev Med Hosp Gen Méx. 2017;80(2):101–5.
25. Chaldakov GN, Fiore M, Ghenev PI, Beltowski J, Rančić G, Tunçel N, Aloe L. Triactome: neuro-immune-adipose interactions. Implication in vascular biology. Front Immunol. 2014;5:130. https://doi.org/10.3389/fimmu.2014.00130.. eCollection 2014
26. Cox AJ, West NP, Cripps AW. Obesity, inflammation, and the gut microbiota. Lancet Diabetes Endocrinol. 2015;3(3):207–15. https://doi.org/10.1016/S2213-8587(14)70134-2.
27. Terrando N, Pavlov VA. Editorial: Neuro-immune interactions in inflammation and autoimmunity. Front Immunol. 2018;9:772. https://doi.org/10.3389/fimmu.2018.00772. eCollection 2018
28. Davy KP, Orr JS. Sympathetic nervous system behavior in human obesity. Neurosci Biobehav Rev. 2009;33(2):116–24. https://doi.org/10.1016/j.neubiorev.2008.05.024.
29. Upadhyay RK. Emerging risk biomarkers in cardiovascular diseases and disorders. J Lipids. 2015;2015:971453. https://doi.org/10.1155/2015/971453.
30. Fidan-Yaylali G, Yaylali YT, Erdogan C, Can B, Senol H, Gedik-Topçu B, Topsakal S. The association between central adiposity and autonomic dysfunction in obesity. Med Princ Pract. 2016;25:442–8. https://doi.org/10.1159/000446915.
31. León-Pedroza JI, González-Tapia LA, del Olmo-Gil E, Castellanos-Rodríguez D, Escobedo G, González-Chávez A. Low-grade systemic inflammation and the development of metabolic diseases: from the molecular evidence to the clinical practice. Cir Cir. 2015;83(6):543–51. https://doi.org/10.1016/j.circir.2015.05.041.
32. Naderpoor N, Shorakae S, Joham A, Boyle J, De Courten B, Teede HJ. Obesity and polycystic ovary syndrome. Minerva Endocrinol. 2015;40(1):37–51.
33. Fontenelle LC, Feitosa MM, Severo JS, Freitas TE, Morais JB, Torres-Leal FL, Henriques GS, do Nascimento Marreiro D. Thyroid function in human obesity: underlying mechanisms. Horm Metab Res. 2016;48(12):787–94.
34. Varghese M, Griffin C, Singer K. The role of sex and sex hormones in regulating obesity-induced inflammation. Adv Exp Med Biol. 2017;1043:65–86. https://doi.org/10.1007/978-3-319-70178-3_5.
35. Grossmann M. Hypogonadism and male obesity: focus on unresolved questions. Clin Endocrinol. 2018;89(1):11–21. https://doi.org/10.1111/cen.13723.
36. Bray GA. Medical consequences of obesity. J Clin Endocrinol Metab. 2004;89:2583–9. https://doi.org/10.1210/jc.2004-0535.

37. Capodaglio P, Castelnuovo G, Brunani A, Vismara L, Villa V, Capodaglio EM. Functional limitations and occupational issues in obesity: a review. Int J Occup Saf Ergon. 2010;16(4):507–23.
38. Gaul D, Mat A, O'Shea D, Issartel J. Impaired visual motor coordination in obese adults. J Obes. 2016;2016:6178575. https://doi.org/10.1155/2016/6178575.
39. Pantalone KM, Hobbs TM, Chagin KM, Kong SX, Wells BJ, Kattan MW, Bouchard J, Sakurada B, Milinovich A, Weng W, Bauman J, Misra-Hebert AD, Zimmerman RS, Burguera B. Prevalence and recognition of obesity and its associated comorbidities: cross-sectional analysis of electronic health record data from a large US integrated health system. BMJ Open. 2017;7(11):e017583. https://doi.org/10.1136/bmjopen-2017-017583.
40. Jacobson BC, Somers SC, Fuchs CS, Kelly CP, Camargo CA Jr. Body-mass index and symptoms of gastroesophageal reflux in women. N Engl J Med. 2006;354(22):2340–8.
41. Chang P, Friedenberg F. Obesity and GERD. Gastroenterol Clin N Am. 2014;43(1):161–73.
42. Delgado-Aros S, Camilleri M, Garcia MA, Burton D, Busciglio I. High body mass alters colonic sensory-motor function and transit in humans. Am J Physiol Gastrointest Liver Physiol. 2008;295(2):G382–8. https://doi.org/10.1152/ajpgi.90286.2008.
43. Ogilvie RP, Patel SR. The epidemiology of sleep and obesity. Sleep Health. 2017;3(5):383–8. https://doi.org/10.1016/j.sleh.2017.07.013.
44. Jarolimova J, Tagoni J, Stern TA. Obesity: its epidemiology, comorbidities, and management. Prim Care Companion CNS Disord. 2013;15(5):PCC.12f01475. https://doi.org/10.4088/PCC.12f01475.
45. Russolillo A, Iervolino S, Peluso R, et al. Obesity and psoriatic arthritis: from pathogenesis to clinical outcome and management. Rheumatology (Oxford). 2013;52(1):62–7.
46. Bliddal H, Leeds AR, Christensen R. Osteoarthritis, obesity and weight loss: evidence, hypotheses and horizons a scoping review. Obes Rev. 2014;15(7):578–86.
47. Qin B, Yang M, Fu H, et al. Body mass index and the risk of rheumatoid arthritis: a systematic review and dose-response meta-analysis. Arthritis Res Ther. 2015;17:86.
48. Whitcomb EL, Lukacz ES, Lawrence JM, Nager CW, Luber KM. Prevalence and degree of bother from pelvic floor disorders in obese women. Int Urogynecol J Pelvic Floor Dysfunct. 2009;20(3):289–94. https://doi.org/10.1007/s00192-008-0765-x.
49. Neto IJFC, Pinto RA, Jorge JMN, Santo MA, Bustamante-Lopez LA, Cecconello I, Nahas SC. Are obese patients at an increased risk of pelvic floor dysfunction compared to non-obese patients? Obes Surg. 2017;27(7):1822–7. https://doi.org/10.1007/s11695-017-2559-z.
50. Hodges PW. Hybrid approach to treatment tailoring for low back pain: a proposed model of care. J Orthop Sports Phys Ther. 2019;49(6):453–63. https://doi.org/10.2519/jospt.2019.8774.
51. Foster NE, Hill JC, O'Sullivan P, Hancock M. Stratified models of care. Best Pract Res Clin Rheumatol. 2013;27(5):649–61. https://doi.org/10.1016/j.berh.2013.10.005.
52. Gibbons SGT, Way CY. The neglected subgroup? Is there plausibility that neurological factors represent a unique subgroup of chronic non-specific low back pain? Submitted. 2019.
53. Gibbons SGT. Are co-morbid medical symptoms associated with poor response to sub-classification based management of chronic low back pain? A retrospective case-control study. Proceedings of: The 10th Interdisciplinary World Congress on Low Back Pain. October 28–31, 2019. Brussels: Antwerp; 2019.
54. Gibbons SGT, Newhook TW, Behm DG. Do core stability exercise types and general exercise have different neurocognitive and sensorimotor requirements for motor skill learning? Proceedings of: The 10th Interdisciplinary World Congress on Low Back Pain. October 28–31, 2019. Brussels: Antwerp; 2019.
55. Puhl RM, Brownell KD. Psychosocial origins of obesity stigma: toward changing a powerful and pervasive bias. Obes Rev. 2003;4(4):213–27.
56. Bocquier A, Verger P, Basdevant A, Andreotti G, Baretge J, Villani P, et al. Overweight and obesity: knowledge, attitudes, and practices of general practitioners in France. Obes Res. 2005;13(4):787–95.

57. Puhl RM, Schwartz MB, Brownell KD. Impact of perceived consensus on stereotypes about obese people: a new approach for reducing bias. Health Psychol. 2005;24(5):517–25.
58. Puhl RM, Brownell KD. Confronting and coping with weight stigma: an investigation of overweight and obese adults. Obesity (Silver Spring). 2006;14(10):1802–15.
59. Puhl RM, Latner JD. Stigma, obesity, and the health of the nation's children. Psychol Bull. 2007;133(4):557–80.
60. Puhl RM, Moss-Racusin CA, Schwartz MB. Internalization of weight bias: implications for binge eating and emotional well-being. Obesity (Silver Spring). 2007;15(1):19–23.
61. Puhl RM, Moss-Racusin CA, Schwartz MB, Brownell KD. Weight stigmatization and bias reduction: perspectives of overweight and obese adults. Health Educ Res. 2008;23(2):347–58.
62. Roehling M, Pilcher S, Oswald F, Bruce T. The effects of weight bias on job-related outcomes: a meta-analysis of experimental studies [paper presented at the Academy of Management Annual Meeting, Anaheim, CA, USA]. 2008.
63. Puhl RM, Heuer CA. The stigma of obesity: a review and update. Obesity (Silver Spring). 2009;17(5):941–64.
64. Courtney M, Townsend JR, Beauchamp D, et al. Sabiston textbook of surgery: the biological basis of modern surgical practice. 18th ed. Philadelphia: Saunders/Elsevier; 2008.
65. Lobera IG, Rios PB. Body image quality of life in eating disorders. Patient Prefer Adherence. 2011;5:109–16.
66. Flegal KM, Graubard BI, Williamson DF, Williamson DF GMH, Gail MH. Excess deaths associated with underweight, overweight, and obesity. JAMA. 2005;293(15):1861–7.
67. Westgaard RH, Bonato P, Westad C. Respiratory and stress-induced activation of low- threshold motor units in the human trapezius muscle. Exp Brain Res. 2006;175(4):689–701.
68. Roman-Liu D, Grabarek I, Bartuzi P, Choromański W. The influence of mental load on muscle tension. Ergonomics. 2013;56(7):1125–33. https://doi.org/10.1080/00140139.2013.798429.
69. Marras WS, Davis KG, Heaney CA, Maronitis AB, Allread WG. The influence of psychosocial stress, gender, and personality on mechanical loading of the lumbar spine. Spine (Phila Pa 1976). 2000;25(23):3045–54.
70. Moseley GL, Nicholas MK, Hodges PW. Pain differs from non-painful attention- demanding or stressful tasks in its effect on postural control patterns of trunk muscles. Exp Brain Res. 2004;156(1):64–71.
71. Fontes MA, Xavier CH, de Menezes RC, Dimicco JA. The dorsomedial hypothalamus and the central pathways involved in the cardiovascular response to emotional stress. Neuroscience. 2011;184:64–74. https://doi.org/10.1016/j.neuroscience.2011.03.018.
72. Dampney RA. Central mechanisms regulating coordinated cardiovascular and respiratory function during stress and arousal. Am J Phys Regul Integr Comp Phys. 2015;309(5):R429–43. https://doi.org/10.1152/ajpregu.00051.2015.
73. Walterfang M, Velakoulis D. Cortical release signs in psychiatry. Aust N Z J Psychiatry. 2005;39(5):317–27. Review
74. Parfrey K, Gibbons SGT, Drinkwater EJ, Behm DG. Head and limb position influence superficial EMG of abdominals during an abdominal hollowing exercise. BMC Musculoskelet Disord. 2014;15:52. https://doi.org/10.1186/1471-2474-15-52.
75. Raji CA, Ho AJ, Parikshak NN, et al. Brain structure and obesity. Hum Brain Mapp. 2010;31(3):353–64.
76. Wang C, Chan JSY, Ren L, Yan JH. Obesity reduces cognitive and motor functions across the lifespan. Neural Plasticity. 2016;2016:2473081. https://doi.org/10.1155/2016/2473081.
77. Liang J, Matheson BE, Kaye WH, Boutelle KN. Neurocognitive correlates of obesity and obesity-related behaviors in children and adolescents. Int J Obes. 2014;38(4):494–506.
78. Prickett C, Brennan L, Stolwyk R. Examining the relationship between obesity and cognitive function: a systematic literature review. Obes Res Clin Pract. 2015;9(2):93–113.
79. Peltonen M, Lindroos AK, Torgerson JS. Musculoskeletal pain in the obese: a comparison with a general population and long-term changes after conventional and surgical obesity treatment. Pain. 2003;104(3):549–57.

80. Hitt HC, McMillen JC, Thornton-Neaves T, Koch K, Cosby AG. Comorbidity of obesity and pain in a general population: results from the southern pain prevalence study. J Pain. 2007;8(5):430–6. https://doi.org/10.1016/j.jpain.2006.12.003.
81. Somers TJ, Wren AA, Keefe FJ. Understanding chronic pain in older adults: abdominal fat is where it is at. Pain. 2011;152(1):8–9. https://doi.org/10.1016/j.pain.2010.09.022.
82. Miscio G, Guastamacchia G, Brunani A, Priano L, Baudo S, Mauro A. Obesity and peripheral neuropathy risk: a dangerous liaison. J Peripher Nerv Syst. 2005;10(4):354–8. https://doi.org/10.1111/j.1085-9489.2005.00047.x.
83. Gautier JF, Chen K, Salbe AD, Bandy D, Pratley RE, Heiman M, et al. Differential brain responses to satiation in obese and lean men. Diabetes. 2000;49:838–46.
84. Park MI, Camilleri M. Gastric motor and sensory functions in obesity. Obes Res. 2005;13:491–500. https://doi.org/10.1038/oby.2005.51.
85. Gardner RM, Salaz V, Reyes B, Brake SJ. Sensitivity to proprioceptive feedback in obese subjects. Percept Mot Skills. 1983;57(3 Pt 2):1111–8. https://doi.org/10.2446/pms.1983.57.3f.1111.
86. Falling C, Mani R. Regional asymmetry, obesity and gender determines tactile acuity of the knee regions: a cross-sectional study. Man Ther. 2016;26:150–7. https://doi.org/10.1016/j.math.2016.08.002.
87. Scarpina F, Castelnuovo G, Molinari E. Tactile mental body parts representation in obesity. Psychiatry Res. 2014;220(3):960–9. https://doi.org/10.1016/j.psychres.2014.08.020.
88. Handrigan GA, Berrigan F, Hue O, Simoneau M, Corbeil P, Tremblay A, Teasdale N. The effects of muscle strength on center of pressure-based measures of postural sway in obese and heavy athletic individuals. Gait Posture. 2012;35(1):88–91. https://doi.org/10.1016/j.gaitpost.2011.08.012.
89. Buschbacher RM. Body mass index effect on common nerve conduction study measurements. Muscle Nerve. 1998;21:1398–404.
90. Mignardot J-B, Olivier I, Promayon E, Nougier V. Origins of balance disorders during a daily living movement in obese: can biomechanical factors explain everything? PLoS One. 2013;8(4):e60491. https://doi.org/10.1371/journal.pone.0060491.
91. Elahi LS, Shamai KN, Abtahie AM, Cai AM, Padmanabhan S, Bremer M, Wilkinson KA. Diet induced obesity alters muscle spindle afferent function in adult mice. PLoS One. 2018;3(5):e0196832. https://doi.org/10.1371/journal.pone.0196832. eCollection 2018
92. Thelen E, Smith LB. A dynamic systems approach to the development of cognition and action. Cambridge, Mass, USA: The MIT Press; 1994.
93. Newell KM. Constraints on the development of coordination. In: Wade M, Whiting HTA, editors. Motor development in children: aspects of coordination and control. Dordrecht, Germany: Martinus Nijhoff; 1986. p. 341–60.
94. Wearing SC, Hennig EM, Byrne NM, Steele JR, Hills AP. The biomechanics of restricted movement in adult obesity. Obes Rev. 2006;7(1):13–24.
95. Mignardot JB, Olivier I, Promayon E, Nougier V. Obesity impact on the attentional cost for controlling posture. PLoS One. 2010;5(12):e14387.
96. Mannix ET, Dempsey JM, Engel RJ, Schneider B, Busk MF. The role of physical activity, exercise and nutrition in the treatment of obesity. In: Goldstein DJ, editor. The role of physical activity, exercise and nutrition in the treatment of obesity, The Management of Eating Disorders and Obesity. Totowa, NJ, USA: Humana Press; 2010. p. 155–72.
97. Corbeil P, Simoneau M, Rancourt D, et al. Increased risk for falling associated with obesity: mathematical modeling of postural control. IEEE Trans Neural Syst Rehabil Eng. 2001;9(2):126–36.
98. Owusu W, Willett W, Ascherio A, et al. Body anthropometry and the risk of hip and wrist fractures in men: results from a prospective study. Obes Res. 1998;6(1):12–9.
99. Menegoni F, Galli M, Tacchini E, Vismara L, Cavigioli M, Capodaglio P. Gender-specific effect of obesity on balance. Obesity (Silver Spring). 2009;17(10):1951–6. https://doi.org/10.1038/oby.2009.82.
100. Parka W, Ramachandranb J, Weismanc P, Jung ES. Obesity effect on male active joint range of motion. Ergonomics. 2010;53(1):102–8.

101. Sibella F, Galli M, Romei M, Montesano A, Crivellini M. Biomechanical analysis of sit-to- stand movement in normal and obese subjects. Clin Biomech (Bristol, Avon). 2003;18(8):745–50.
102. Galli M, Crivellini M, Sibella F, Montesano A, Bertocco P, Parisio C. Sit-to-stand movement analysis in obese subjects. Int J Obes Relat Metab Disord. 2000;24(11):1488–92.
103. Gilleard W, Smith T. Effect of obesity on posture and hip joint moments during a standing task, and trunk forward flexion motion. Int J Obes. 2007;31:267–27.
104. Vismara L, Menegoni F, Zaina F, Galli M, Negrini S, Capodaglio P. Effect of obesity and low back pain on spinal mobility: a cross sectional study in women. J Neuro Eng Rehabilit. 2010;7:3.
105. Berrigan F, Simoneau M, Tremblay A, Hue O, Teasdale N. Influence of obesity on accurate and rapid arm movement performed from a standing posture. Int J Obes. 2006;30(12):1750–7.
106. Messier SP. Osteoarthritis of the knee and associated factors of age and obesity: effects on gait. Med Sci Sports Exerc. 1994;26:1446–52.
107. Ling CG, Brotherton SS, Smith SO. Review of the literature regarding gait and class III obesity. J Exerc Physiol Online. 2009;12(5):51–61.
108. Bezzoli E, Andreotti D, Pianta L, Mascheroni M, Piccinno L, Puricelli L, Cimolin V, Salvatori A, Codecasa F, Capodaglio P. Motor control exercises of the lumbar-pelvic region improve respiratory function in obese men. A pilot study. Disabil Rehabil. 2018;40(2):152–8. https://doi.org/10.1080/09638288.2016.1244292.
109. Melo LC, Silva MA, Calles AC. Obesity and lung function: a systematic review. Einstein (Sao Paulo). 2014;12(1):120–5.
110. Koenig SM. Pulmonary complications of obesity. Am J Med Sci. 2001;321:249–79.
111. Kress JP, Pohlman AS, Alverdy J, et al. The impact of morbid obesity on oxygen cost of breathing (VO(2RESP)) at rest. Am J Respir Crit Care Med. 1999;160:883–6.
112. Hodges P, Heijnen I, Gandevia SC. Postural activity of the diaphragm is reduced in humans when respiratory demand increases. J Physiol. 2001;537(Pt 3):999–1008. https://doi.org/10.1111/j.1469-7793.2001.00999.x.
113. Kocjan J, Adamek M, Gzik-Zroska B, Czyżewski D, Rydel M. Network of breathing. Multifunctional role of the diaphragm: a review. Adv Respir Med. 2017;85(4):224–32. https://doi.org/10.5603/ARM.2017.0037.
114. Tomlinson DJ, Erskine RM, Morse CI, Winwood K, Onambe'le-Pearson G. The impact of obesity on skeletal muscle strength and structure through adolescence to old age. Biogerontology. 2016;17:467–83. https://doi.org/10.1007/s10522-015-9626-4.
115. Maffiuletti NA, Ratel S, Sartorio A, Martin V. The impact of obesity on in vivo human skeletal muscle function. Curr Obes Rep. 2013;2:251–60.
116. Bollinger LM. Potential contributions of skeletal muscle contractile dysfunction to altered biomechanics in obesity. Gait Posture. 2017;56:100–7.
117. Rodacki AL, Fowler NE, Provensi CL, et al. Body mass as a factor in stature change. Clin Biomech. 2005;20(8):799–805.
118. Frilander H, Solovieva S, Mutanen P, et al. Role of overweight and obesity in low Back disorders among men: a longitudinal study with a life course approach. BMJ Open. 2015;5:e007805. https://doi.org/10.1136/bmjopen-2015-007805.
119. Wannamethee SG, Shaper AG, Peter H, Whincup PH. Body fat distribution, body composition, and respiratory function in elderly men. Am J Clin Nutr. 2005;82:996–1003.
120. Rossi AP, Watson NL, Newman AB, Harris TB, Kritchevsky SB, Bauer DC, Satterfield S, Goodpaster BH, Zamboni M. Effects of body composition and adipose tissue distribution on respiratory function in elderly men and women: the health, aging, and body composition study. J Gerontol A Biol Sci Med Sci. 2011;66A(7):801–8. https://doi.org/10.1093/gerona/glr059.
121. Hunskaar S, Arnold EP, Burgio K, Diokno AC, Herzog AR, Mallett VT. Epidemiology and natural history of urinary incontinence. Int Urogynecol J. 2000;11:301–19.
122. Hodges PW, Sapsford R, Pengel LHM. Postural and respiratory functions of the pelvic floor muscles. Neurourol Urodyn. 2007;26:362–71. https://doi.org/10.1002/nau2007.

123. Sapsford R. Rehabilitation of pelvic floor muscles utilizing trunk stabilization. Man Ther. 2004;9:3–12.
124. Gibbons SGT, Comerford MJ, Emerson P. Rehabilitation of the stability function of psoas major. Orthopaed Div Rev. 2002;18:63–75.
125. Lerner ZF, Board WJ, Browning RC. Effects of obesity on lower extremity muscle function during walking at two speeds. NIH Public Access. 2014;39(3):978–84.
126. Hooper MM, Stellato TA, Hallowell PT, Seitz BA, Moskowitz RW. Musculoskeletal findings in obese subjects before and after weight loss following bariatric surgery. Int J Obes. 2007;31:114–20.
127. Smith SM, Sumar B, Dixon KA. Musculoskeletal pain in overweight and obese children. Int J Obes. 2014;38(1):11–5. https://doi.org/10.1038/ijo.2013.187.
128. Andersen RE, Crespo CJ, Bartlett SJ, Bathon JM, Fontaine KR. Relationship between body weight gain and significant knee, hip, and back pain in older Americans. Obes Res. 2003;11(10):1159–62.
129. Okifuji A, Hare BD. The association between chronic pain and obesity. J Pain Res. 2015;8:399–408.
130. Messier SP, Pater M, Beavers DP, Legault C, Loeser RF, Hunter DJ, DeVita P. Influences of alignment and obesity on knee joint loading in osteoarthritic gait. NIH Public Access. 2014;22(7):912–7.

6 Respiratory Exercises and Noninvasive Ventilation

Emanuela Bezzoli, Paolo Fanari, and Franco Codecasa

Key Points

- Ventilation is noticeably affected by fat deposition, which limits movement and function of the diaphragm.
- Sleep apnea is a very frequent complaint, involving oxidative capacity and therefore weight loss and also engagement in physical activity programs.
- Rehabilitation program for obese people with respiratory problems should encompass weight loss, aerobic exercise, noninvasive ventilation for OSAS, respiratory muscle strengthening and motor control exercises for the lumbar-pelvic muscles, and psychological support if dyspnea generates apprehension.
- Enhancing coordination, on top of strength, of the lumbar-pelvic muscles and correcting posture can improve respiratory function.

The dramatic raising in global obesity prevalence, associated with a growing number of persons with chronic respiratory diseases, leads to an increase in subjects involved in respiratory rehabilitation [1]. In addition, more and more people with obesity-related respiratory disorders such as "obesity hypoventilation syndrome" and "obstructive sleep apnea syndrome" may be included in rehabilitation programs if they are affected by functional limitations [2]. For this kind of patient, respiratory-rehabilitation-specific interventions including physical exercise, nutrition education, weight loss, psychological support, and noninvasive ventilation training are recommended [2]. Most literature compares obese with normal-weight subjects and

E. Bezzoli (✉) · P. Fanari · F. Codecasa
Respiratory Rehabilitation Unit and Sleep Medicine Unit, Istituto Auxologico Italiano, Piancavallo, Italy
e-mail: e.bezzoli@auxologico.it; p.fanari@auxologico.it; f.codecasa@auxologico.it

P. Capodaglio (ed.), *Rehabilitation Interventions in the Patient with Obesity*,
https://doi.org/10.1007/978-3-030-32274-8_6

obese patients with respiratory disorders recognized as an indication for respiratory rehabilitation (e.g., chronic obstructive pulmonary disease, COPD) [3]. Obesity per se is not a usual criteria for pulmonary rehabilitation. The main reason for that is the not clearly defined impact of obesity on respiratory pathology [3]. There are no guidelines explaining what exercises/training should be prescribed to an obese patient with respiratory problems [4]. It is common practice to rely on the expert's opinions, based on the physiopathology and the clinical experience [4]. Obesity may occur in various respiratory diseases, although many of these are associated in the long term with reduced body weight or even cachexia (e.g., asthma, cystic fibrosis, interstitial pathologies), and the effect of overweight is not mentioned in the most recent systematic reviews on training in different respiratory diseases [5–7].

6.1 Pathophysiological Changes

Obesity has long been recognized as a negative factor on respiratory function. This topic has been studied thoroughly, and there are now clear patterns of how obese subjects breathe: they are inclined to breathe rapidly and superficially with an high respiratory rate [8–11] and lower tidal volume (V_t) [9–11]. Minute ventilation is increased [8, 12, 13]. It is not very clear how patients change their breathing pattern; the increased respiratory rate means that respiratory time is reduced [8]. The augmented activity of chest wall receptors or a change in central breathing timing could result in reduced inspiratory time [8]. The shortening of expiratory times may depend on the increase in expiratory flow rate due to reduced compliance or persistent expiratory diaphragm activity [8]. In obesity, the compliance of the respiratory system is reduced [14–16]. Whether this depends on the chest wall or the lung itself is still controversial in the literature; however, both are likely to contribute to lower the compliance of the respiratory system. Due to the reduction in lung volumes, the lung may present micro-atelectasis [16]. It is important to observe the thoracic cage conformation and how adiposity is distributed [17]; in subjects with a high waist-to-hip ratio (WHR) the reduction in compliance may be more pronounced [18]. One of the most consistent effects of obesity on lung volumes is the decrease in expiratory reserve volume (ERV) [19–28] which is inversely correlated to body mass index (BMI) [19, 24, 26, 28]. There is an equally consistent negative correlation between obesity and functional residual capacity (FRC), although the changes are less dramatic than ERV [24, 28, 29]. BMI's effect on residual volume (RV) is modest, with the consequence that FRC's reduction is largely due to ERV's reduction [13]. If obesity reduces ERV and FRC, we might expect a similar effect on total lung capacity (TLC), but TLC is usually not affected if patients are not extremely obese [30].

The effect of obesity on lung volumes is attributable to the cranial displacement of the diaphragm caused by abdominal fat and viscera [31]. This is supported by studies in which the lung volumes were correlated with high WHR values [32].

Fat deposition has a compression effect on the chest with a lung volume reduction [31]. Similar mechanisms have been observed measuring lung volumes with elastic straps on the chest [33]; fat mass seems to act as an elastic load [34].

With the exception of patients with severe obesity, spirometry is generally not characterized by low values of forced expiratory volume in the first second (FEV1) and forced vital capacity (FVC). The ratio of FEV1/FVC is conserved [12, 22, 26, 28, 30].

The airway resistance is usually increased due to the reduced volume of the lung, which leads to the collapse of smaller airways [22, 23, 29]. However, there was no difference between normal-weight and obese subjects adjusting the airway conductance for lung volumes [22].

In some cases, obese patients may have normal blood oxygenation [15, 35, 36] or may be slightly hypoxemic [12, 21, 26]; a slight hypercapnia can also be found in the presence of obesity hypoventilation syndrome [14]. This is probably caused by a mismatch of ventilation-perfusion: when the subject is in sitting position [37] or supine [38], the pulmonary bases are over-perfused and under-ventilated due to the closure of small airways in the gravity-dependent lung area [39].

Gas exchange at diffusing capacity of the lung for carbon monoxide test (DLCO) seems to be well preserved in subjects with obesity [15, 25, 39, 40]; factors such as high WHR values negatively affect gas exchanges [36].

The spirometric values return to normality after weight loss, and this is proof that obesity per se causes these changes [21, 27, 35, 41–43]. Concerning ERV [43], FRC, and TLC [21, 27, 35, 41], even modest weight losses lead to significant improvements.

Many changes associated with obesity seem to be influenced exactly by fat distribution and body composition. Other factors should be considered, apart from BMI, such as WHR and [18, 36] fat-free body mass. Interesting is the result of a large study showing a linear inverse correlation between WHR, FEV1, and FVC [44].

6.2 Dyspnea and Exercise Capacity

All these changes lead to dyspnea and intolerance to effort. A fundamental basis for respiratory rehabilitation is physical exercise; in fact, it is essential to improve exercise tolerance, exercise dyspnea, fatigue, and activity of daily living (ADL) impairment in subjects with chronic respiratory disease according to the official guidelines of the American Thoracic Society and European Respiratory Society [2].

Respiratory rehabilitation provides different types of interventions (e.g., treatment of abnormalities in body composition, pharmacological and non-pharmacological therapy, education in self-management, psychological support) in which physical exercise represents an essential element [4]. It has been observed that respiratory rehabilitation improves physical performance in patients with chronic respiratory diseases (e.g., COPD), and it has also been suggested in management of the obese subject [4]. However, regular physical exercise in obese subjects is difficult to perform due to the association of pathophysiological changes in respiratory function. Also, the hypothesis that there is a preexisting impairment of physical performance must also be taken into account [3].

Obese patients often refer dyspnea [45], some of them having shortness of breath without significant coexisting clinical conditions [46]. In the presence of respiratory abnormalities, we should search the cause, but in the absence of a true respiratory condition, abnormalities can occur because of deconditioning or obesity per se [4, 18, 46]. Perception of dyspnea occurs especially during physical activity when the demand for ventilation increases; the changes in pulmonary volumes at rest are also reflected during exercise [47].

Abdominal fat occludes small airways, resulting in a cranial displacement of the diaphragm [48, 49]. It significantly decreases ERV and FRC, forcing obese patients to breathe at lower lung volumes [18, 28], although during exercise partial pressure of oxygen (PaO_2) improves [50], as there is still an increase in tidal volumes that helps the recruitment of closed lung areas [51]. The increased work of the inspiratory muscles to expand the lungs and chest wall against the fat load [52–54], as well as the reduction of compliance of the lung and chest wall [14], can also contribute to the increased oxygen cost of breathing during exercise [47, 55, 56] and to the characteristic pattern of rapid and shallow breathing [14, 57, 58].

Another consequence of lower lung volumes operating during exercise is the risk of developing an expiratory flow limitation, which might conversely increase dyspnea [59].

Therefore, the respiratory muscles and their regulation play a fundamental role during effort [60] in the generation of dyspnea; drive is increased, while strength is reduced [10, 61, 62]. It has been shown that obese subjects yield an increase in inspiratory muscle activity during exercise, which predisposes to exercise-dependent fatigue of respiratory muscles [62]. Also, fat distribution seems to be a fundamental point for the tendency of breathing rapidly and superficially [63] as fat mass can reduce diaphragm excursion making it unable to increase the inspired volumes [18]. In normal-weight subjects, as in obese subjects under stress, the inspired volume and respiratory frequency increase, but the need for more oxygen increases the minute ventilation even more than in normal-weight subjects; therefore, respiratory rate increases significantly, but the volumes not so [57, 63, 64].

Another reason for the reduced exercise performance is the increase in dead space ventilation, which hinders an adequate ventilation [18].

Rapid and shallow breathing may be an appropriate compensatory response to minimize the mechanical effects of elastic loading, which may help to reduce respiratory distress in obese subjects [65, 66], but there is evidence that compensatory hyperventilation is insufficient in obese subjects during exercise [67]. Even during effort, the respiratory system's compliance is reduced.

The reduction of compliance, on one hand, from the chest wall due to the adipose mass and, on the other hand, from the lung due to the volume reduction with the consequent atelectasis overloads the respiratory muscles [14, 17, 18]. Reducing compliance, however, means that the respiratory muscles of obese subjects need more strength to ventilate the same amount of air.

As for the relation between dyspnea and respiratory muscles, it appears that the subjects presenting dyspnea have higher oxygen costs of breathing with the same values at pulmonary tests [55]. In another study with obese patients with similar BMI but with different dyspnea perception, it was observed that those with more symptoms also had lower values of TLC, FRC, and ERV and higher respiratory drive [42].

Other investigations attribute more importance to psychophysiological differences, independent from respiratory variables and body composition; some subjects have increased afferent feedback to the respiratory control center. The threshold for awareness generation of respiratory stimulant may be influenced by mood status, negative emotions, or past experiences [68].

For a person who has shortness of breath with even mild-to-moderate exercise [56], the increase in daily physical activity may be difficult. The adherence to exercise programs in obese patients can be poor for musculoskeletal factors or pain [69]. The effects of obesity is even more visible in older age, with consequent impairment in daily activities [70, 71].

Obesity has traditionally been associated with a decrease in exercise capacity measured by the VO_2 peak during cardiorespiratory testing, but studies on healthy obese adults show that most of them do not show cardiorespiratory deconditioning [49, 72, 73].

A severe limit of obesity in terms of physical performance is the high metabolic cost required for a given exercise level. This was demonstrated in weight-supported exercise (e.g., cycling), in which energy expenditure per unit of workload was significantly increased in obese subjects [64]. These observations imply that obese individuals work closer to their maximum performance than normal-weight subjects, both during weight-supported and non-weight-supported exercises, even in daily activities that would normally require sub-maximal effort [3]. Obese subjects have a higher basal metabolism than normal, so that oxygen consumption during exercise is increased at any work rate [40, 57, 58], and even ventilation for a given work rate is higher [48, 57, 64, 66, 74, 75], due to the increased metabolic demand to move the limbs [76]. Further, if we add the oxygen cost of breathing, the values are much higher than in normal subjects [52, 53, 62]. Partial pressure of carbon dioxide ($PaCO_2$) remains within the normal limits, while the PaO_2 is normal or only slightly reduced in the obese subjects; the diffusion of the gasses is slightly altered due to the mismatch of the perfusion ventilation due to the occlusion of the small airways in the dependent gravity zones [18, 37, 64, 67]. It has been shown that an abdominal fat distribution increases the need for oxygen, and in these subjects, the anaerobic threshold is lower [63].

6.3 Obstructive Sleep Apnea and Noninvasive Ventilation

Obstructive sleep apnea (OSA) is a common disorder: its prevalence in the general population is 3–7% for men and 2–5% for women [77]. For obese subjects, the percentages are much higher. Patients with OSA, on the other hand, are at risk of obesity and vice versa; inadequate sleep and daytime sleepiness predispose to

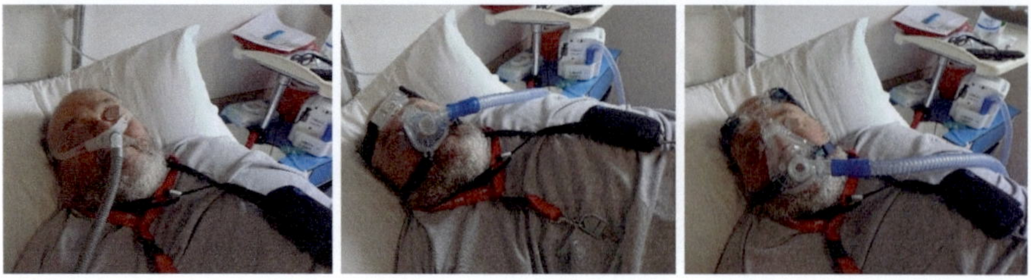

Fig. 6.1 Example of CPAP masks: from left to right, nasal pillow mask, nasal mask, and facial mask

weight gain [78]. OSA is characterized by complete or partial obstruction of the airways during sleep, resulting in intermittent hypoxia, hypercapnia, sleep fragmentation and increased sympathetic drive, high blood pressure, and increased cardiovascular risk [79].

The occurrence of excessive daytime sleepiness, morning headache, decreased libido, attention deficit, decreased concentration, neurocognitive damage, irritability, and depression is common in subjects with OSA, and work efficiency significantly reduced [80, 81]. The apnea-hypopnea index (AHI) measures the number of episodes of apnea and hypopnea per hour of monitored sleep and evaluates the severity of OSA. Mild, moderate, and severe OSA is defined with an AHI between 5 and 15 and 15 and 30 and more than 30 events/h, respectively [75, 79]. Continuous positive airway pressure (CPAP) (Fig. 6.1) is considered the gold standard treatment for moderate-to-severe OSA [82]. OSA is a chronic condition that requires a long treatment period. Patient adherence, however, can affect treatment efficacy. For selected patients, surgery or oral appliance treatment may be successful [82]. Patients can also benefit from lifestyle changes such as exercise and diet control [83].

Physical activity can reduce the severity of OSA by acting on body weight and abdominal fat. A 10% decrease in the BMI has been shown to be associated with a 30% decrease in AHI [84, 85]. It is still necessary to define well the mechanisms by which physical exercise attenuates OSA. The beneficial effects of physical exercise on OSA patients have long been believed to be related purely to weight loss; however, experimental and clinical studies have shown that the benefits of exercise are independent from weight loss [86, 87]. Low physical exercise levels are often associated with OSA's severity [88, 89]. It is plausible that patients with OSA are not motivated to perform exercise either physically or psychologically. The lack of physical activity not only increases the chances of OSA, but sleep apnea itself is a possible cause for physical inactivity due to drowsiness and daytime fatigue [89]. Several studies have shown that treatment with CPAP also has beneficial effects on physical activity [90], but other studies have shown that CPAP users do not increase the level of exercise significantly despite improvements in quality of life, psychological well-being, and subjective and objective daytime sleepiness [91, 92]. Intolerance to effort in obese subjects with OSAS can be explained not only as a combination of factors including respiratory mechanics and drive deficit but also as a combination of cardiovascular and muscular cardiovascular factors that affect aerobic capacity. In addition to the conventional training program, noninvasive ventilation (NIV) was proposed during training to reduce respiratory work and improve exercise tolerance in OSAS subjects with restrictive problems such as obesity [93].

In patients with different respiratory diseases, including restrictive problems [94, 95], NIV improves exercise capacity. In particular, proportional assist ventilation (PAV) is capable of discharging both the resistive and elastic load [96], which in obese subjects is known to be important. Furthermore, PAV generates pressures that depend on the inspirational demand of the patient [96], making this mode particularly suitable for supporting physical activity. If so, PAV could be considered as a new treatment option for enhancing exercise capacity in obese patients and thus substantially support weight loss initiation and maintenance.

6.4 Posture and Ventilation

Respiratory inefficiency of obese patients is correlated to the weakness of the respiratory muscles. The international guidelines of pulmonary rehabilitation recommend strengthening of the respiratory muscles in order to improve their efficiency [2, 97], as the reduced ability to generate inspiratory pressure contributes to both intolerance to exercise and perception of dyspnea. Using devices that impose a resistive or threshold load is the most common approach to inspiratory muscle training [98]. We have proposed a different approach to reinforce the respiratory muscles in obese subjects [99], as pathophysiology is different from that of COPD subjects. The increase in body weight affects posture [100, 101] as the center of mass shifts forward [102, 103], and a compensatory posture with lumbar extension occurs to maintain the center of mass in the base of support [102–104], causing an imbalance between anterior and posterior muscles of the trunk. The muscles of the pelvic cylinder (the diaphragm, transverse abdomen, and pelvic floor) modulate the intra-abdominal pressure, which is essential for breathing as well as for spinal stability. This activity improves the inspiratory action of the diaphragm on the thoracic cage by means of two components: the insertion force, which is the force directly applied by the diaphragm fibers to the ribs, and the special force or lateral force due to the transmission of abdominal pressure to the lower ribs where the diaphragm area is located [105, 106]. The appositional diaphragm area (Fig. 6.2) is the anatomical region in which the diaphragm overlaps the lower part of the thoracic cage: the larger it is, the greater the mechanical efficacy of the respiratory action, with a wider movement on the frontal as compared to the sagittal plane [107]. Especially the last ribs are raised and externally rotated [108]. If the lumbar-pelvic muscles are active during inhalation, the abdominal pressure slightly pushes the diaphragm cranially, thus increasing the appositional area and making a larger chest expansion [107].

Intra-abdominal pressure, together with postural control, contributes to load reduction on the spine [109–111]. It has been suggested that poor coordination of the diaphragm can hinder spinal stability [112] and, conversely, the defective stability of the lumbar spine due to poor postural alignment could have a negative effect

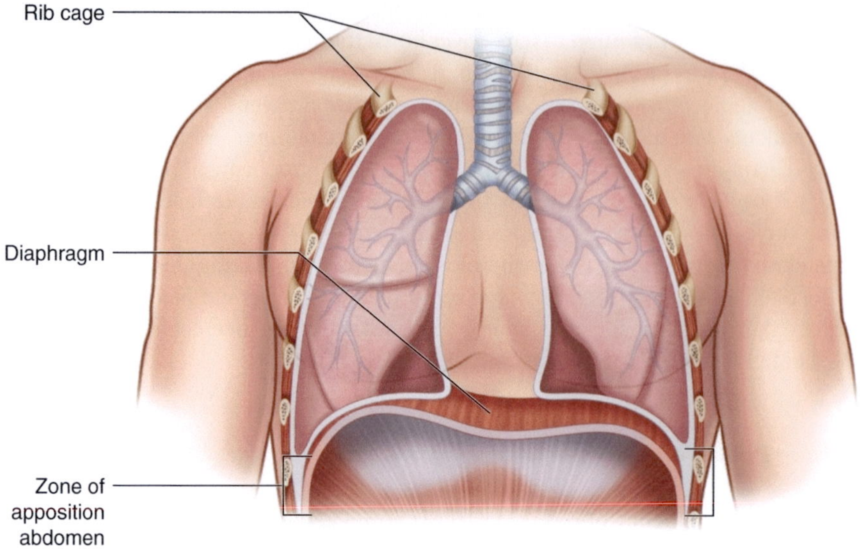

Fig. 6.2 Diaphragm appositional area

on respiratory function. It has been shown that spinal stability depends more on activating large axial muscles when ventilation demand increases [113]. The resulting superficial muscle overactivity can interfere with breathing by inhibiting the lumbar-pelvic musculature and decreasing rib cage mobility [114]. The lumbar-pelvic region requires sensory-motor and cognitive processing to coordinate muscle activation [115]. Body perception disturbances can lead to inconsistencies between predicted and actual proprioceptive feedback [116], making breath control economic and efficient and postural control difficult. It has been shown that the increase in adipose tissue influences the cutaneous and proprioceptive receptors resulting in a modified representation of the body [115].

In line with the concepts of SmartRehab (see The Motor Control Training chapter), our proposal is to teach our patients how to activate the muscles of the lumbar-pelvic cylinder while maintaining both breathing and neutral lumbar posture in the supine and sitting and standing positions. The neutral position can be defined as the position where the head, thorax, and pelvis are aligned with the gravity line without significant superficial muscle co-contraction (Fig. 6.3). There is evidence that the adoption of neutral lumbar-pelvic positions in a sitting and standing position automatically facilitates deep muscle activity without activating the large superficial muscles [117–121].

In a recent study from our group [99], we compared motor control exercises (Fig. 6.4) aimed at the lumbar-pelvic cylinder with a traditional protocol for muscle strengthening, in addition to diet and aerobic activity for both groups. Specific motor control exercises obtained significant results, improving respiratory parameters, such as FVC, maximal voluntary ventilation (MVV), maximal expiratory

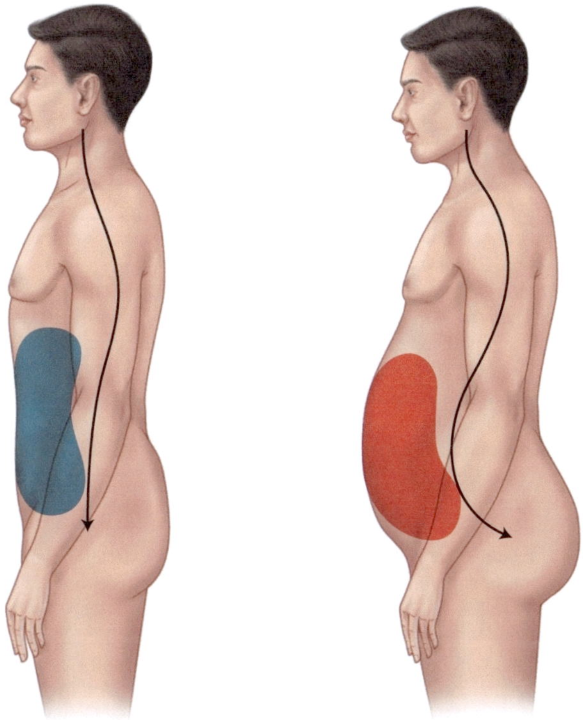

Fig. 6.3 Example of neutral posture and the classic attitude with obese anterior pelvic tilt

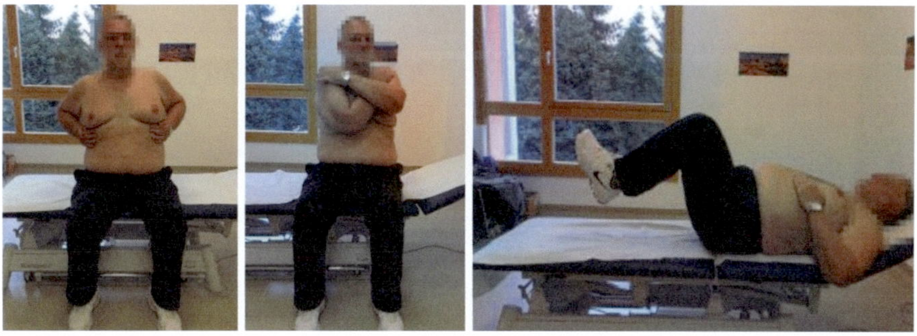

Fig. 6.4 Examples of exercises used in the motor control group: from left to right, diaphragmatic respiration, thoracic rotation, and hip and knee flexion in supine

pressure (MEP), and RV-to-TLC ratio, as well as six minute walking test (6MWT), dyspnea in oxygen cost diagram (OCD) scales, and thoracic excursion. Even anthropometric parameters improved with respect to the control group in both weight loss and WHR, which, as previously reported, is a key factor for respiratory parameters.

References

1. Velasco R, Pirraglia PA, Casserly B, Nici L. Influence of body mass index on changes in disease-specific quality of life of veterans completing pulmonary rehabilitation. J Cardiopulm Rehabil Prev. 2010;30(5):334–9.
2. Spruit MA, Singh SJ, Garvey C, et al. An official American Thoracic Society/European Respiratory Society statement: key concepts and advances in pulmonary rehabilitation. Am J Respir Crit Care Med. 2013;188(8):e13–64.
3. Dreher M, Kabitz H-J. Impact of obesity on exercise performance and pulmonary rehabilitation. Respirology. 2012;17(6):899–907.
4. Nici L, Donner C, Wouters E, et al. American Thoracic Society/European Respiratory Society statement on pulmonary rehabilitation. Am J Respir Crit Care Med. 2006;173(12):1390–413.
5. Bradley J, Moran F. Physical training for cystic fibrosis. Cochrane Database Syst Rev. 2008;1:CD002768.
6. Ram FS, Robinson SM, Black PN, Picot J. Physical training for asthma. Cochrane Database Syst Rev. 2005;4:CD001116.
7. Holland A, Hill C. Physical training for interstitial lung disease. Cochrane Database Syst Rev. 2008;4:CD006322.
8. Sampson MG, Grassino AE. Load compensation in obese patients during quiet tidal breathing. J Appl Physiol Respir Environ Exerc Physiol. 1983;55(4):1269–76.
9. Pankow W, Podszus T, Gutheil T, Penzel T, Peter J, Von Wichert P. Expiratory flow limitation and intrinsic positive end-expiratory pressure in obesity. J Appl Physiol (1985). 1998;85(4):1236–43.
10. Chlif M, Keochkerian D, Choquet D, Vaidie A, Ahmaidi S. Effects of obesity on breathing pattern, ventilatory neural drive and mechanics. Respir Physiol Neurobiol. 2009;168(3):198–202.
11. Lourenço RV. Diaphragm activity in obesity. J Clin Invest. 1969;48(9):1609–14.
12. Barnett TB, Rasmussen B. Ventilatory regulation in eucapnic morbid obesity. Am Rev Respir Dis. 1984;130(6):1188.
13. Kryger MH. Sleep apnea. From the needles of dionysius to continuous positive airway pressure. Arch Intern Med. 1983;143(12):2301–3.
14. Naimark A, Cherniack RM. Compliance of the respiratory system and its components in health and obesity. J Appl Physiol. 1960;15:377–82.
15. Sharp JT, Henry JP, Sweany SK, Meadows WR, Pietras RJ. The total work of breathing in normal and obese men. J Clin Invest. 1964;43:728–39.
16. Hedenstierna G, Santesson J. Breathing mechanics, dead space and gas exchange in the extremely obese, breathing spontaneously and during anaesthesia with intermittent positive pressure ventilation. Acta Anaesthesiol Scand. 1976;20(3):248–54.
17. Pelosi P, Croci M, Ravagnan I, Vicardi P, Gattinoni L. Total respiratory system, lung, and chest wall mechanics in sedated-paralyzed postoperative morbidly obese patients. Chest. 1996;109(1):144–51.
18. Littleton SW. Impact of obesity on respiratory function. Respirology. 2012;17(1):43–9.
19. Ladosky W, Botelho MA, Albuquerque JP. Chest mechanics in morbidly obese non-hypoventilated patients. Respir Med. 2001;95(4):281–6.
20. Kelly TM, Jensen RL, Elliott CG, Crapo RO. Maximum respiratory pressures in morbidly obese subjects. Respiration. 1988;54(2):73–7.
21. Thomas PS, Cowen ER, Hulands G, Milledge JS. Respiratory function in the morbidly obese before and after weight loss. Thorax. 1989;44(5):382–6.
22. Rubinstein I, Zamel N, DuBarry L, Hoffstein V. Airflow limitation in morbidly obese, nonsmoking men. Ann Intern Med. 1990;112(11):828–32.
23. Zerah F, Harf A, Perlemuter L, Lorino H, Lorino AM, Atlan G. Effects of obesity on respiratory resistance. Chest. 1993;103(5):1470–6.
24. Collet F, Mallart A, Bervar JF, et al. Physiologic correlates of dyspnea in patients with morbid obesity. Int J Obes. 2007;31(4):700–6.

25. Ray CS, Sue DY, Bray G, Hansen JE, Wasserman K. Effects of obesity on respiratory function. Am Rev Respir Dis. 1983;128(3):501–6.
26. Biring MS, Lewis MI, Liu JT, Mohsenifar Z. Pulmonary physiologic changes of morbid obesity. Am J Med Sci. 1999;318(5):293–7.
27. Emirgil C, Sobol BJ. The effects of weight reduction on pulmonary function and the sensitivity of the respiratory center in obesity. Am Rev Respir Dis. 1973;108(4):831–42.
28. Jones RL, Nzekwu MM. The effects of body mass index on lung volumes. Chest. 2006;130(3):827–33.
29. Watson RA, Pride NB. Postural changes in lung volumes and respiratory resistance in subjects with obesity. J Appl Physiol (1985). 2005;98(2):512–7.
30. Watson RA, Pride NB, Thomas EL, et al. Reduction of total lung capacity in obese men: comparison of total intrathoracic and gas volumes. J Appl Physiol (1985). 2010;108(6):1605–12.
31. Koenig SM. Pulmonary complications of obesity. Am J Med Sci. 2001;321(4):249–79.
32. Collins LC, Hoberty PD, Walker JF, Fletcher EC, Peiris AN. The effect of body fat distribution on pulmonary function tests. Chest. 1995;107(5):1298–302.
33. Caro CG, Butler J, Dubois AB. Some effects of restriction of chest cage expansion on pulmonary function in man: an experimental study. J Clin Invest. 1960;39:573–83.
34. Sharp JT, Henry JP, Sweany SK, Meadows WR, Pietras RJ. Effects of mass loading the respiratory system in man. J Appl Physiol. 1964;19:959–66.
35. Vaughan RW, Cork RC, Hollander D. The effect of massive weight loss on arterial oxygenation and pulmonary function tests. Anesthesiology. 1981;54(4):325–8.
36. Zavorsky GS, Murias JM, Kim DJ, Gow J, Sylvestre JL, Christou NV. Waist-to-hip ratio is associated with pulmonary gas exchange in the morbidly obese. Chest. 2007;131(2):362–7.
37. Holley HS, Milic-Emili J, Becklake MR, Bates DV. Regional distribution of pulmonary ventilation and perfusion in obesity. J Clin Invest. 1967;46(4):475–81.
38. Hurewitz AN, Susskind H, Harold WH. Obesity alters regional ventilation in lateral decubitus position. J Appl Physiol (1985). 1985;59(3):774–83.
39. Douglas FG, Chong PY. Influence of obesity on peripheral airways patency. J Appl Physiol. 1972;33(5):559–63.
40. Salvadori A, Fanari P, Mazza P, Fontana M, Clivati A, Longhini E. Breathing pattern during and after maximal exercise testing in young untrained subjects and in obese patients. Respiration. 1993;60(3):162–9.
41. Weiner P, Waizman J, Weiner M, Rabner M, Magadle R, Zamir D. Influence of excessive weight loss after gastroplasty for morbid obesity on respiratory muscle performance. Thorax. 1998;53(1):39–42.
42. El-Gamal H, Khayat A, Shikora S, Unterborn JN. Relationship of dyspnea to respiratory drive and pulmonary function tests in obese patients before and after weight loss. Chest. 2005;128(6):3870–4.
43. Babb TG, Wyrick BL, Chase PJ, et al. Weight loss via diet and exercise improves exercise breathing mechanics in obese men. Chest. 2011;140(2):454–60.
44. Canoy D, Luben R, Welch A, et al. Abdominal obesity and respiratory function in men and women in the EPIC-Norfolk Study, United Kingdom. Am J Epidemiol. 2004;159(12):1140–9.
45. Plan and operation of the Third National Health and Nutrition Examination Survey, 1988–94. Series 1: programs and collection procedures. Vital Health Stat 1. 1994;32:1–407.
46. Bhatt DV, Kocheril AG. Submaximal cardiopulmonary exercise testing for the evaluation of unexplained dyspnea. South Med J. 2014;107(3):144–9.
47. Bernhardt V, Wood HE, Moran RB, Babb TG. Dyspnea on exertion in obese men. Respir Physiol Neurobiol. 2013;185(2):241–8.
48. DeLorey DS, Wyrick BL, Babb TG. Mild-to-moderate obesity: implications for respiratory mechanics at rest and during exercise in young men. Int J Obes. 2005;29(9):1039–47.
49. Babb TG, DeLorey DS, Wyrick BL, Gardner PP. Mild obesity does not limit change in end-expiratory lung volume during cycling in young women. J Appl Physiol (1985). 2002;92(6):2483–90.

50. Whipp BJ, Davis JA. The ventilatory stress of exercise in obesity. Am Rev Respir Dis. 1984;129(2 Pt 2):S90–2.
51. Sood A. Altered resting and exercise respiratory physiology in obesity. Clin Chest Med. 2009;30(3):445–54, vii
52. Kress JP, Pohlman AS, Alverdy J, Hall JB. The impact of morbid obesity on oxygen cost of breathing (VO(2RESP)) at rest. Am J Respir Crit Care Med. 1999;160(3):883–6.
53. Cherniack RM. Respiratory effects of obesity. Can Med Assoc J. 1958;80(8):613–6.
54. Milic-Emili J, Orzalesi MM. Mechanical work of breathing during maximal voluntary ventilation. J Appl Physiol (1985). 1998;85(1):254–8.
55. Babb TG, Ranasinghe KG, Comeau LA, Semon TL, Schwartz B. Dyspnea on exertion in obese women: association with an increased oxygen cost of breathing. Am J Respir Crit Care Med. 2008;178(2):116–23.
56. Bernhardt V, Babb TG. Exertional dyspnoea in obesity. Eur Respir Rev. 2016;25(142):487–95.
57. Babb TG, Korzick D, Meador M, Hodgson JL, Buskirk ER. Ventilatory response of moderately obese women to submaximal exercise. Int J Obes. 1991;15(1):59–65.
58. Salvadori A, Fanari P, Mazza P, Agosti R, Longhini E. Work capacity and cardiopulmonary adaptation of the obese subject during exercise testing. Chest. 1992;101(3):674–9.
59. Tantucci C. Expiratory flow limitation definition, mechanisms, methods, and significance. Pulm Med. 2013;2013:749860.
60. Scano G, Stendardi L, Bruni GI. The respiratory muscles in eucapnic obesity: their role in dyspnea. Respir Med. 2009;103(9):1276–85.
61. Steier J, Jolley CJ, Seymour J, Roughton M, Polkey MI, Moxham J. Neural respiratory drive in obesity. Thorax. 2009;64(8):719–25.
62. Chlif M, Keochkerian D, Feki Y, Vaidie A, Choquet D, Ahmaidi S. Inspiratory muscle activity during incremental exercise in obese men. Int J Obes. 2007;31(9):1456–63.
63. Li J, Li S, Feuers RJ, Buffington CK, Cowan GS. Influence of body fat distribution on oxygen uptake and pulmonary performance in morbidly obese females during exercise. Respirology. 2001;6(1):9–13.
64. Dempsey JA, Reddan W, Balke B, Rankin J. Work capacity determinants and physiologic cost of weight-supported work in obesity. J Appl Physiol. 1966;21(6):1815–20.
65. Ora J, Laveneziana P, Ofir D, Deesomchok A, Webb KA, O'Donnell DE. Combined effects of obesity and chronic obstructive pulmonary disease on dyspnea and exercise tolerance. Am J Respir Crit Care Med. 2009;180(10):964–71.
66. Ofir D, Laveneziana P, Webb KA, O'Donnell DE. Ventilatory and perceptual responses to cycle exercise in obese women. J Appl Physiol (1985). 2007;102(6):2217–26.
67. Zavorsky GS, Hoffman SL. Pulmonary gas exchange in the morbidly obese. Obes Rev. 2008;9(4):326–39.
68. von Leupoldt A, Chan PY, Esser RW, Davenport PW. Emotions and neural processing of respiratory sensations investigated with respiratory-related evoked potentials. Psychosom Med. 2013;75(3):244–52.
69. Calenzani G, Santos FFD, Wittmer VL, Freitas GKF, Paro FM. Prevalence of musculoskeletal symptoms in obese patients candidates for bariatric surgery and its impact on health related quality of life. Arch Endocrinol Metab. 2017;61(4):319–25.
70. Vincent HK, Vincent KR, Lamb KM. Obesity and mobility disability in the older adult. Obes Rev. 2010;11(8):568–79.
71. Salvadego D, Lazzer S, Busti C, et al. Gas exchange kinetics in obese adolescents. Inferences on exercise tolerance and prescription. Am J Phys Regul Integr Comp Phys. 2010;299(5):R1298–305.
72. Babb TG, Wyrick BL, DeLorey DS, Chase PJ, Feng MY. Fat distribution and end-expiratory lung volume in lean and obese men and women. Chest. 2008;134(4):704–11.
73. Bernhardt V, Stickford JL, Bhammar DM, Babb TG. Aerobic exercise training without weight loss reduces dyspnea on exertion in obese women. Respir Physiol Neurobiol. 2016;221:64–70.

74. Salvadori A, Fanari P, Tovaglieri I, et al. Ventilation and its control during incremental exercise in obesity. Respiration. 2008;75(1):26–33.
75. Bernhardt V, Mitchell GS, Lee WY, Babb TG. Short-term modulation of the ventilatory response to exercise is preserved in obstructive sleep apnea. Respir Physiol Neurobiol. 2017;236:42–50.
76. Bhammar DM, Stickford JL, Bernhardt V, Babb TG. Effect of weight loss on operational lung volumes and oxygen cost of breathing in obese women. Int J Obes. 2016;40(6):998–1004.
77. Lurie A. Obstructive sleep apnea in adults: epidemiology, clinical presentation, and treatment options. Adv Cardiol. 2011;46:1–42.
78. Gami AS, Caples SM, Somers VK. Obesity and obstructive sleep apnea. Endocrinol Metab Clin N Am. 2003;32(4):869–94.
79. Lee W, Nagubadi S, Kryger MH, Mokhlesi B. Epidemiology of Obstructive Sleep Apnea: a Population-based Perspective. Expert Rev Respir Med. 2008;2(3):349–64.
80. Bradley TD, Floras JS. Obstructive sleep apnoea and its cardiovascular consequences. Lancet. 2009;373(9657):82–93.
81. Somers VK, White DP, Amin R, et al. Sleep apnea and cardiovascular disease: an American Heart Association/American College of Cardiology Foundation Scientific Statement from the American Heart Association Council for High Blood Pressure Research Professional Education Committee, Council on Clinical Cardiology, Stroke Council, and Council on Cardiovascular Nursing. J Am Coll Cardiol. 2008;52(8):686–717.
82. Rotenberg BW, Vicini C, Pang EB, Pang KP. Reconsidering first-line treatment for obstructive sleep apnea: a systematic review of the literature. J Otolaryngol Head Neck Surg. 2016;45:23.
83. Andrade FM, Pedrosa RP. The role of physical exercise in obstructive sleep apnea. J Bras Pneumol. 2016;42(6):457–64.
84. Peppard PE, Young T, Palta M, Dempsey J, Skatrud J. Longitudinal study of moderate weight change and sleep-disordered breathing. JAMA. 2000;284(23):3015–21.
85. Newman AB, Foster G, Givelber R, Nieto FJ, Redline S, Young T. Progression and regression of sleep-disordered breathing with changes in weight: the Sleep Heart Health Study. Arch Intern Med. 2005;165(20):2408–13.
86. Schwartz AR, Gold AR, Schubert N, et al. Effect of weight loss on upper airway collapsibility in obstructive sleep apnea. Am Rev Respir Dis. 1991;144(3 Pt 1):494–8.
87. Awad KM, Malhotra A, Barnet JH, Quan SF, Peppard PE. Exercise is associated with a reduced incidence of sleep-disordered breathing. Am J Med. 2012;125(5):485–90.
88. Simpson L, McArdle N, Eastwood PR, et al. Physical inactivity is associated with moderate-severe obstructive sleep apnea. J Clin Sleep Med. 2015;11(10):1091–9.
89. Peppard PE, Young T. Exercise and sleep-disordered breathing: an association independent of body habitus. Sleep. 2004;27(3):480–4.
90. Jean RE, Duttuluri M, Gibson CD, et al. Improvement in physical activity in persons with obstructive sleep apnea treated with continuous positive airway pressure. J Phys Act Health. 2017;14(3):176–82.
91. Diamanti C, Manali E, Ginieri-Coccossis M, et al. Depression, physical activity, energy consumption, and quality of life in OSA patients before and after CPAP treatment. Sleep Breath. 2013;17(4):1159–68.
92. Bamberga M, Rizzi M, Gadaleta F, Grechi A, Baiardini R, Fanfulla F. Relationship between energy expenditure, physical activity and weight loss during CPAP treatment in obese OSA subjects. Respir Med. 2015;109(4):540–5.
93. Dreher M, Kabitz HJ, Burgardt V, Walterspacher S, Windisch W. Proportional assist ventilation improves exercise capacity in patients with obesity. Respiration. 2010;80(2):106–11.
94. Tsuboi T, Ohi M, Chin K, et al. Ventilatory support during exercise in patients with pulmonary tuberculosis sequelae. Chest. 1997;112(4):1000–7.
95. Borel JC, Wuyam B, Chouri-Pontarollo N, Deschaux C, Levy P, Pépin JL. During exercise non-invasive ventilation in chronic restrictive respiratory failure. Respir Med. 2008;102(5):711–9.

96. Younes M, Puddy A, Roberts D, et al. Proportional assist ventilation. Results of an initial clinical trial. Am Rev Respir Dis. 1992;145(1):121–9.
97. Miller MB, Pearcey GE, Cahill F, et al. The effect of a short-term high-intensity circuit training program on work capacity, body composition, and blood profiles in sedentary obese men: a pilot study. Biomed Res Int. 2014;2014:191797.
98. Eastwood PR, Hillman DR. A threshold loading device for testing of inspiratory muscle performance. Eur Respir J. 1995;8(3):463–6.
99. Bezzoli E, Andreotti D, Pianta L, et al. Motor control exercises of the lumbar-pelvic region improve respiratory function in obese men. A pilot study. Disabil Rehabil. 2018;40(2):152–8.
100. Corbeil P, Simoneau M, Rancourt D, Tremblay A, Teasdale N. Increased risk for falling associated with obesity: mathematical modeling of postural control. IEEE Trans Neural Syst Rehabil Eng. 2001;9(2):126–36.
101. Gilleard W, Smith T. Effect of obesity on posture and hip joint moments during a standing task, and trunk forward flexion motion. Int J Obes. 2007;31(2):267–71.
102. Clark K. Balance and strength training for obese individuals. ACSM'S Health Fitness J. 2004;8:14–20.
103. Fabris SM, Valezi AC, de Souza SA, Faintuch J, Cecconello I, Junior MP. Computerized baropodometry in obese patients. Obes Surg. 2006;16(12):1574–8.
104. Rossi AP, Watson NL, Newman AB, et al. Effects of body composition and adipose tissue distribution on respiratory function in elderly men and women: the health, aging, and body composition study. J Gerontol A Biol Sci Med Sci. 2011;66(7):801–8.
105. De Troyer A, Boriek AM. Mechanics of the respiratory muscles. Compr Physiol. 2011;1(3):1273–300.
106. De Troyer A, Wilson TA. Mechanism of the increased rib cage expansion produced by the diaphragm with abdominal support. J Appl Physiol (1985). 2015;118(8):989–95.
107. Estenne M, De Troyer A. Relationship between respiratory muscle electromyogram and rib cage motion in tetraplegia. Am Rev Respir Dis. 1985;132(1):53–9.
108. Loring SH, Mead J. Action of the diaphragm on the rib cage inferred from a force-balance analysis. J Appl Physiol Respir Environ Exerc Physiol. 1982;53(3):756–60.
109. Hodges PW, Gandevia SC. Changes in intra-abdominal pressure during postural and respiratory activation of the human diaphragm. J Appl Physiol (1985). 2000;89(3):967–76.
110. Hodges PW, Gurfinkel VS, Brumagne S, Smith TC, Cordo PC. Coexistence of stability and mobility in postural control: evidence from postural compensation for respiration. Exp Brain Res. 2002;144(3):293–302.
111. Hodges PW, Eriksson AE, Shirley D, Gandevia SC. Intra-abdominal pressure increases stiffness of the lumbar spine. J Biomech. 2005;38(9):1873–80.
112. Malátová R, Drevikovská P. Testing procedures for abdominal muscles using the muscle dynamometer SD02. Proc Inst Mech Eng H. 2009;223(8):1041–8.
113. Hodges PW, Heijnen I, Gandevia SC. Postural activity of the diaphragm is reduced in humans when respiratory demand increases. J Physiol. 2001;537(Pt 3):999–1008.
114. Key J. 'The core': understanding it, and retraining its dysfunction. J Bodyw Mov Ther. 2013;17(4):541–59.
115. Mignardot JB, Olivier I, Promayon E, Nougier V. Obesity impact on the attentional cost for controlling posture. PLoS One. 2010;5(12):e14387.
116. McCabe CS, Blake DR. An embarrassment of pain perceptions? Towards an understanding of and explanation for the clinical presentation of CRPS type 1. Rheumatology (Oxford). 2008;47(11):1612–6.
117. O'Sullivan PB, Beales DJ, Beetham JA, et al. Altered motor control strategies in subjects with sacroiliac joint pain during the active straight-leg-raise test. Spine (Phila Pa 1976). 2002;27(1):E1–8.
118. O'Sullivan PB, Dankaerts W, Burnett AF, et al. Effect of different upright sitting postures on spinal-pelvic curvature and trunk muscle activation in a pain-free population. Spine (Phila Pa 1976). 2006;31(19):E707–12.

119. Pinto RZ, Ferreira PH, Franco MR, et al. The effect of lumbar posture on abdominal muscle thickness during an isometric leg task in people with and without non-specific low back pain. Man Ther. 2011;16(6):578–84.
120. Claus AP, Hides JA, Moseley GL, Hodges PW. Different ways to balance the spine: subtle changes in sagittal spinal curves affect regional muscle activity. Spine (Phila Pa 1976). 2009;34(6):E208–14.
121. Reeve A, Dilley A. Effects of posture on the thickness of transversus abdominis in pain-free subjects. Man Ther. 2009;14(6):679–84.

Balance Training

7

Stefano Corna, Elif Kirdi, Cinzia Parisio, and Paolo Capodaglio

Key Points

- Obesity negatively affects balance, but balance exercises are often neglected in rehabilitation programs.
- Evidence exists that majority of patients with obesity complain of dizziness, but they seem to underestimate the risk of fall.
- Assessment of balance with self-reported measures, clinical scales, or static and dynamic posturography is key to quantify unbalance, define effective rehabilitation program, and evaluate outcomes.
- Considering the increased risk of fall, balance exercises for the patient with obesity should be implemented even in the absence of specific balance disorders.

During everyday life, even to perform a simple motor task, we continuously need to counteract gravity. In order to successfully complete this task, we may have to make a conscious effort to keep from falling. Balance is the skill required to maintain upright posture of the body on a gravitational environment. Dizziness is the common symptom to describe a difficulty in controlling our balance. It is commonly

---

S. Corna (✉)
Istituti Clinici Scientifici Maugeri IRCCS, Veruno, Novara, Italy
e-mail: stefano.corna@icsmaugeri.it

E. Kirdi
Department Physical Therapy and Rehabilitation, Hacettepe University, Ankara, Turkey
e-mail: elifkaragul@hacettepe.edu.tr

C. Parisio · P. Capodaglio
Istituto Auxologico Italiano IRCCS, Piancavallo, Verbania, Italy
e-mail: p.capodaglio@auxologico.it

P. Capodaglio (ed.), *Rehabilitation Interventions in the Patient with Obesity*,
https://doi.org/10.1007/978-3-030-32274-8_7

encountered in the general population. Secondary to labyrinth, cardiac, neurological, endocrinological, and psychological dysfunctions, dizziness can lead to balance disorders with a significant impact on quality of life and ability to work [1] and can become permanent [2]. Balance disorders increase risk of falls [3]. A recent review [4] reports a lifetime prevalence of dizziness 17–30%. Bisdorff [5] using a more analytic survey for vertigo, dizziness, and unsteadiness, resulting from a range of vestibular and non-vestibular conditions, found a 1-year prevalence of 48.3%, 35.6%, and 39.1%, respectively.

Obesity is currently regarded as one of the major health challenges of the developed world and is a growing concern in developing countries. Large evidence exists that obesity negatively affects balance [6], yet little is known about evaluation and rehabilitation of balance capacity in the patient with obesity.

7.1 Physiology

To move our body around an environment, we exploit a combination of biomechanical characteristics, specific sensory inputs, and central nervous system integration of all these information combined with a feedforward and backward control. This complex system produces postural tone, postural stability, and postural orientation [7]. Postural tone corresponds to the active and passive muscle tone of extensor muscles aimed at counteracting gravity. Further biomechanical constraints, such as muscle strength and range of motion, also play an important role in postural control. Postural stability refers to balance, the condition in which the projection of the center of mass (CoM), named center of pressure (CoP), is contained within the boundaries of the base of support (BoS). Postural orientation is the position of the body segments with respect to each other and the environment. In order to make a voluntary postural task, we need an integrating multiple sensory inputs from the somatosensory, vestibular, and visual systems to determine the relative orientation of body segments and position relative to the environment. To achieve the desired postural target, we often apply also anticipatory postural adjustments and automatic postural responses. Control of *limits of stability* (referred to the area within which a person can move his CoP without changing BoS) and *verticality* (internal representation of the body alignment in space that comes from the vestibular otoliths, proprioceptors, and visual system) is an essential contribution to avoid falls in any postural task.

The visual system allows recognition and detection of orientation and movement of objects in the environment. The vestibular system is specialized for the control of postural orientation and balance. It can detect both linear and rotational accelerations of the head in space. It is involved in balance and motor control as well as in perception of spatial self-motion [8, 9]. Afferents from the otolith organs (the utricle and saccule) and the semicircular canals converge with optokinetic, somatosensory, and motor-related signals in the vestibular nuclei, which are reciprocally interconnected with the vestibulocerebellar cortex and deep cerebellar nuclei [10]. The reflexes relayed through the vestibular nuclei are strongly involved in balance and movement and are grouped into three categories. The vestibulospinal reflex modulates muscle tone of the limbs and trunk muscles, the vestibulo-collic reflex is involved in head and neck posture and movement, and the vestibulo-ocular reflex regulates the position of the eyes in the orbits in order to compensate for movements of the head. Since the visual and the vestibular systems are located in the head, they do not provide direct information about body orientation in space. This important information comes from somatosensors featured all over the body, such as muscle spindles, Golgi tendon organs, and cutaneous mechanoreceptor, pressure receptor, and joint receptor.

All inputs are integrated in the central nervous system. The integration of sensory information produces an internal representation of the position and movements of the body (kinesthesia). The sensory inputs converge in the spinal cord, vestibular nuclei, brainstem, thalamus, and cerebral cortex, allowing their interaction [11]. The cerebellum is involved in the control of limb movements, balance, and motor learning [12]. An abnormal sensorimotor integration by the cerebellum produces ataxia, a discoordination of movements. The basal ganglia are involved in the planning, initiation, and control of voluntary movements. The basal ganglia have important projections to the upper brainstem nuclei which control trunk and proximal musculature for balance and gait [13].

To control balance during movement, two other mechanisms are involved: anticipatory postural adjustments and automatic postural responses. Before or simultaneously a voluntary movement, there is time for sensory feedback to elicit postural responses. Anticipatory postural adjustments are dependent on predictive, feedforward control, as the postural muscles are activated prior to or at the same time as the muscles, the prime movers for voluntary movement [14, 15]. Automatic postural responses are triggered in response to external perturbations to the body and produce a continuum of strategies that may or may not involve changes in the bases of support with a step or reach [16, 17]. Automatic postural responses are ankle strategy, generated in response to small perturbations experienced when standing on a firm, wide surface, and hip strategy, generated in response to larger perturbations. Different blends of ankle and hip strategies can be used depending on the characteristics of the perturbation. Stepping is one example of a change in support strategy that is used for very large or fast perturbations [18].

More complex is the balance and postural control of the body during gait. It involves continuous control of the trunk and body center of mass, primarily in the lateral direction and during single limb support [19]. People use preparatory strategies for proper foot placement to initiate walking, increase ground clearance, change speed and direction, and stop walking.

The cognitive contributions to balance are also important, which include attention and psychological factors. In fact, many studies have shown that even quiet stance in healthy subjects involves attentional resources because sway increases with divided attention. Psychological factors such as fear of falling have also been found to associate with poor postural stability, functional decline, decreased quality of life, and institutionalization [20, 21].

7.2 Postural Characteristics in the Patient with Obesity

Previous studies have already demonstrated that obesity produces a greater forward displacement of the CoP during dynamic balance activities while standing [22]. Excessive body weight affects posture linearly with the increase of BMI [6, 23]. The center of mass shifts forward, the lumbar lordosis increases together with the pelvic forward tilt, and dorsal kyphosis and secondary cervical lordosis become more pronounced. Frequently, internal rotation of the hips, knee valgism, and flat feet coexist [24]. The feet tend to splay apart during standing to optimize the center of gravity and for stability. Body mass distribution usually shows gender differences (gynoid and android shape). Whether shape induces possible gender-specific consequences on balance is still controversial. An increased body mass contributes to an increased ankle torque (anteroposterior destabilization) in both genders, but the android shape involves a greater amount of mass/load over the hips, which could account for the increased medial-lateral center of pressure excursion. Also, a different mass distribution has an effect on the center of mass, the imaginary point where we can assume the total body mass is concentrated, and the stabilization of its spatial position, previously proposed as the goal of postural responses [6]. The relationship between dizziness and falls in the obese population is a relatively unexplored but important issue, given the prevalence of obesity worldwide.

7.3 Assessment of Balance Disorders

Assessment of balance is mandatory in order to measure unbalance, define effective rehabilitation program of intervention, and evaluate outcomes. In the last decades, several balance tools have been developed. We can divide them in questionnaires, clinical scales, and instrumental balance evaluation devices. Often they are also utilized for training purposes. Below we report the assessment schema in use for patients with obesity.

7.3.1 Self-Reported Measures

A recent review [25] describes the Dizziness Handicap Inventory (DHI) as the most widely used and accepted self-reported measure for dizziness, translated into fourteen languages. The DHI was developed to evaluate the self-perceived impairment induced by conditions affecting the vestibular system, but it was also utilized in geriatric, brain-injured, and multiple sclerosis patients. It includes 25 items with a total score ranging between 0 and 100. DHI can be further divided into physical (DHI-P, 28 points), functional (DHI-F 36 points), and emotional (DHI-E 36 points) sub-scores. The DHI has been reported to have high test-retest reliability (interclass correlation coefficient [ICC] 0.72–0.97), internal consistency reliability (Cronbach

$\alpha = 0.72–0.89$), and responsiveness [26, 27]. In a recent paper, we used the DHI self-questionnaire tool in an obese population. We demonstrated that in our sample (239 subjects), almost 70% of subjects complain dizziness, but they seem to underestimate risk of fall due to unsteadiness [28].

7.3.2 Clinical Assessment

A considerable number of scales designed to help therapists to identify impaired postural control have been completed. To evaluate postural stability in a more functional context, these clinical scales would appear to be more appropriate than simple tests of postural stability. The Berg Balance Scale (BBS) [29] is one of the most widely used tools for balance assessment [30]. Its psychometric properties have been well assessed, and the scale has shown to be a valid and reliable measure of balance [31]. However, some important limitations of the BBS have been described, such as the need for some rescoring of the rating scale [32], a ceiling effect, and relatively low responsiveness [33]. Moreover, dynamic balance (i.e., reacting to a perturbation, gait) is unexplored by the BBS. Recently, a new clinical tool for assessing balance impairments has been presented, the Balance Evaluation Systems Test (BESTest) [34], and the Mini-BESTest includes important aspects of dynamic balance control, such as the capability to react to postural perturbations, to stand on a compliant or inclined surface, and to walk while performing a cognitive task. All of these features of balance control are known to be important in assessing balance disorders in different types of patients and reflect balance challenges during activities of daily living [35]. See also www.bestest.us for details.

7.3.3 Instrumental Evaluation

More sophisticated tools for balance and posture analysis have been developed. Generally, they are divided in platforms that analyze balance in the upright position and mobile platforms that analyze body reaction to external perturbations, besides gait analyses. Also, a combination of them has been developed: the computerized dynamic posturography (EquiTest®, NeuroCom, USA). It is an assessment equipment to objectively measure postural control: it isolates and quantifies the functional contributions of different sensory systems (somatosensory, visual and vestibular input) and the mechanisms for integrating these sensory inputs for maintaining balance. It is a valuable tool for investigating sensory, motor, and central adaptive impairments. It can quantify postural strategies to static and dynamic perturbations and provides an objective assessment of postural control. However, it is also expensive and not portable. Thus, it is intended to complement, not replace, existing clinical measures that categorize the mechanisms of balance disorders.

7.4 Balance Training and Rehabilitation

7.4.1 Customized Training

As already demonstrated by many studies, balance training can improve balance and reduce falls [36]. Several approaches are possible. One of these considers necessary to design a customized treatment intervention to address any specific impairment field pointed out by the assessment. In this case, six different aspects of balance control are explored:

1. Treatment of biomechanical constraints. It is imperative to address balance problems including weakness, reduced range of motion, reduced flexibility, and improper postural alignment. Most strength training interventions last for at least 12 weeks [37, 38].
2. Many patients with balance problems show reduced limits of stability as reflected by decreased functional reach distance [39] or reduced movement velocity and excursion distance measured by limits of stability posturography. Weight-shifting exercise training with a balance master has been shown to increase limits of stability [40].
3. Sensory orientation can be enhanced by habituation and/or compensation. Excessive visual motion sensitivity can be habituated by gradually exposing a subject to a moving visual surround. Compensation would encourage subjects to use alternative sensory information. Several tools such as computerized dynamic posturography, optokinetic stimulation, and virtual reality can be used to manipulate visual feedback. Sensory biofeedback is another tool for sensory retraining of balance control [41].
4. Training of anticipatory postural adjustments is focused on improving postural preparation for transition from one position to another, such as sit-to-stand single-leg stance, step initiation, and compensatory forward stepping.
5. Enhance appropriate postural responses to perturbations in order to promote proper strategies. For the ankle strategy, postural responses using a broad, stable surface and movement at the ankles without movement at the hips or knees should be facilitated. For the hip strategy, use narrow surfaces where the ability to generate ankle torque is reduced. The stepping strategy is taking the weight off the stepping leg during gait initiation and moving the CoM outside the BoS. To enhance postural responses, use an unstable support surface such as foam [42] and the sudden start or stop of a treadmill [43].
6. Dynamic stability during gait can be enhanced using the speed-dependent treadmill, obstacle pathways [44, 45], and walking in different directions and environments. The use of a dual-task paradigm may also help to make balance a more automatic process, as attention must be diverted to the secondary task rather than being focused on keeping balance.

7.4.2 Rehabilitation Protocols

Patients with obesity have intrinsically reduced postural stability and balance than their normal-weight counterparts. This reduced stability increases linearly with BMI. They are at increased risk of falling at any age, even before puberty [46]. Although many studies investigated the risk of falling in obese individuals, balance exercises in these individuals are often not implemented in the rehabilitation program. After conventional rehabilitation with exercises, obese patients improve their balance control. Furthermore, they need to perform training to ameliorate their balance in everyday life and to avoid risk of falls. Maffiuletti et al. [47] showed that just 4-min of specific balance training incorporated into the physical exercise routine improved postural stability in patients with severe obesity. The recommended exercise program for patient with obesity is a multicomponent 90-min exercise program that includes 15-min balance training, 15-min flexibility, 30-min aerobic exercise, and 30-min high-intensity resistance training [48]. A few examples of balance exercises for patients with obesity without specific balance problems are shown in the Fig. 7.1.

Often protocols are designed and prescribed only for a specific balance problem. For instance, dizziness and unsteadiness, resulting from a range of vestibular and non-vestibular conditions, have a high prevalence. Vestibular patients who underwent a rehabilitation program to avoid movements that can trigger vertigo reported no improvement in balance control [49, 50], but evidence exists [51, 52] that improvements can be obtained when appropriate rehabilitation protocols were used. Rehabilitation training can be based on standard protocol such as the Cawthorne-Cooksey exercises [53] or vestibular habituation training [54, 55]. The functional gain achieved through those exercises supposedly relies on adaptation, that is, modification of the gain of the relevant vestibulo-oculomotor and vestibule-spinal circuits [56] and habituation [57, 58], a central process of learning that is independent from sensory adaptation and motor fatigue [59]. Cawthorne-Cooksey exercises are widely used in dizziness. Recently, a Cochrane review reported moderate to strong evidence for patients with peripheral vestibular dysfunction [60]. The exercise protocol includes training of the eye movement, practicing balance in everyday situation, practicing head movements that cause dizziness, improving general coordination, and encouraging natural unprompted movements (see also www.wsh.nhs.uk for full explanation of the protocol).

7.4.3 Instrumental Rehabilitation

As already mentioned, often instrumental platforms made for balance assessment include also the possibility of performing training and rehabilitation programs: from the simple visual feedback, where the patient actively moves his CoP following a

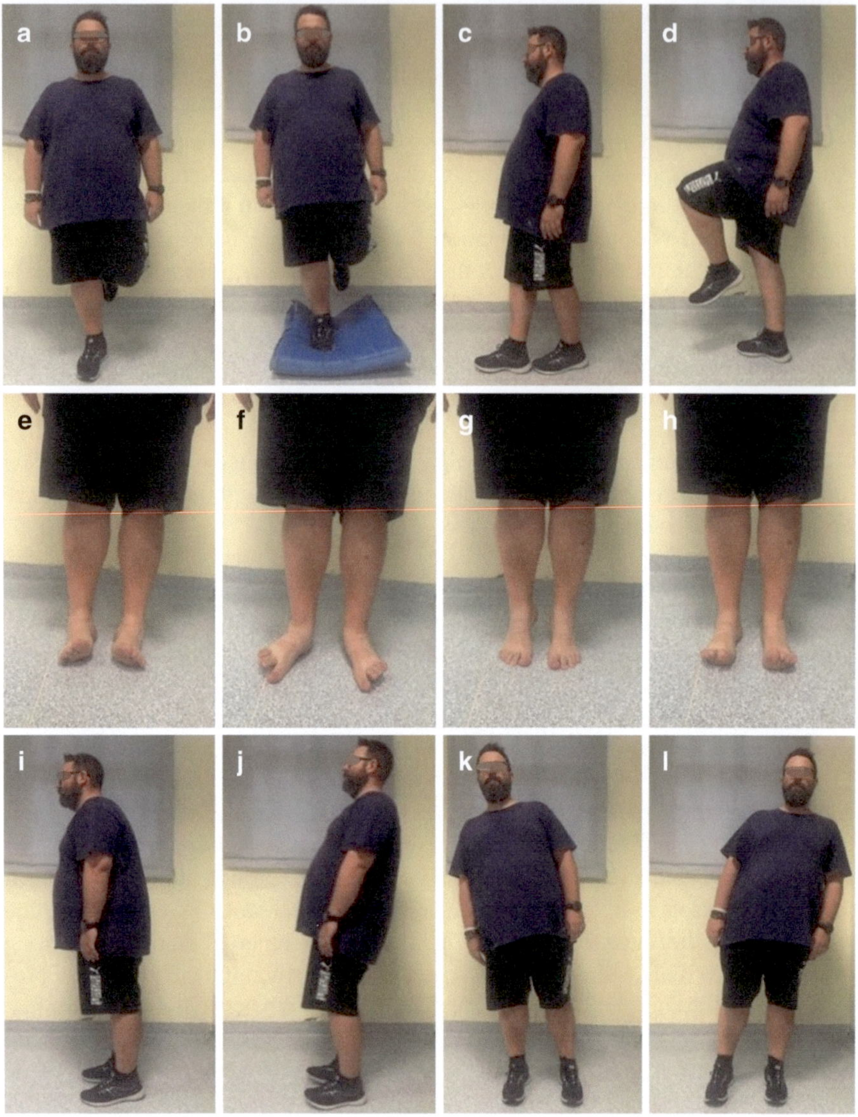

Fig. 7.1 Examples of balance exercises for patients with obesity without any specific vestibular disorders. (**a**) Single-leg standing (eyes open); (**b**) single-leg standing on foam surface (eyes open); (**c**) heel-to-toe walking on a line; (**d**) soldier march exercise; (**e**) foot inversion; (**f**) foot eversion; (**g**) bilateral heel rise; (**h**) isolated toe movements; (**i**) anterior weight shifting; (**j**) posterior weight shifting; (**k**) right side weight shifting; (**l**) left side weight shifting

target on the screen, to more sophisticated moving platforms challenging balance control, where the patient has to contrast the platform displacement to avoid fall.

In dizzy patients, we have developed a protocol using a platform continuously moving in an anteroposterior direction [61]. This kind of perturbation induces predictable postural displacements of the legs, trunk, and head; these displacements have to be appropriately counteracted and anticipated [62]. Further, when the balance perturbation is provided in a periodic fashion, as in a continuously moving platform, subjects can anticipate the appropriate postural adjustment [63]. A platform moving according to a sinusoidal program requires subjects to use sensory input both in a feedback and feedforward mode to produce an adequate motor output [64]. We compared the effectiveness of vestibular rehabilitation by using Cawthorne-Cooksey exercises with instrumental rehabilitation. We demonstrate that both Cawthorne-Cooksey and instrumental rehabilitation are effective for treating balance disorders of vestibular origin. Improvement affects both control of body balance and performance of activities of daily living. The larger decrease in body sway and greater improvement of DHI after instrumental rehabilitation suggest that it is more effective than Cawthorne-Cooksey exercises in improving balance control [65].

7.4.4 Vestibular Disorders in the Obese Patients

With regard to rehabilitation of dizziness, very few has been made in obese population. To understand if the Cawthorne-Cooksey protocol is effective in obese patients, we have made a pilot study (unpublished data) on a sample of 12 vestibular obese patients (BMI between 35 and 56 kg/m^2). They were evaluated prior and after rehabilitation training with Dizziness Handicap Inventory, Mini-BESTest, stabilometry, and EquiTest®. Despite the small size of our sample, we found statistical significance either in the DHI with a reduction of 14 points of the total score. Also the Mini-BESTest demonstrated a significant modification of the score (from prior 22–26 after treatment). Due to the high variability of the data in the sample, stabilometry failed to demonstrate modifications. Instead, EquiTest® sensory organization test (SOT) showed improvement in the more challenging dynamic conditions. Also the "composite equilibrium score" showed a significant score increasing from 63 prior to 72 after rehabilitation. In conclusion, despite their different posture characteristics, obese vestibular patients improve their balance control after conventional rehabilitation with Cawthorne-Cooksey exercises.

References

1. Yardley L, Owen N, Nazareth I, Luxon L. Prevalence and presentation of dizziness in a general practice community sample of working age people. Br J Gen Pract. 1998;48(429):1131–5.
2. Skøien AK, Wilhemsen K, Gjesdal S. Occupational disability caused by dizziness and vertigo: a register-based prospective study. Br J Gen Pract. 2008;58(554):619–23.
3. Agrawal Y, Carey JP, Della Santina CC, Schubert MC, Minor LB. Disorders of balance and vestibular function in US adults: data from the National Health and Nutrition Examination Survey, 2001-2004. Arch Intern Med. 2009;169(10):938–44.
4. Murdin L, Schilder AG. Epidemiology of balance symptoms and disorders in the community: a systematic review. Otol Neurotol. 2015;36(3):387–92.

5. Bisdorff A, Bosser G, Gueguen R, Perrin P. The epidemiology of vertigo, dizziness, and unsteadiness and its links to co-morbidities. Front Neurol. 2013;4:29.
6. Menegoni F, Galli M, Tacchini E, Vismara L, Cavigioli M, Capodaglio P. Gender-specific effect of obesity on balance. Obesity. 2009;17(10):1951–6.
7. Horak F, MacPherson JM. Postural orientation and equilibrium. In: Handbook of physiology exercise: regulation and integration of multiple systems neural control of movement. New York: Oxford University Press; 1996. p. 255–92.
8. St George RJ, Fitzpatrick RC. The sense of self-motion, orientation and balance explored by vestibular stimulation. J Physiol. 2011;589(4):807–13.
9. Dieterich M, Brandt T. The bilateral central vestibular system: its pathways, functions, and disorders. Ann N Y Acad Sci. 2015;1343(1):10–26.
10. Green AM, Angelaki DE. Internal models and neural computation in the vestibular system. Exp Brain Res. 2010;200(3–4):197–222.
11. Manzoni D. The cerebellum and sensorimotor coupling: looking at the problem from the perspective of vestibular reflexes. Cerebellum. 2007;6(1):24.
12. Synofzik M, Ilg W. Motor training in degenerative spinocerebellar disease: ataxia-specific improvements by intensive physiotherapy and exergames. Biomed Res Int. 2014;2014:583507.
13. Pahapill PA, Lozano AM. The pedunculopontine nucleus and Parkinson's disease. Brain. 2000;123(9):1767–83.
14. Crenna P, Frigo C, Massion J, Pedotti A. Forward and backward axial synergies in man. Exp Brain Res. 1987;65(3):538–48.
15. Oddsson L, Thorstensson A. Fast voluntary trunk flexion movements in standing: motor patterns. Acta Physiol Scand. 1987;129(1):93–106.
16. Horak FB, Henry SM, Shumway-Cook A. Postural perturbations: new insights for treatment of balance disorders. Phys Ther. 1997;77(5):517–33.
17. Maki BE, McIlroy WE. The role of limb movements in maintaining upright stance: the "change-in-support" strategy. Phys Ther. 1997;77(5):488–507.
18. Horak FB, Nashner LM. Central programming of postural movements: adaptation to altered support-surface configurations. J Neurophysiol. 1986;55(6):1369–81.
19. Winter DA. Human balance and posture control during standing and walking. Gait Posture. 1995;3(4):193–214.
20. Deschamps T, Beauchet O, Annweiler C, Cornu C, Mignardot J-B. Postural control and cognitive decline in older adults: position versus velocity implicit motor strategy. Gait Posture. 2014;39(1):628–30.
21. Adkin AL, Frank JS, Jog MS. Fear of falling and postural control in Parkinson's disease. Mov Disord. 2003;18(5):496–502.
22. Berrigan F, Simoneau M, Tremblay A, Hue O, Teasdale N. Influence of obesity on accurate and rapid arm movement performed from a standing posture. Int J Obes. 2006;30(12):1750.
23. Hue O, Simoneau M, Marcotte J, Berrigan F, Doré J, Marceau P, et al. Body weight is a strong predictor of postural stability. Gait Posture. 2007;26(1):32–8.
24. De Souza SAF, Faintuch J, Valezi AC, Sant'Anna AF, Gama-Rodrigues JJ, de Batista Fonseca IC, et al. Postural changes in morbidly obese patients. Obes Surg. 2005;15(7):1013–6.
25. Mutlu B, Serbetcioglu B. Discussion of the dizziness handicap inventory. J Vestib Res. 2013;23(6):271–7.
26. Jacobson GP, Newman CW. The development of the dizziness handicap inventory. Arch Otolaryngol Head Neck Surg. 1990;116(4):424–7.
27. Cattaneo D, Jonsdottir J, Repetti S. Reliability of four scales on balance disorders in persons with multiple sclerosis. Disabil Rehabil. 2007;29(24):1920–5.
28. Corna S, Aspesi V, Cau N, Scarpina F, Valdes NG, Brugliera L, et al. Dizziness and falls in obese inpatients undergoing metabolic rehabilitation. PLoS One. 2017;12(1):e0169322.
29. Berg KO, Wood-Dauphinee SL, Williams JI, Maki B. Measuring balance in the elderly: validation of an instrument. Can J Public Health. 1992;83(Supp 2):7–11.

30. Tyson S, Connell L. How to measure balance in clinical practice. A systematic review of the psychometrics and clinical utility of measures of balance activity for neurological conditions. Clin Rehabil. 2009;23(9):824–40.
31. Blum L, Korner-Bitensky N. Usefulness of the Berg Balance Scale in stroke rehabilitation: a systematic review. Phys Ther. 2008;88(5):559–66.
32. Kornetti DL, Fritz SL, Chiu Y-P, Light KE, Velozo CA. Rating scale analysis of the Berg Balance Scale. Arch Phys Med Rehabil. 2004;85(7):1128–35.
33. Pardasaney PK, Latham NK, Jette AM, Wagenaar RC, Ni P, Slavin MD, et al. Sensitivity to change and responsiveness of four balance measures for community-dwelling older adults. Phys Ther. 2012;92(3):388–97.
34. Horak FB, Wrisley DM, Frank J. The balance evaluation systems test (BESTest) to differentiate balance deficits. Phys Ther. 2009;89(5):484–98.
35. Horak FB. Postural orientation and equilibrium: what do we need to know about neural control of balance to prevent falls? Age Ageing. 2006;35(suppl_2):ii7–ii11.
36. Gillespie LD, Gillespie WJ, Robertson MC, Lamb SE, Cumming RG, Rowe BH. Interventions for preventing falls in elderly people. Cochrane Database Syst Rev. 2003;4:CD000340.
37. Falvo MJ, Schilling BK, Earhart GM. Parkinson's disease and resistive exercise: rationale, review, and recommendations. Mov Disord. 2008;23(1):1–11.
38. Orr R. Contribution of muscle weakness to postural instability in the elderly. Eur J Phys Rehabil Med. 2010;46(2):183–220.
39. Newton RA. Validity of the multi-directional reach test: a practical measure for limits of stability in older adults. J Gerontol Ser A Biol Med Sci. 2001;56(4):M248–52.
40. Jessop RT, Horowicz C, Dibble LE. Motor learning and Parkinson disease: refinement of movement velocity and endpoint excursion in a limits of stability balance task. Neurorehabil Neural Repair. 2006;20(4):459–67.
41. Yelnik AP, Le Breton F, Colle FM, Bonan IV, Hugeron C, Egal V, et al. Rehabilitation of balance after stroke with multisensorial training: a single-blind randomized controlled study. Neurorehabil Neural Repair. 2008;22(5):468–76.
42. Bayouk J-F, Boucher JP, Leroux A. Balance training following stroke: effects of task-oriented exercises with and without altered sensory input. Int J Rehabil Res. 2006;29(1):51–9.
43. Protas EJ, Mitchell K, Williams A, Qureshy H, Caroline K, Lai EC. Gait and step training to reduce falls in Parkinson's disease. NeuroRehabilitation. 2005;20(3):183–90.
44. Missaoui B, Rakotovao E, Bendaya S, Mane M, Pichon B, Faucher M, et al. Posture and gait abilities in patients with myotonic dystrophy (Steinert disease). Evaluation on the short-term of a rehabilitation program. Ann Phys Rehabil Med. 2010;53(6–7):387–98.
45. Ashburn A, Fazakarley L, Ballinger C, Pickering R, McLellan LD, Fitton C. A randomised controlled trial of a home based exercise programme to reduce the risk of falling among people with Parkinson's disease. J Neurol Neurosurg Psychiatry. 2007;78(7):678–84.
46. McGraw B, McClenaghan BA, Williams HG, Dickerson J, Ward DS. Gait and postural stability in obese and nonobese prepubertal boys. Arch Phys Med Rehabil. 2000;81(4):484–9.
47. Maffiuletti N, Agosti F, Proietti M, Riva D, Resnik M, Lafortuna C, et al. Postural instability of extremely obese individuals improves after a body weight reduction program entailing specific balance training. J Endocrinol Investig. 2005;28(3):2–7.
48. Mathus-Vliegen EM, Basdevant A, Finer N, Hainer V, Hauner H, Micic D, et al. Prevalence, pathophysiology, health consequences and treatment options of obesity in the elderly: a guideline. Obes Facts. 2012;5(3):460–83.
49. Herdman S. Vestibular rehabilitation therapy. Philadelphia, PA: FA Davis; 1994.
50. Norre M, De Weerdt W. Treatment of vertigo based on habituation: 2. Technique and results of habituation training. J Laryngol Otol. 1980;94(9):971–7.
51. Hecker HC, Haug CO, Herndon JW. Treatment of the vertiginous patient using Cawthorne's vestibular exercises. Laryngoscope. 1974;84(11):2065–78.
52. Robertson D, Ireland D. Evaluation and treatment of uncompensated unilateral vestibular disease. Otolaryngol Clin N Am. 1997;30(5):745–57.

53. Cooksey F. Rehabilitation in vestibular injuries. Thousand Oaks, CA: SAGE Publications; 1946.
54. Norré ME, Beckers AM. Vestibular habituation training: specificity of adequate exercise. Arch Otolaryngol Head Neck Surg. 1988;114(8):883–6.
55. Norré ME. Rationale of rehabilitation treatment for vertigo. Am J Otolaryngol. 1987;8(1):31–5.
56. Herdman SJ. Role of vestibular adaptation in vestibular rehabilitation. Otolaryngol Head Neck Surg. 1998;119(1):49–54.
57. Shepard NT, Telian SA, Smith-Wheelock M. Habituation and balance retraining therapy: a retrospective review. Neurol Clin. 1990;8(2):459–75.
58. Cawthorne T. The physiological basis for head exercises. J Char Soc Physiother. 1944;3:106–7.
59. Thompson RF, Spencer WA. Habituation: a model phenomenon for the study of neuronal substrates of behavior. Psychol Rev. 1966;73(1):16.
60. McDonnell MN, Hillier SL. Vestibular rehabilitation for unilateral peripheral vestibular dysfunction. Cochrane Database Syst Rev. 2015;1:CD005397.
61. Nardone A, Corna S, Grasso M, Tarantola J, Schieppati M. Posturo-kinetic coordination on a continuously moving platform: role of proprioceptive and vestibular informations. In: Proceedings of the International Symposium on Gait Disorders. Prague: Galén; 1999. p. 189–90.
62. Corna S, Tarantola J, Nardone A, Giordano A, Schieppati M. Standing on a continuously moving platform: is body inertia counteracted or exploited? Exp Brain Res. 1999;124(3):331–41.
63. Nardone A, Grasso M, Tarantola J, Corna S, Schieppati M. Postural coordination in elderly subjects standing on a periodically moving platform. Arch Phys Med Rehabil. 2000;81(9):1217–23.
64. Buchanan JJ, Horak FB. Emergence of postural patterns as a function of vision and translation frequency. J Neurophysiol. 1999;81(5):2325–39.
65. Corna S, Nardone A, Prestinari A, Galante M, Grasso M, Schieppati M. Comparison of Cawthorne-Cooksey exercises and sinusoidal support surface translations to improve balance in patients with unilateral vestibular deficit. Arch Phys Med Rehabil. 2003;84(8):1173–84.

The Post-acute Patient

8

Natalia Gattini and Paolo Capodaglio

Key Points

- Obesity associated with reduced mortality and hemorrhagic transformation after stroke ("obesity paradox," probably due to reduction of post-stroke pro-inflammatory state); however, weight reduction in obese patients still recommended for primary stroke prevention.
- Functional disability after acute ischemic stroke does not differ significantly in obese and normal-weight patients.
- No prognostic meaning of BMI after intravenous thrombolysis with regard to functional outcome, death, or occurrence of symptomatic intracranial hemorrhage.
- After orthopedic surgery, increased risk of infections and other, pre-, intra-, and postsurgical complications; longer hospital stay; and greater hospital costs, but rehabilitation efficiency similar to normal-weight patients.
- Multidimensional approach needed for optimal disease management, guidelines for rehabilitation in the post-acute patient with obesity are needed.

N. Gattini
Hospital Clínico Universidad de Chile, Santiago, Chile

P. Capodaglio (✉)
Rehabilitation Unit and Research Laboratory in Biomechanics and Rehabilitation, Istituto Auxologico Italiano IRCCS, Piancavallo, Italy
e-mail: p.capodaglio@auxologico.it

P. Capodaglio (ed.), *Rehabilitation Interventions in the Patient with Obesity*,
https://doi.org/10.1007/978-3-030-32274-8_8

8.1 Stroke

Obesity is an established risk factor for the development of vascular diseases such as stroke. A meta-analysis [1] evaluated data from more than 2.2 million participants to address the relationship between excess body weight and stroke incidence. Overweight and obesity were significantly associated with a progressively increasing risk of ischemic stroke. It has been shown that each unit increase of BMI was associated with a significant 6% increase in the adjusted relative risk of stroke [2]. The association between BMI and risk of ischemic stroke was linear, similar in men and women and regardless of race [3, 4].

8.1.1 Clinical Outcomes After Stroke

While obesity is an established risk factor for stroke, its influence on clinical outcome, mortality, and thrombolysis in acute ischemic stroke is still under debate. Several studies indicated that overweight and obese patients with heart failure have significantly lower mortality rates (both cardiovascular death and all-cause mortality) as compared to the normal-weight counterparts. The in-hospital mortality for patients with decompensated heart failure has been reported to be 10% lower with each 5-unit increase in BMI [5]. A meta-analysis of 40 studies involving more than 250,000 patients with coronary artery disease showed that total and cardiovascular mortality was lowest among overweight patients [6]. Meanwhile, many studies suggest better outcomes for obese patients in other diseases or interventions such as chronic heart failure, coronary revascularization, chronic kidney disease, rheumatoid arthritis, chronic obstructive lung disease, or advanced cancers [7, 8–11]. The counterintuitive relationship observed between higher BMI and improved survival after stroke has been described as an "obesity paradox" and is seen in other disease states such as heart failure and myocardial infarction [12, 13]. Hemorrhagic transformation occurrence after stroke was found to be decreased with obesity [14]. Some prospective studies have observed lower mortality after stroke in persons with obesity compared with those with normal weight [15], but others have not [16]. The obesity paradox seems to exist also in patients with intracerebral hemorrhage: being overweight or obese was associated with favorable functional outcome after adjustment for established predictors [17]. Aparicio et al. [18] investigated overweight, obesity, and survival after stroke in the Framingham Heart Study, comparing all-cause mortality in participants stratified by pre-stroke weight. Overweight and mildly obese participants had better 10-year survival after ischemic stroke compared with normal-weight participants, even after excluding persons with recent pre-stroke weight loss. The authors concluded that there may be unknown protective factors associated with a moderately increased body weight before stroke. This is in line with Doehner [19], who found that overweight and obese patients with stroke or TIA have better survival and better combined outcomes of survival and nonfatal functional status than patients with BMI of 25 kg/m^2. They also found that obesity predicted a decreased risk of severe disability. Sun et al. [20] did not find any outcome advantage associated with being overweight or obese at the time of experiencing an acute ischemic stroke. The risks of death and functional disability in overweight and obese patients did not differ significantly from normal-weight patients. However, underweight patients consistently had the worst outcomes after ischemic stroke. Although no significant differences of survival and functional were found, their results still support the recommendation of current guidelines to strive for normal weight after stroke, given the association between weight loss and improvements in major cardiovascular risk factors, including dyslipidemia, diabetes, and hypertension. According to a systematic review aiming at assessing the clinical outcome of obese patients after stroke and the impact of obesity on acute stroke treatment by thrombolysis [1], the results hint to an obesity paradox in stroke in terms of higher survival rates and better functional outcome in stroke patients with an excess in body weight. From a biological point of view, obesity paradox could be explained by the potentially protective effects of adipose tissue, which is now increasingly acknowledged as a major endocrine organ. Adipose tissue secretes soluble TNF-α receptors and may so neutralize the biologic impact of TNF-α. Moreover, obese individuals have increased levels of serum lipid levels which could bind and detoxify endotoxin-lipoproteins and consequently block the release of inflammatory cytokines. Both mechanisms may impede the poststroke pro-inflammatory state [21]. Most observational data indicate a survival benefit of obese patients after stroke, but a number of methodological concerns exist. Obesity is a well-proven independent risk factor for occurrence of stroke, and weight reduction in overweight or obese patients is still recommended for primary stroke prevention. It is also advisable to stick to the same recommendation in younger patients after occurrence of stroke (secondary prevention) with respect to longer life expectancy and detrimental cardiovascular effects of obesity over the years.

8.1.2 Clinical Outcomes After Intravenous Thrombolysis

There are challenging studies concerning intravenous thrombolysis in stroke and obesity. According to the systematic review of Oesch [1], no obesity paradox was observed for acute stroke patients treated with intravenous thrombolysis, whereas no data were available for intra-arterial thrombolysis or mechanical thrombectomy. Sarikaya et al. [22] aimed to compare the clinical outcome and safety after intravenous thrombolysis in obese and nonobese patients with ischemic stroke. They found that obesity is an independent predictor of unfavorable clinical outcome and mortality in acute ischemic stroke treated with intravenous thrombolysis. Gensicke [23], in a large study investigating the impact of BMI in intravenous thrombolysis-treated stroke patients, reported that BMI had no prognostic meaning with regard to 3-month functional outcome, death, or occurrence of symptomatic intracranial hemorrhage. Funda Bas [24] found that obesity was not to have any significant role on clinical course and outcome of patients treated with intravenous recombinant tissue-type plasminogen activator. No obesity paradox was observed in patients after intravenous thrombolysis; thus there is no need to change the current dosage scheme of alteplase in obese patients. However, there is still a need for well-designed and adequately powered randomized controlled trials assessing the effects of weight reduction on stroke occurrence and recurrence in obese patients.

8.1.3 Functional Outcomes After Stroke

Despite the volume of research reviewing the relationship between obesity, acute medical care outcome, and functional capacity, few data exist concerning the relationship between obesity and stroke rehabilitation outcome. In fact, the impact of obesity on a person undergoing rehabilitation after an acute stroke is still a controversial topic. Several small studies have explored the relationship between BMI and rehabilitation after a stroke. Kalichman et al. [25] studied patients treated for 3 months. They found that after 12 weeks of rehabilitation, a significant negative correlation was present between relative improvement of FIM score and BMI. A large study [26] among patients admitted to an acute rehabilitation hospital for stroke rehabilitation found that overweight patients had better functional progress than did patients in the other weight categories. For 819 patients, BMI was compared with FIM score changes per day (FIM efficiency). After adjusting for age and sex, the FIM efficiency differed by BMI: the underweight group had the lowest FIM efficiency, followed by the obese and normal-weight subgroups. The overweight group had the highest FIM efficiency when compared with the obese subgroup. These findings suggested an inverse U-shaped curve, with the worst performance among those with the lowest and highest BMIs and the best among those with normal weight or overweight. According to this relatively large study, among patients who had been hospitalized in an acute inpatient rehabilitation facility with a diagnosis of acute stroke, the overweight recovered more quickly than the remaining groups. Age differed by weight category and was a significant determinant of outcome. After adjusting for age, the overweight group did better than the other groups. Jang et al. [27] examined whether BMI was a predictor of functional independence measure (FIM) at 6 months after the ischemic stroke onset while adjusting for stroke risk factors and covariates, and stratifying by age group. They found that extreme obesity was a predictor of a good 6-month FIM, especially in patients with ischemic stroke who were at least 65 years of age.

Padwal et al. [28] found that severe obesity was an independent predictor of total length of stay, rehabilitation length of stay, and health expenditures, but not of FIM efficiency in 84 severely obese subjects undergoing post-acute rehabilitation in a population-based, publically funded rehabilitation center. 62% of those subjects had been admitted after orthopedic surgery, 19% after admission for acute medical illness, and 19% following stroke, brain, or spinal cord injury. Patients with obesity experienced increased lengths of stay and incurred in greater hospital costs, but had similar rehabilitation efficiency compared to nonobese controls. The findings from this study prompt clinicians and decision makers to clarify the reasons for this increased length of stay and hospital costs, in order to develop strategies to mitigate these effects. The findings of this study also support considering modifying rehabilitation equipment so that traditional components of post-acute rehabilitation can be safely delivered in the severely obese (i.e., implementing activities such as water-based exercises or whole-body vibration). Multidisciplinary case management, with specific attention paid to the challenges and complexities found in severely obese subjects, may also help to optimize care and prevent complications and setbacks.

8.2 Orthopedic Surgery

Obesity is associated with significantly younger age at the time of primary total hip arthroplasty (THA) and total knee arthroplasty (TKA) [29].

8.2.1 Weight Loss Before Orthopedic Surgery

It has recently become a common accepted practice to encourage weight management before orthopedic surgery in morbidly obese subjects. Weight loss could be encouraged through pharmacological therapies, restrictive diets, or, in selected cases, bariatric surgery before orthopedic surgery. Current data on the efficacy of bariatric surgery in reducing risks associated with total joint arthroplasty in the morbidly obese is still controversial and based mostly on retrospective studies [30]. One of the largest studies to date by Werner et al. [31] compared more than 11,000 morbidly obese patients who underwent TKA with 219 morbidly obese who had bariatric surgery before their TKA. The group that had the bariatric surgery first had reduced rates of major (OR 0.45) and minor (OR 0.61) complications. But a meta-analysis of subjects who underwent bariatric surgery before TKA, compared with obese control subjects who did not go through bariatric surgery before the arthroplasty, found no statistical difference in infections, venous thromboembolism, or revision surgery [32]. Thus, considering that obesity increases the risk for perioperative complications following orthopedic surgery, especially when BMI exceeds 40 kg/m^2, bariatric surgery before orthopedic surgery could help reduce these risks. However, further studies are needed to better evaluate the effect bariatric surgery has on orthopedic surgery outcomes and determine the optimal timing for both procedures.

8.2.2 Preoperative Risks

Obesity-related medical comorbidities should be taken into account when preparing for surgery [33]. If there is any history of apnea, the patient should be positioned in such a way to minimize the risk of decreased ventilation, avoiding the supine position if possible. The presence of arrhythmias and the use of anticoagulants must be considered, and special planning must be made to minimize the risk of excessive intraoperative bleeding [34]. Diabetic patients also require further preparation as optimal glycemic control is desired to minimize the risk of complications, including wound healing and infection [35]. A HbA1c <7% in type 2 diabetes could be a valid set point as values above that have shown, for example, an increased risk of retear after arthroscopic rotator cuff repair [36].

8.2.3 Intraoperative Complications

Most surgical beds have weight limits; thus selection of an appropriate operative bed to withstand the weight of the patient is important [33]. Also, the operating team must consider that the excess weight will cause pressure on the soft tissue over bony structures, and may produce pressure ulcers, especially in procedures exceeding 2 h, or even nerve injuries. There have been case reports describing lateral femoral cutaneous nerve palsy in obese patients after shoulder surgery in the beach chair position, due to pannus compression of the nerve [37]. In arthroscopic surgery, bony landmarks must be identified in order to guide accurate portal placement and prevent neurovascular injury. However, in the obese patient, excess adipose tissue may decrease the ability to palpate these bony landmarks [38]. In addition to this, hip arthroscopy in obese patients requires longer instruments and more difficult methods of hip distraction [39], which may in turn result in decreased precision and more complications. Jibodh et al. [40] found that obese patients who underwent THA (84 obese of 188 patients) had longer mean operative times and higher mean intraoperative blood loss, with a trend toward more complications, but no significant difference in functional recovery and hospital use.

8.2.4 Postoperative Complications

Obesity is a risk factor for deep vein thrombosis (DVT) in the general population [41]. Pulmonary hypertension, chronic inflammation, and impaired fibrinolysis increase the risk of thrombosis in the patient with obesity, and venous stasis caused by limited mobility increases this risk even more [42]. Elevated BMI appears to be a minor risk factor for DVT following knee arthroscopy [43]. However, literature is lacking in regard to a specific rate following orthopedic surgeries in general. At least after hip or knee arthroscopy, no significant increase in asymptomatic or symptomatic DVT or pulmonary embolism has been established in the obese population [44]. But early mobilization, mechanical prophylaxis, and use of unfractionated heparin or low-molecular-weight heparin with weight-based doing should be used to mitigate any increased risk [42].

Obesity has also been associated to increased early and late wound infection and poor healing [45]. This has been demonstrated in both THA and TKA [46] as well as arthroscopic surgery. Based on a study of 126 subjects who underwent multiligamentous knee arthroscopy, Ridley et al. [47] found that for every 1 unit increase in BMI, the odds ratio of complication rate, including wound infection, increased by 9.2%. In fact, the results of a large, multicenter, multi-category study [48] show that being overweight or obese significantly increased the risk of postsurgical infection in a number of orthopedic and non-orthopedic surgical categories. This increase in risk persisted even after adjustment for other risk factors, including the degree of wound contamination, the preoperative physical status of the patient, and the duration of the operation. Obese surgical patients have been shown to have reduced subcutaneous tissue oxygenation and to require a greater fraction of inspired oxygen to achieve the same arterial oxygen tension as normal-weight patients, thus predisposing them to surgical site infection (SSI) [49]. Wound hypoxia impairs healing by a number of potential mechanisms; healing wounds have high metabolic demands, and insufficient oxygen will slow the healing process. Immune cells also have high oxygen demands, requiring oxygen for the formation of microbicidal reactive oxygen species [50]. In addition to poor tissue oxygenation, adequate tissue levels of prophylactic antibiotics may be harder to achieve in obese patients [51]. Antimicrobials show different pharmacokinetics when administered to obese patients, with both hydrophilic and hydrophobic compounds generally having a higher volume of distribution, requiring a higher dose to reach the same plasma drug concentrations as for nonobese patients [51]. Hepatic clearance may also be increased in obese patients [52]. Therefore, obese patients may need to be dosed differently from nonobese patients. A recent cohort study comparing patients undergoing joint replacements 6 months before bariatric surgery with patients undergoing joint replacements 6 months after bariatric surgery failed to show a significant difference in the 30-day joint infection rate, suggesting that weight loss prior to surgery may not improve SSI outcomes [53]. This effect is likely to continue to increase with the rising rates of obesity in the general population, and new approaches are therefore needed to both understand the pathophysiology of the increase in infection rates in obese surgical patients and develop means of reducing rates of infection. The specific needs of these patients could be addressed by an increased focus on weight loss programs in the time before elective surgery. A key approach is to ensure that antimicrobial prophylaxis is adequate. Current guidelines for the prevention of SSI do not make specific recommendations about the prevention of SSI in obese patients [54]. Guidance on antibiotic prophylaxis is limited to recommending that prophylactic agents are administered within 1 h prior to incision and to administer repeat doses in operations of extended duration. Further research may provide evidence to refine the current guidelines. Research into improving other factors such as oxygenation, skin preparation, and glycemic control in overweight people is also needed. Continued surveillance of SSI is also essential to provide a means of monitoring the impact of the changing obesity rate on postsurgical wound infection, and interventions introduced to counteract the effects of obesity on the risk of infection.

Other than infections and the previously mentioned complications, obese patients that undergo THA are at an increased risk for dislocation. According to a study done by Davis et al. [55] on 1617 subjects, patients with BMI over 35 kg/m^2 have 4.42 times higher rate of dislocation than those with a BMI lower than 25 kg/m^2. At BMI over 40 kg/m^2 dislocation is even more likely, and the mechanism behind this relies on the fact that there is a laterally directed force on the prosthesis that arises from thigh-to-thigh contact during hip adduction that finally pushes the femoral head from the cup [56]. Therefore, weight management also becomes an important issue when trying to prevent dislocation of hip prosthesis in obese patients. In general, higher BMIs put higher mechanical strain on an implanted prosthesis, and this could also lead to increased wear, shorter survivorship, and increased need for revision due to aseptic failure [45]. A large meta-analysis that included 20 studies and a total of 15,276 TKA established an overall revision odds ratio of 1.3 for obese subjects [57]. Meta-analysis data of 5137 THA patients also show similar results, with higher revision rates for aseptic loosening in obese subjects with BMI over 30 kg/m^2 (OR 0.6) favoring less revision in nonobese subjects [58].

8.2.5 Clinical Outcomes After Orthopedic Surgery

Apart from increasing the risk of developing stroke and cardiovascular disease, obesity also increases the risk of musculoskeletal disease, including osteoarthritis, tendinopathy, osteoporosis, and sarcopenia [59]. The resultant damage and pain associated with these conditions are caused in part by the low-level systemic inflammation, the articular load applied by the higher body weight, and the reduced ability to withstand loading due to sarcopenia [60]. In obesity, the need for orthopedic surgery to manage these musculoskeletal problems is more common. In middle-aged women, the risk of having a hip or knee replacement increases with increasing BMI [61]. Also, obesity is associated with significantly younger age at the time of primary THA [29]. But apart from requiring more orthopedic surgery, obese patients present different pre-, intra-, and postoperative risk profiles than their lean counterparts, which may imply difficulties in their rehabilitation process.

8.2.6 Functional Outcomes After Orthopedic Surgery

Obesity has been linked to poor outcome measures in many studies, but results are inconsistent. Obese patients that underwent arthroscopic rotator cuff repair had worse functional outcomes measured through specific functional scores (American Shoulder and Elbow Surgeons Score and University of Pennsylvania Score) [62]. Dowsey et al. [63] found that patients with morbid obesity who underwent TKA also had poorer functional outcomes measured with the International Knee Society score. Dewan et al. [64] stated that patients with BMI > 40 that underwent TKA had less strength and range of movement, with more patellofemoral symptoms at 5 years, and thus needed more monitoring and rehabilitation.

Vincent et al. [65] reviewed 177 cases of consecutive obese and nonobese patients with diagnosis of either primary or revision THA. They found a curvilinear relationship between BMI and FIM efficiency, with the best efficiency in the overweight group and the worst in the severely obese. The same authors found that the FIM efficiency was lowest in the severely obese as compared with the remaining groups and that the severely obese group had higher total, physical and occupational therapy, and pharmacy charges than did the remaining groups. Finally, among patients who underwent primary TKA, the greatest FIM efficiency was found in the overweight and moderately obese groups.

In contrast, Stevens-Lapsley et al. [66] looked at 140 patients with BMIs ranging from 21 to 40 kg/m^2 that were followed up over the first 6 months after unilateral TKA, and found no meaningful relationships between BMI and functional performance in the subacute (1 and 3 months) and intermediate (6 months) stages of recovery. Unver et al. [67] found that obesity did not impact inpatient's rehabilitation outcomes such as function (Iowa Level of Assistance Scale and Iowa Ambulation Velocity Scale), range of movement, and pain after TKA.

But given the numerous instruments that have been used across studies to measure functional outcome, it is difficult to draw conclusions or much less define guidelines of rehabilitation in obese patients that undergo an orthopedic procedure. Considering that a group of these studies suggest poorer functional outcomes associated with obesity, new studies are needed that use standardized function measures, ideally obesity-specific function measures, to correctly identify these difficulties. Capodaglio et al. [68] studied the impact of a 4-week multidisciplinary rehabilitation inpatient protocol for obese patients with orthopedic conditions and motor disability. The group of 464 patients improved function measured by the Functional Independence Measure, the Visual Analogue Scale for functioning, and the Timed-Up-and-Go test and reduced disability as measured by a validated obesity-specific disability scale (TSD-OC).

Also, describing results according to the obesity class may help clarifying in which obese populations functional outcomes are worse, which in turn will help define guidelines that consider different approaches depending on BMI categories. Timing of rehabilitation is also a question worth considering. Robbins et al. [69], in a retrospective study on obese patients who underwent total joint arthroplasty, compared those who performed self-reported preoperative exercise to those who did not and found that the first ones had better early mobility and were more likely to be discharged home earlier. This underlines that rehabilitation efforts may be more successful if started before the surgery takes place.

8.2.7 Final Considerations

As obesity rates around the world increase, patients with obesity are more likely to be seen in rehabilitation units requiring inhospital rehabilitation after an acute event [70]. Obesity has been shown to be associated with longer rehabilitation length of stay and higher hospital costs [28]. As a response to this, more literature has been published to better understand this scenario. Up to now, there are still no published guidelines on how best to treat patients with obesity that require hospital rehabilitation. Seida et al. [70] conducted a scoping review looking to explore the evidence on rehabilitation for hospitalized patients with obesity. They included 39 studies with patients who underwent rehabilitation after orthopedic surgery, neurological conditions, acute medical illnesses, and other procedures. However, they found that most studies compared functional outcomes across patients in different BMI categories, but only few actually studied the effectiveness of the rehabilitation program. Of those that did, there was only one randomized controlled trial that compared two different rehabilitation interventions, as to be able to develop knowledge on the best treatment approach toward hospitalized obese patients. Also, the rehabilitation intervention was poorly described in many of the studies that were included. The authors concluded that the evidence to guide rehabilitation for patients with obesity is sparse and more rigorous comparative studies are needed to create evidence-based guidelines. A position paper of the European Society of Physical and Rehabilitation Medicine on the role of rehabilitation in patients with obesity has been published in 2017 [71]. On this basis, and in the wake of the WHO recommendations for developing guidelines and the Cochrane GRADE method, a panel of international experts under the aegis of the International Society of Physical and Rehabilitation Medicine (ISPRM) is presently working on the development of guidelines for rehabilitation in patients with obesity. Post-acute rehabilitation units should be structurally and ergonomically adequate and safe for obese patients and staff alike with availability of a number of bariatric lifting/transferring aids proportionate to the number of obese inpatients [71]. Also the rehabilitation equipment and the program's components should adapt to the needs of severely obese patient. A multidimensional approach by a multidisciplinary team should be able to provide assessment, risk stratification, and disease management. For that purpose, the integration of several medical specialties, including clinical nutrition, endocrinology, psychiatry, rehabilitation medicine, and different health professionals, including dietitians, psychologists, physiotherapists, occupational therapists, and nurses, is required. Specific staff training to avoid weight bias is needed, and adapted equipment may be necessary to promote patient and healthcare provider safety, and optimal patient quality care [70].

References

1. Oesch L, Tatlisumak T, Arnold M, Sarikaya H. Obesity paradox in stroke—myth or reality? A systematic review. PLoS One. 2017;12(3):e0171334. https://doi.org/10.1371/journal.pone.0171334.
2. Strazzullo P, D'Elia L, Cairella G, Garbagnati F, Cappuccio FP, Scalfi L. Excess body weight and incidence of stroke: meta-analysis of prospective studies with 2 million participants. Stroke. 2010;41:e418–26. https://doi.org/10.1161/STROKEAHA.109.576967. PMID: 20299666.
3. Bazzano LA, Gu D, Whelton MR, Wu X, Chen CS, Duan X, et al. (2010) Body mass index and risk of stroke among Chinese men and women. Ann Neurol 67: 11–20. https://doi.org/10.1002/ana.21950 . PMID: 20186847.
4. Yatsuya H, Folsom AR, Yamagishi K, North KE, Brancati FL, Stevens J, et al. Race- and sex-specific associations of obesity measures with ischemic stroke incidence in the Atherosclerosis Risk in Communities (ARIC) study. Stroke. 2010;41:417–25. https://doi.org/10.1161/STROKEAHA.109.566299. PMID: 20093637.
5. Fonarow GC, Srikanthan P, Costanzo MR, Cintron GB, Lopatin M, Committee ASA, et al. An obesity paradox in acute heart failure: analysis of body mass index and inhospital mortality for 108,927 patients in the Acute Decompensated Heart Failure National Registry. Am Heart J. 2007;153:74–81.

6. Romero-Corral A, Montori VM, Somers VK, Korinek J, Thomas RJ, Allison TG, et al. Association of bodyweight with total mortality and with cardiovascular events in coronary artery disease: a systematic review of cohort studies. Lancet. 2006;368:666–78. https://doi.org/10.1016/S0140-6736(06)69251-9. PMID: 16920472.
7. Escalante A, Haas RW, del Rincon I. Paradoxical effect of body mass index on survival in rheumatoid arthritis: role of comorbidity and systemic inflammation. Arch Intern Med. 2005;165:1624–9. https://doi.org/10.1001/archinte.165.14.1624. PMID: 16043681.
8. Hastie CE, Padmanabhan S, Slack R, Pell AC, Oldroyd KG, Flapan AD, et al. Obesity paradox in a cohort of 4880 consecutive patients undergoing percutaneous coronary intervention. Eur Heart J. 2010;31:222–6. https://doi.org/10.1093/eurheartj/ehp317. PMID: 19687163.
9. Kalantar-Zadeh K, Block G, Humphreys MH, Kopple JD. Reverse epidemiology of cardiovascular risk factors in maintenance dialysis patients. Kidney Int. 2003;63:793–808. https://doi.org/10.1046/j.15231755.2003.00803.x. PMID: 12631061.
10. Landbo C, Prescott E, Lange P, Vestbo J, Almdal TP. Prognostic value of nutritional status in chronic obstructive pulmonary disease. Am J Respir Crit Care Med. 1999;160:1856–61. https://doi.org/10.1164/ajrccm.160.6.9902115. PMID: 10588597.
11. Kalantar-Zadeh K, Horwich TB, Oreopoulos A, Kovesdy CP, Younessi H, Anker SD, et al. Risk factor paradox in wasting diseases. Curr Opin Clin Nutr Metab Care. 2007;10:433–42. https://doi.org/10.1097/MCO.0b013e3281a30594. PMID: 17563461.
12. Doehner W, Clark A, Anker SD. The obesity paradox: weighing the benefit. Eur Heart J. 2010;31:146–8. https://doi.org/10.1093/eurheartj/ehp339. PMID: 19734553.
13. Amundson DE, Djurkovic S, Matwiyoff GN. The obesity paradox. Crit Care Clin. 26:583–96. https://doi.org/10.1016/j.ccc.2010.06.004. PMID: 20970043.
14. Kim CK, Ryu WS, Kim BJ, Lee SH. Paradoxical effect of obesity on hemorrhagic transformation after acute ischemic stroke. BMC Neurol. 2013;13:123. https://doi.org/10.1186/1471-2377-13-123.
15. Vemmos K, Ntaios G, Spengos K, Savvari P, Vemmou A, Pappa T, Manios E, Georgiopoulos G, Alevizaki M. Association between obesity and mortality after acute first-ever stroke: the obesity-stroke paradox. Stroke. 2011;42:30–6.
16. Dehlendorff C, Andersen KK, Olsen TS. Body mass index and death by stroke: no obesity paradox. JAMA Neurol. 2014;71:978–84.
17. Dangayach NS, et al. Does the obesity paradox predict functional outcome in intracerebral hemorrhage? J Neurosurg. 2017;129:1125–9.
18. Aparicio HJ, et al. Overweight, obesity, and survival after stroke in the Framingham Heart Study. J Am Heart Assoc. 2017;6:e004721. https://doi.org/10.1161/JAHA.116.004721.
19. Doehner W, et al. Overweight and obesity are associated with improved survival, functional outcome, and stroke recurrence after acute stroke or transient ischaemic attack: observations from the TEMPiS trial. Eur Heart J. 2013;34:268–77. https://doi.org/10.1093/eurheartj/ehs340.
20. Sun W, et al. Association of body mass index with mortality and functional outcome after acute ischemic stroke. Sci Rep. 2017;7:2507. https://doi.org/10.1038/s41598-017-02551-0.
21. Oreopoulos A, Padwal R, Kalantar-Zadeh K, Fonarow GC, Norris CM, McAlister FA. Body mass index and mortality in heart failure: a meta-analysis. Am Heart J. 2008;156:13–22. https://doi.org/10.1016/j.ahj.2008.02.014. PMID: 18585492.
22. Sarikaya H, et al. Impact of obesity on stroke outcome after intravenous thrombolysis. Stroke. 2011;42:2330–2.
23. Gensicke H, et al. Impact of body mass index on outcome in stroke patients treated with intravenous thrombolysis. Eur J Neurol. 2016;12:1–8.
24. Funda Bas D, Ozdemir AO. The effect of metabolic syndrome and obesity on outcomes of acute ischemic stroke patients treated with systemic thrombolysis. J Neurol Sci. 2017;383:1–4.
25. Kalichman L, Rodrigues B, Gurvich D, Israelov Z, Spivak E. Impact of patient's weight on stroke rehabilitation results. Am J Phys Med Rehabil. 2007;86:650–5.
26. Burke DT, et al. Effect of body mass index on stroke rehabilitation. Arch Phys Med Rehabil. 2014;95(6):1055–9. https://doi.org/10.1016/j.apmr.2014.01.019. Epub 2014 Feb 4.

27. Jang SY, Shin Y, Young Kim D, et al. Effect of obesity on functional outcomes at 6 months post-stroke among elderly Koreans: a prospective multicentre study. BMJ Open. 2015;5:e008712. https://doi.org/10.1136/bmjopen-2015-008712.
28. Padwal RS et al. The impact of severe obesity on post-acute rehabilitation efficiency, length of stay, and hospital costs. J Obes 2012, 972365, 7. https://doi.org/10.1155/2012/972365.
29. Haynes J, Nam D, Barrack RL. Obesity in total hip arthroplasty: does it make a difference? Bone Joint J. 2017;99-B(1 Suppl A):31–6. https://doi.org/10.1302/0301-620X.99B1.BJJ-2016-0346.R1.
30. Hooper JM, Deshmukh AJ, Schwarzkopf R. The role of bariatric surgery in the obese total joint arthroplasty patient. Orthop Clin N Am. 2018;49:297–306.
31. Werner BC, Kurkis GM, Gwathmey FW, et al. Bariatric surgery prior to total knee arthroplasty is associated with fewer postoperative complications. J Arthroplast. 2015;30(9):81–5.
32. Smith TO, Aboelmagd T, Hing CB, MacGregor A. Does bariatric surgery prior to total hip or knee arthroplasty reduce post-operative complications and improve clinical outcomes for obese patients? Systematic review and meta-analysis. Bone Joint J. 2016;98-B:1160–6.
33. Prodromo J, Rackley J, Mulcahey MK. A review of important medical and surgical considerations for obese patients undergoing arthroscopic surgery. Phys Sportsmed. 2016;44:231.
34. Ortel TL. Perioperative management of patients on chronic antithrombotic therapy. Hematology Am Soc Hematol Educ Program. 2012;2012:529–35. https://doi.org/10.1182/asheducation-2012.1.529.
35. DeMaria EJ, Carmody BJ. Surgical clinics of North America. Perioperative management of special populations: obesity. Surg Clin North Am. 2005;85(6):1283–9.
36. Cho NS, Moon SC, Jeon JW, Rhee YG. The influence of diabetes mellitus on clinical and structural outcomes after arthroscopic rotator cuff repair. Am J Sports Med. 2015;43(4):991–7.
37. Satin AM, DePalma AA, Cuellar J, Gruson KI. Lateral femoral cutaneous nerve palsy following shoulder surgery in the beach chair position: a report of 4 cases. Am J Orthop (Belle Mead NJ). 2014;43(9):E206–9.
38. Paxton ES, Backus J, Keener J, Brophy RH. Shoulder arthroscopy: basic principles of positioning, anesthesia, and portal anatomy. J Am Acad Orthop Surg. 2013;21(6):332–42.
39. Khanduja V, Villar RN. Arthroscopic surgery of the hip: current concepts and recent advances. J Bone Joint Surg Br. 2006;88(12):1557–66.
40. Jibodh SR, Gurkan I, Wenz JF. In-hospital outcome and resource use in hip arthroplasty: influence of body mass. Orthopedics. 2004;27:594–601.
41. Holst AG, Jensen G, Prescott E. Risk factors for venous thromboembolism: results from the Copenhagen City Heart Study. Circulation. 2010;121(17):1896–903.
42. Spitler CA, Hulick RM, Graves ML, Russell GV, Bergin PF. Obesity in the polytrauma patient. Orthop Clin N Am. 2018;49:307–15.
43. Sun Y, Chen D, Xu Z, et al. Incidence of symptomatic and asymptomatic venous thromboembolism after elective knee arthroscopic surgery: a retrospective study with routinely applied venography. Arthroscopy. 2014;10(7):818–22.
44. Djerbi I, Chammas M, Mirous MP, et al. French Society For Shoulder and Elbow (SOFEC). Impact of cardiovascular risk factor on the prevalence and severity of symptomatic full thickness rotator cuff tears. Orthop Traumatol Surg Res. 2015;101(6 Suppl):S269–73.
45. Bookman JS, Schwarzkopf R, Rathod P, Iorio R, Deshmukh AJ. Obesity; the modifiable risk factor in total joint arthroplasty. Orthop Clin N Am. 2018;49:291–6.
46. Gage MJ, Schwarzkopf R, Abrouk M, et al. Impact of metabolic syndrome on perioperative complication rates after total joint arthroplasty surgery. J Arthroplast. 2014;29(9):1842–5.
47. Ridley TJ, Cook S, Bollier M, et al. Effect of body mass index on patients with multiligamentous knee injuries. Arthroscopy. 2014;30:1447–52.
48. Thelwall P, Harrington E, Sheridan, Lamagni T. Impact of obesity on the risk of wound infection following surgery: results from a nationwide prospective multicentre cohort study in England. Microbiol Infect. 2015;21:1008.e1–8.
49. Kabon B, Nagele A, Reddy D, Eagon C, Fleshman JW, Sessler DI, et al. Obesity decreases perioperative tissue oxygenation. Anesthesiology. 2004;100:274–80.

50. Sen CK. Wound healing essentials: let there be oxygen. Wound Repair Regen. 2009;17:1–18.
51. Falagas ME, Karageorgopoulos DE. Adjustment of dosing of antimicrobial agents for body weight in adults. Lancet. 2010;375:248–51.
52. Chopra T, Zhao JJ, Alangaden G, Wood MH, Kaye KS. Preventing surgical site infections after bariatric surgery: value of perioperative antibiotic regimens. Expert Rev Pharmacoecon Outcomes Res. 2010;10:317–28.
53. Kulkarni A, Jameson SS, James P, Woodcock S, Muller S, Reed MR. Does bariatric surgery prior to lower limb joint replacement reduce complications? Surgeon. 2011;9:18–21.
54. National Collaborating Centre for Women's and Children's Health Surgical site infection—prevention and treatment of surgical site infection. Clinical Guideline. NICE; 2008. Available at: http://www.nice.org.uk/nicemedia/pdf/CG74FullGuideline.pdf [accessed 06.11.12] Journal of Surgical Research 174, 7–11 (2012).
55. Davis AM, Wood AM, Keenan ACM, et al. Does body mass index affect clinical outcome postoperatively and at five years after primary unilateral total hip replacement performed for osteoarthritis? A multivariate analysis of prospective data. J Bone Joint Surg Br. 2011; 93(9):1178–82.
56. Elkins JM, Daniel M, Pedersen DR, et al. Morbid obesity may increase dislocation in total hip patients: a biomechanical analysis. Clin Orthop Relat Res. 2013;471(3):971–80.
57. Kerkhoffs GMMJ, Servien E, Dunn W, et al. The influence of obesity on the complication rate and outcome of total knee arthroplasty. J Bone Joint Surg Am. 2012;94(20):1839–44.
58. Haverkamp D, Klinkenbijl MN, Somford MP, et al. Obesity in total hip arthroplasty—does it really matter? A meta-analysis. Acta Orthop. 2011;82(4):417–22.
59. Finkelstein EA, Chen H, Prabhu M, et al. The relationship between obesity and injuries among U.S. adults. Am J Health Promot. 2007;13(5):460–8.
60. Collins KH, Herzog W, MacDonlad GZ, et al. Obesity, metabolic syndrome, and musculoskeletal disease: common inflammatory pathways suggest a central role for loss of muscle integrity. Front Physiol. 2018;9:112.
61. Liu B, Balkwill A, Banks E, et al. Relationship of height, weight and body mass index to the risk of hip and knee replacements in middle-aged women. Rheumatology (Oxford). 2007;46:861–7.
62. Warrender WJ, Brown OL, Abboud JA. Outcomes of arthroscopic rotator cuff repairs in obese patients. J Shoulder Elb Surg. 2011;20:961–7.
63. Dowsey MM, Liew D, Stoney JD, et al. The impact of preoperative obesity on weight change and outcome in total knee replacement: a prospective study of 529 consecutive patients. . [Erratum appears in J Bone Joint Surg Br. 2010 Jun;92(6):902]. J Bone Joint Surg Br. 2010;92:513–20.
64. Dewan A, Bertolusso R, Karastinos A, et al. Implant durability and knee function after total knee arthroplasty in the morbidly obese patient. J Arthroplast. 2009;24:89–94.
65. Vincent HK, Weng JP, Vincent KR. Effect of obesity on inpatient rehabilitation outcomes after total hip arthroplasty. Obesity (Silver Spring). 2007;15:522–30.
66. Stevens-Lapsley JE, Petterson SC, Mizner RL, Snyder-Mackler L. Impact of body mass index on functional performance after total knee arthroplasty. J Arthroplast. 2010;25:1104–9.
67. Unver B, Karatosun V, Bakirhan S. Effects of obesity on inpatient rehabilitation outcomes following total knee arthroplasty. Physiotherapy. 2008;94:198–203.
68. Capodaglio P, Cimolin V, Tacchini E, et al. Effectiveness of in-patient rehabilitation in obesity-related orthopedic conditions. J Endocrinol Investig. 2013;36:628–31.
69. Robbins CE, Bono JV, Ward DM, et al. Effect of preoperative exercise on postoperative mobility in obese total joint replacement patients. Orthopedics. 2010;33:666.
70. Seida JC, Sharma AM, Johnson A, Forhan M. Hospital rehabilitation for patients with obesity: a scoping review. Disabil Rehabil. 2016;40:125.
71. Capodaglio P, Ilieva E, Oral A, Kiekens C, Negrini S, Varela Donoso E, Christodoulou N, the UEMS-PRM EBPP Methodological Group. Evidence-based position paper on physical and rehabilitation medicine (PRM) professional practice for people with obesity and related comorbidities. The European PRM position (UEMS PRM section). Eur J Phys Rehabil Med. 2017;53(4):611–24.

9 Lower Limb Lymphedema

Maurizio Ricci, Francesco Federighi, and Paolo Capodaglio

Key Points

- Lymphedema is a chronic progressive condition frequently correlated to obesity.
- Lymphedema leads to disability, whose severity is important to assess.
- Clinical examination and differential diagnosis are key to define appropriate treatment protocols.
- Centimetric or volumetric measures of limb circumferences are important to assess clinical severity of lymphedema and rehabilitation outcomes.
- Combined treatment of lymphedema is recommended, including physical exercise programs, decongestive manual techniques, multilayered compression with short-stretch bandages, wound and skin care, and teaching of self-management techniques; preliminary evidence about the effectiveness of TECAR in reducing edema exists.

Lymphedema (LE) is frequently correlated to obesity. It is a chronic progressive condition involving not only cutaneous and subcutaneous tissues but also muscles, bones, nerves, joints, and internal organs, leading to disability [1]. A differential diagnosis with lipedema, lipodystrophy, and obesity is mandatory and clinical examination allows per se the diagnosis. In obesity, an increase of intracellular and extracellular liquid compound is evident with bioelectric impedance analysis

M. Ricci (✉)
Rehabilitation Medicine, Ospedali Riuniti di Ancona, Ancona, Italy
e-mail: Maurizio.Ricci@ospedaliriuniti.marche.it

F. Federighi · P. Capodaglio
Rehabilitation Unit and Research Laboratory of Biomechanics and Rehabilitation, S Giuseppe Hospital, Istituto Auxologico Italiano IRCCS, Piancavallo, Italy

P. Capodaglio (ed.), *Rehabilitation Interventions in the Patient with Obesity*,
https://doi.org/10.1007/978-3-030-32274-8_9

measures, especially in the lower limbs [2]. The obesity-related edema presents the same features of LE: a high-protein compound due to functional impairment of the lymphatic vessels. The lower limb lymphatic system is hindered by reduced muscle strength related to the limited mobility and the encumbrance of the inertial masses in the lower limbs of the patient with obesity. The fat mass can also compress the lymphatic vessels at groin level. The chronic progression of LE has physical, psychological, and economical repercussions on the patient, leading to disability [3].

According to WHO, there are 300 million persons affected by LE worldwide. Half of them consist of primary LE, following congenital dysplasia of lymphatic vessels and nodes. Of the other half, secondary LE, 70 million have a parasitic origin (i.e., filaria bancrofti, in the tropical and subtropical areas of the planet), 60 million are postsurgical after lymph node dissection, and 20 million are secondary to deep phlebothrombosis of the lower limb or overload of the lymphatic circulation [1]. Primary LE is genetically caused by an incomplete development of the lymphatic system. Family LE (Milroy syndrome) represents 3% of all primary LE and is linked to well-known genetic loci. Sporadic primary LE represents 93% and syndromic LE 4% of the primary LE.

An example of the latter is the Prader-Willi syndrome, where metabolic disorders, obesity, general hypotonia, and behavioral or psychiatric disorders are often present.

Secondary LE is caused by damage of the lymphatic system following surgery, radiotherapy, cortisone injections, metastasis, filaria infections, and large trauma, whereas minor trauma can unveil a latent primary LE.

Secondary LE has a centrifugal development, from the groin to the distal part of the limb. Stemmer's sign is generally negative, but it can become positive when fibrotic development occurs. The natural history of LE is to persist indefinitely after the onset. Progression is, more frequently, slow, but can be in other cases rapid with intermittence. If not adequately treated, LE progressively worsens. Malignant LE, due to a metastasis, is the only form with rapid evolution and presents always with a soft edema. Protein concentration in subcutaneous tissues associated with relative local immunodeficiency due to the reduced lymphatic flow favors hypodermic infections. Lymphangitis sets on acutely and is due to common germs (*Streptococcus viridans*, aureus, or beta-hemolytic) proliferating because of poor local hygiene.

Epidemiological studies show that in Italy secondary LE is more frequent (58%) than primary forms (42%). Females are mostly affected and the onset is more often in the III–IV decades of life. This is in relation to the surgical treatment of breast cancer. 25% of cases of axillary dissection associated with breast quadrantectomy develop LE of the upper limb. This percentage rises to 30% when radiotherapy is associated. In Italy, it is estimated that there are at least 200,000 patients with secondary LE and more than 150,000 with a primary form [1]. A correct treatment of LE is important to prevent lymphatic stasis as a cause of serious complications, the most frequent of which is lymphangitis, but we must consider also the rare occurrence of lymphangiosarcoma [3].

9.1 The Lymphatic System

The lymphatic system has the function of draining the lymph from the interstitial space and bringing it back to the venous circulation passing through some filters (lymph nodes) that are arranged along its vessels. The amount of lymph that is produced every day in the body is variable from 2 to 20 L depending on the needs of cellular metabolism. The regulation of this production depends on pressure gradients defined by the Starling equation:

$$F = K_{\mathrm{f}}\left(\mathrm{PI} - \mathrm{PT}\right) - d\left(\mathrm{PCO_c} - \mathrm{PCO_t}\right)$$

F is the quantity of lymph (F) drained by the lymphatic capillary in the unit of time. The leakage is determined by the hydrostatic pressure (PI) in the blood vessels, contrasted by the interstitial pressure (PT). The filtration coefficient (K_f) represents the filtration capacity of the individual arterial capillary in that district (hydraulic conductance). Proteins have the capacity to retain water with the colloid osmotic pressure (COP). The proteins inside the capillary lumen (PCO_c) limit the leakage of liquid while those in the interstitial space attract liquid (PCO_t). Proteins migrate through the cell membrane depending on the reflection coefficient (*d*). This coefficient is very low in the liver, for example, and because of that albumin is able to move freely through the membranes. On the contrary, in the renal glomerulus, this coefficient is high causing impossibility for the proteins to pass the capillary membrane. In the patient with obesity, this equation depends also on the presence of adipose tissue around the capillaries. Of all the lymph coming from the arterial capillaries, 90% is drained by the venous circulation and only 10% by the lymphatic system. The latter originates from capillaries formed by a thin layer of endothelial cells lining their lumen (Fig. 9.1) that favors filtration of the lymph into the vessels

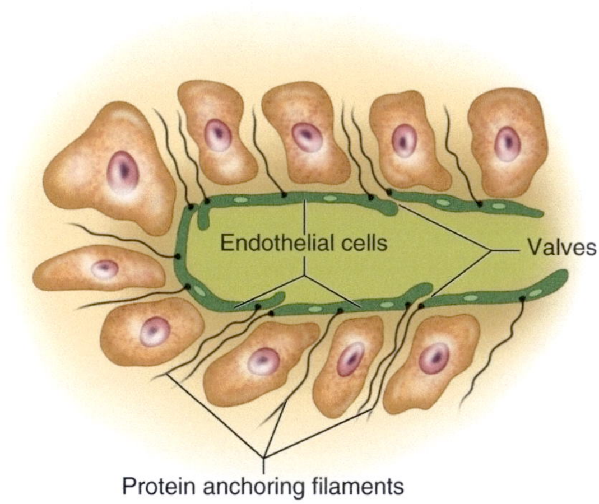

Fig. 9.1 Lymphatic capillary

due to the differential pressure between interstitium and lumen [4]. Capillaries progressively form larger lymphatic vessels with a three-layer wall (*intima*, composed by endothelium laid on a basal membrane; *tunica media*, with muscle fibers that contribute to the lymph flow; *tunica adventitia*, which represents an anchor to the interstitial connective tissue). A one-way valvular system supports lymph progression. The segment of lymphatic way between two valves has an independent capacity to contract and acts as a functional unit [4]. The main lymphatic vessels return then the lymph to the blood circulation system at supraclavicular level (*terminus* point). The large vessels of the upper limb converge with those coming from the head and neck near the *terminus* point on the right part of the body. On the left, the large vessels of the upper limb converge with those from the thoracic duct and the head near the *terminus* point. The thoracic duct is a large vessel (up to 4 mm of diameter) originating from the *cisterna chyli* at the level of the second lumbar vertebra in the retroperitoneal space, formed by the large lymphatic vessels from the lower limbs. From here, the thoracic duct branches to the subclavia region. Approximately 600 lymph nodes are dotted all along the lymphatic system throughout the body. Their inner core is populated by lymphocytes, macrophages, and plasma cells, which serve to purify the lymph passing through.

This lymph circulates in the subcutaneous space between skin and muscle fascia where adipose tissue is also present. This explains why it is sometimes difficult to differentiate edema and lipedema. The lymph flows at a speed of around 120 mL/h (the lymph produced at foot level reaches the terminus in less than 10 min). The lymph propulsion is generated by 10 contractions/min of the functional unit, but the contractile activity can be more if interstitial and intracapillary pressures increase [4]. Depending on the latter, the lymphatic flow can increase up to 10–12 times the basal flow until the maximal flow capacity is reached. Beyond that maximal point lymphatic functional failure and a high-flow LE occur. Compensatory mechanisms, like collateral circulation and increase in contractile activity of the vessel walls, can support lymphatic flow increases. Failure of such mechanisms determines the onset of LE. Two types of failures exist: dynamic and mechanical [4]. The first one is secondary to increase of the lymphatic load with a low-protein (0.1–0.5 g/100 mL) edema (type I Foldi). The second one is low-flow, high-protein edema (type II Foldi edema) and is due to drainage failure, secondary to an obstruction to the lymph flow. The mechanical failure can be extrinsic (post-radiotherapy or surgery) or intrinsic (metastasis, filaria, relapsing lymphangitis). Mechanical failure induces a self-maintaining mechanism of LE because of the interstitial high protein content. Erysipelas, a skin condition due to beta-hemolytic Streptococcus of Group A, presents with both mechanisms (type III Foldi edema): initially, a dynamic failure, due to phlogosis and increase in interstitial proteins, and then a mechanical failure, due to macrophages and germs obstructing the lymphatic capillaries. Erysipelas appears suddenly, like a localized, painful lymphangitis with formation of a vividly red raised step skin, high fever, and tendency to progress to the whole limb (Fig. 9.2).

Lymphangitis can set on suddenly or following a trauma with skin lesion and infiltration of germs superimposed on a previous condition of LE, or even after

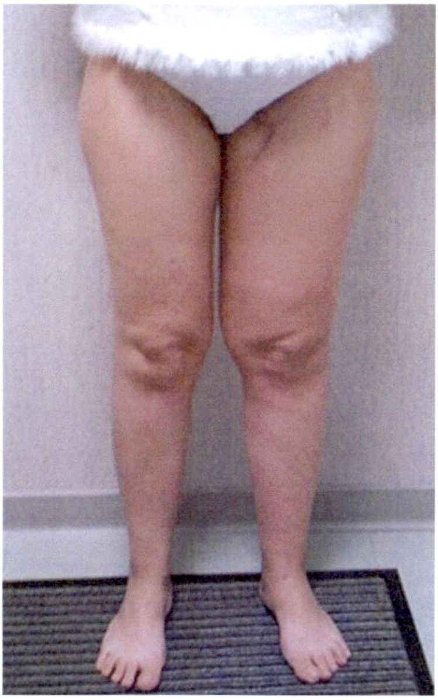

Fig. 9.2 Erysipelas

manual lymphatic drainage maneuvers. Sterile hypodermitis with painless and stable over time edema should be excluded first. This is often linked to the obesity-related panniculopathy (cellulitis). Lymphangitis calls for adequate antibiotic therapy and suspension of the manual treatment. Penicillin, clavulanic acid, and fluoroquinolones are the most used antibiotics. In case of frequent relapses, benzathine penicillin intramuscular injections 1,200,000 U.I. every 3 weeks for at least 6 months are recommended.

9.2 Clinical Examination

The diagnosis of LE is clinical and instrumental examination per se is insufficient for a correct diagnosis [5]. Medical history is of paramount importance: modality of onset and progression of edema indicate whether LE is of primary or secondary origin. Primary LE initiates distally and progresses proximally, while secondary LE starts where there is an interruption of the lymphatic vessel and proceeds distally from there (Fig. 9.3). Postsurgical LE develops some weeks after surgery (usually, 6–12), which represents the time lapse for the lymph to accumulate near the surgical scar and progress distally to become clinically sound. In some cases, a vascular component can be relevant (phlebolymphedema): the limb volume usually increases towards evening and after prolonged standing position.

Clinical examination can document the progression of LE, entity of edema, presence of irregularities, and dysmorphism in the limb and if they were present before the onset of LE. The skin is always pale; other rashes suggest the presence of inflammatory, infectious disorders. Sores or fissures represent a doorway for infections

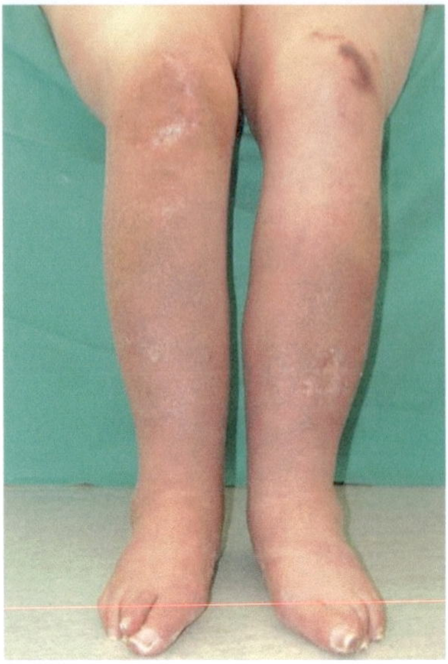

Fig. 9.3 Secondary lymphedema

that can complicate LE. When palpating, uncomplicated LE is "cold." Elasticity, softness, or hardness of the subcutaneous tissues relates to the protein content of the edema and, therefore, to the LE phase. Stemmer's sign is always positive in primary LE with recent onset, while, in secondary LE, its positivity appears only in persisting LE with infectious complications. LE is not painful. If pain is present, LE secondary to vasculopathies or lipedema should be suspected. In lipedema, digital pressure or skin pinching is always painful because of the edematous-fibrosclerotic adipose panniculus. Surgical scares should always be assessed since they tend to alter the lymphatic circulation and provide indications on the possible alternative lymph circulation. Fovea sign, obtained by prolonged digital pressure, is a characteristic of LE that should always be checked. When pressure ceases, the fingerprint can either remain or disappear to the *quo ante* subcutaneous conditions. Depth and persistence of the fovea are related to the amount of liquid present and mobilized by digital pressure. When proteins are present in the subcutaneous tissue, fovea can be minimal or just detectable. It will be absent when lipedema is present, since adipose tissue is uncompressible and has an immediate elastic reaction.

Phlebedema and phlebolymphedema are two clinical pictures deriving from venous insufficiency of the lower limbs. Usually due to vasodilation (primary or secondary varicose veins), an increase in hydrostatic pressure at capillary level occurs, which causes increase in the interstitial liquid. When lymphatic mechanisms become unable to compensate, the accumulated lymph produces phlebedema, which is low in proteins and soft. The skin becomes cyanotic and digital pressure is painful. Phlebolymphedema is harder and is generated by the persistence of venous and lymphatic insufficiency, inducing an increase of interstitial proteins. From this stage on, edema becomes irreversible and LE can progress. The other differential diagnosis is lipedema, a condition where adipose tissue accumulates in the lower limbs, except the feet. Fat accumulation is associated with an increase in interstitial liquid and often venous insufficiency is also present. Pressure is painful, more than in phlebedema, but feet are normal and no fovea is present. The two conditions affect exclusively female patients from the second decade on, and are often associated to obesity. Patients with obesity and lipedema who lose weight have shown to reduce adipose accumulation in the body but to maintain large lower limb volumes. The progression of lipedema gradually impairs the lymphatic system leading to lympholipedema. The Streeten test can help discriminate simple liquid retention. After pharmacological washout of diuretic and hormone-based drugs in the last 24 h, the patient's weight is recorded the day before the test. The patient is then asked to drink 20 ml of water/kg of body weight in 20 min. In the following 4 h, urine samples are taken and body weight is recorded again. Urinary retention is present when the total urine sampled is 60% less than the liquids introduced or if body weight is significantly higher.

9.2.1 Measures of LE

Measuring limb circumferences is important for assessing clinical severity of LE. The latter is related to the magnitude of the functional damage in the lymphatic system rather than to the limb volume per se, which depends also on the time of formation and persistence of LE. Volumes can be measured in different modalities: centimetric, volumetric, photographic, and impedentiometric. Water displacement is considered the gold standard for limb volume measurement. It is based on the Archimedes' principle according to which the water volume moved by an object equals the object's volume and it provides a direct measure of the limb volume. According to this method, the lower extremity is submerged in a tank of water whose displacement is measured to determine the volume of the leg. Despite its accuracy, this method is not commonly used by clinicians for practical reasons and it does not detect where edema is more evident at different stages of the therapeutic intervention.

Photography in different stages allows to detect the limb volume and differences in between. It can provide objective feedback and indicate limb's dysmorphism.

The most widely used method in clinical practice is the circumferential measurement using a flexible measure tape. The leg volume is obtained using an indirect method as it is computed using a geometrical approximation (frustum formula). The whole leg is divided into sections, usually ten, with each section representing a truncated cone. The final volume is determined by summing up the volumes of the different sections. This method presents with the advantages of being simple, inexpensive, and accurate; however, it is operator dependent and its reliability depends on the operator's skills. As the formula used for the volume calculation assumes that the leg is approximated to a truncated cone, it does not capture information regarding leg shape (i.e., gibbousness or localized swelling). The body landmarks for the lower limb are the inferior margin of the internal malleolus, the condylus femoris, and the great trochanter. Based on those, other intermediate points are determined.

Another indirect volume measure is the bio-impedance method, which measures the tissue resistance to an electrical current in order to determine extracellular fluid volume [6]. When a current is applied to the body through surface electrodes, it is transmitted through water-containing component within the tissues and a value of impedance can be calculated. The latter can be converted into an index score, which reflects volume measurement. This method is consistent and measures small water variations.

A recent study [7] supports the use of a new technique for an accurate and reliable measurement of body segments based on 3D portable laser scanner method. It is a fast modality, presenting the advantage of detecting gibbousness and uneven limb shapes which can be overlooked by centimetric evaluation. It should always be borne in mind that the volume of the limb can vary due to associated endocrinological or renal conditions. Contralateral measurements and clinical examination will discriminate those conditions.

9.2.2 LE Stages

The International Society of Lymphology [5] describes four stages for LE progression:

Stage 0, or Stage Ia, where edema is subclinical in patients who underwent lymph node dissection.

Stage I or Ib, when an initial accumulation of high-protein liquid is present. Limb elevation can reduce it and it is more evident in the evening than in the morning. Fovea is always present.

Stage II, when limb elevation does not reduce edema and limb volume remains consistent throughout the day, even with a tendency to progress as day goes by. Fovea can be negative because subcutaneous proteins can create an elastic gel-like layer.

Stage III refers to elephantiasis. The volume of the limb's segments has lost its normal anatomical shape due to edema, subcutaneous thickness, and adiposity. Irregularities of the skin surface can appear, differentiating into stages IIIa and IIIb.

Often, in the same limb, two different LE stages can be observed. A LE classification which takes into account etiopathogenesis, inheritability, and clinical aspects has been proposed [8].

9.2.3 Disability in LE

According to the International Society of Lymphology, LE is a chronic progressive condition involving not only cutaneous and subcutaneous tissues but also muscles, bones, nerves, joints, and internal organs, leading to disability. The widely used FIM scale or Barthel Index cannot capture the effect of LE on disability. SF-36 can document the individual changes in quality of life due to LE. In 2009, a LE-specific disability scale [9] was proposed to assess individual needs of patients with LE (Fig. 9.4). The scale has 5 levels (from 0—no disability to 4—complete disability), where every level is identified with a disability index composed of 14 ICF items with 5 levels each. The 14 ICF items concern the activities of daily living which are mostly affected by the presence of LE.

DISABILITY SCALE IN LYMPHEDEMA		
DEGREE	DEFINITION	DESCRIPTION
0	No Disability	The patient has a value of index between 0 and 0,5.
1	Low Disability	" " 0,6 and 1,5.
2	Low Disability	" " 1,6 and 2,5.
3	High Disability	" " 2,6 and 3,5.
4	Total Disability	" " 3,6 and 4.

Fig. 9.4 Disability scale

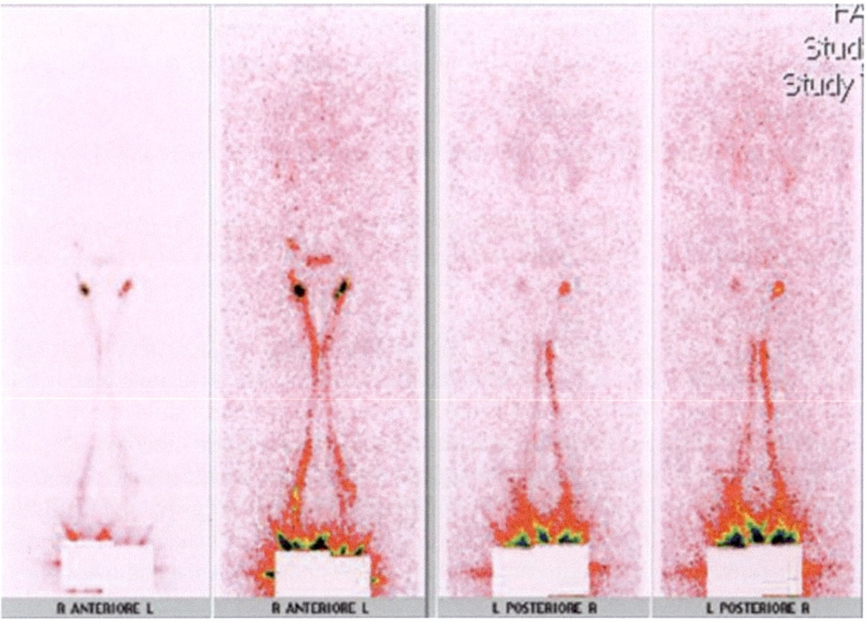

Fig. 9.5 Lymphoscintigraphy

9.2.4 Instrumental Evaluation

LE diagnosis is basically clinical but diagnostic tests can support the diagnosis and staging of LE phases, providing clinicians relevant information.

9.2.4.1 Lymphoscintigraphy

It is considered the gold standard for instrumental diagnosis of LE (Fig. 9.5). This test should be performed at least once in the lifetime of a LE patient. This minimally invasive test uses albumin tagged with Technetium-99m, injected between the second interdigital space of the hands or feet. These proteins are captured by the lymphatic system and transported to the bloodstream. Radioactivity captured by a gamma camera can help tracking the lymphatic system, highlighting the presence of lymphatic glands and of eventual dermal backflows.

Among the pros of lymphoscintigraphy are a sensibility of 73–100% and a specificity of 100%. The cons are high costs, time required for the test (around 3 h), and the anatomic resolution, which is noticeably weaker than that of other tests, so that discrimination between a primitive and secondary LE is not possible.

9.2.4.2 Echography

High-frequency (10–14 Hz) probes directly applied on the lymphedema can highlight the lymphatic collectors and allow to determine, through longitudinal and sagittal scans, the morphological and structural characteristics of the cutaneous and subcutaneous tissue and to measure the thickness of the fascia and the under-fascial tissues, which is of paramount importance to document changes after treatment. Quantification of tissue compressibility can help differentiate LE from lymphedema.

9.2.4.3 Echo-Doppler

Echo-Doppler in addition to echography allows to investigate the blood circulation system. This is particularly useful in cases of fast-developing edema in a LE patient who was previously asymptomatic and where phlebothrombosis has to be excluded.

9.3 Treatment

Existing guidelines on LE [1] recommend the combined use of manual and instrumental techniques. Therapy of LE is based on four cornerstones: skin care, manual decongestive lymphatic drainage, elastocompression, and kinesis therapy. The use of monotherapy is not considered enough for an effective treatment of LE and its prescription should be avoided [5]. A combined use of decongestive manual lymphatic drainage, multilayered compression with short-stretch bandages, sequential pressotherapy, wound and skin care, teaching of self-management techniques, physical exercise programs, and kinesis therapy is therefore recommended.

In the first intensive treatment phase, decongestive therapy protocols address edema reduction. Then, less intensive treatments aimed at maintaining the benefits obtained in the first phase and achieving patient's educational goals and self-maintenance.

9.3.1 Skin Care

Thorough cleaning of the interdigital spaces, skin folds, and areas involved by LE, where formation of bacterial flora is likely to occur, is crucial. If bacteria are present, antibiotic therapy should be started immediately. Educating patients on the use of devices such as elastic socks or gloves which can protect the sensitive areas preventing skin scratches or cuts or hydrate skin when sunbathing is important.

9.3.2 Manual Lymphatic Drainage

This manual technique is performed in the presence of lymphatic stasis to drain the interstitial fluid and proteins into the lymphatic system. A gentle pressure performed on the edema area and on the anatomical path of the lymphatic vessels allows the opening of the lymphatic capillaries and the entrance of the stagnating fluids. Such massage should be applied on areas where lymphatic stations of alternative lymphatic pathways are present. The maneuvers consist of light pressures that stimulate the lymphangions and the lymph flow.

Several lymphatic drainage techniques exist, such as Vodder, Leduc, and Casley Smith [5]. They all teach different maneuvers to achieve the same goals. Knowledge of the anatomy of the lymphatic system is always fundamental and instruments like the lymphofluoroscopy can provide some support, specially for identifying lymphatic routes that may compensate for the surgically removed ones. All of the drainage maneuvers involve light pressures (30–40 mmHg) with a frequency that recalls the physiological lymphangion's contractile activity (around 10 pressures/min). While performing the manual drainage it is always important to familiarize the patient with diaphragmatic breathing, which helps directing the fluids from the limbs to the abdomen and thoracic area.

Lymphatic drainage is contraindicated in case of neoplasia localized in the area to be treated that has invaded the blood or the lymphatic system.

9.3.3 Elastocompression

Elastocompression consists of the application of an elastic force on the limb affected by LE with the purpose to drain stagnant liquid and proteins from the extremity of the limb.

It can be applied with two methods: a multilayer anelastic compression bandage applied by the therapist for 24 h (generally it is well tolerated by the patient at night), and a compression sheath that takes dynamic advantage from the muscular activity of the patient while performing daily activities and is therefore considered an active treatment.

To maintain the goals obtained during the phase of intense treatment, the use of specific orthosis such as sleeves, gloves, tights, and knee-highs is recommended. These orthoses can be customized, according to the limb's anatomy, with a flat or circular texture. Circular texture is more likely to exert excessive pressure particularly on the skin folds and hinder the lymph flow. Flat texture, which is also less likely to irritate the patient's skin, is usually preferred.

The four classes of compression are first class (light) 18–21 mmHg, second class (moderate) 23–32 mmHg, third class (strong) 34–46 mmHg, and fourth class (very strong) 49 mmHg. The pressure should not be consistent through all the length of the orthosis and the highest pressure should always be on the distal extremity to guarantee the lymphatic drainage.

9.3.4 Kinesis Therapy

This is a milestone in the treatment of LE. Despite the fact that muscular contraction does not act directly on the lymphatic system because the pathological alteration is located over the fascial tissue, its effect on the vascular component is crucial for the drainage of the interstitial tissues.

The patient has to be educated on the importance of wearing its orthosis/bandage/sheath during exercise and daily living, because it enhances the drainage of the interstitial fluid.

Isotonic exercises for the improvement of the muscle trophism combined to diaphragmatic breathing and respiratory exercises are recommended to enhance the effects on the lymphatic and blood circulation.

9.3.5 Pressotherapy

Pressotherapy consists of instrumental lymphatic drainage induced by a pressure wave generated by a compressor. The therapist places a pneumatic sleeve around the patient's limb affected by LE. The pneumatic bags forming the sleeve have to be longitudinally aligned along the limb and partially overlapped to generate consistent pressure on the limb. The higher the number of bags, the higher the decongestive effect. Compression is alternated to allow refilling of the lymphatic vessels. Pressure should be lower than 60 mmHg [10]. Pressotherapy should not be prolonged without complementing it with manual lymphatic drainage [11]. Absolute contraindications are heart failure and recent phlebothrombosis, while a relative contraindication is skin infection.

Sound wave drainage is performed with very-low-frequency impulses (infrasound) aimed to activate the resonance phenomenon on the interstitial proteins [12]. This therapy is strongly contraindicated in patients with implanted pacemaker or metallic implants.

9.3.6 Physical Agents

The intensive phase of the treatment is followed by the maintenance phase consisting of the daily use of standard or individually sized compression garments. Various physical agents are traditionally used for reducing edema. Treatment of this chronic condition, however, becomes costly in the long term. Optimizing treatment modalities and defining cost-effective protocols for reducing edema and duration of cyclic treatments appear as important goals in the rehabilitation of LE. A recent study [13] investigated the effects of TECAR in reducing edema in patients with obesity and LE. The authors suggested that, due to reduced pressure on resources (i.e., physiotherapists and long-term use of compressive bandages), implementation of TECAR may be promising in offering cost savings in the treatment of LE. Also, being operator independent, it may allow the treatment of more patients simultaneously, further reducing pressure on resources.

9.3.7 Surgical Therapy

Microsurgical therapy can be beneficial both for draining the lymphatic fluid and for repairing/reconstructing the damaged/removed part of the lymphatic system. In both cases, delicate microsurgery techniques are applied. In the *derivative* technique, the main goal is to ensure contact between the lymphatic and the venous circulation before the block causing LE. Surgery can basically provide multiple anastomoses close to the lymphatic interruption or along the lymphatic vessel. The *reconstructive* technique is aimed at restoring the lymphatic system bypassing the interruption with an autologous venous segment. It is also used to remove lymphatic glands and implant them in the area affected by LE. It appears (Grade B recommendation) that microsurgery has an important role in the first stages of LE: in fact, the long-term outcome is strongly related to the stage of LE and to the surgeon's skills [1]. The lymphatic surgery has always to be accompanied by other therapies previously described (kinesis therapy, manual lymphatic drainage, and elastic compression), both before and after surgery to guarantee the effectiveness of the drainage.

References

1. Atto della Conferenza Stato Regioni Linee di indirizzo sul linfedema. 2016.
2. Pereira de Godoy JM, Pereira de Godoy LM, Pereira de Godoy AC, Guerreiro Godoy MF. Bariatric surgery and the evaluation of subclinical systemic lymphedema. J Surg Case Rep. 2019;(2):rjz028. https://doi.org/10.1093/jscr/rjz028.
3. Ricci M. Disability and lymphedema intern. Angiology. 2011;XXX(Suppl 1 to n° 6):14–5.
4. Cavezzi A, Michelini S. Il flebolinfedema. Bologna: Edizioni P.R; 1997.
5. The Diagnosis and Treatment of Peripheral Lymphedema: 2016 Consensus Document of the International Society of Lymphology. Lymphology. 2016;49(4):170–84.
6. Ricci M, Serrani R, Foglia AP L'impedenziometria come mezzo predittivo di insorgenza di linfedema post-operatorio. In atti XXXVII Congresso SIMFER Campobasso 2009. Eur Med Phys 2009; 45(Suppl. 1 to n° 3).
7. Cau N, Corna S, Aspesi V, Postiglione F, Galli M, Tacchini E, Brugliera L, Cimolin V, Capodaglio P. Circumferential versus hand-held laser scanner method for the evaluation of lower limb volumes in Normal-weight and obese subjects. J Nov Physiother. 2016;6(4):2–6.
8. Gasbarro V, Michelini S, Antignani PL, Tsolaki E, Ricci M, Allegra C. The CEAP-L classification for lymphedemas of the limbs: the Italian experience. Int Angiol. 2009;28(4):315–24.
9. Ricci M, Michelini S, Cossu M, Bufalini C, Pinto M, Antonelli P, Onorato A, Leone A, Carle F, Sandroni L. Efficacy of Ricci's Disability Index (RDI). In atti XI EFRR Congress Riva del Garda 26–28.05.2011. Eur J Phys Rehab Med 2011; 47 (Suppl. 1 to n° 2).
10. Cossu M, Ricci M. Approccio clinico riabilitativo al linfedema ed al flebolinfedema. Trattato di Medicina Fisica e Riabilitazione. Utet Div. Scienze Mediche. 2010. Vol IV, cap. n. 149: 1–20. ISBN: 8802078963.
11. Ricci M, Michelini S, Boccardo F, Belgrado JP, Baroncelli T, Aluigi L. Pressoterapia: Consensus conference. Ancona 11.06.2008.
12. Fulgenzi G, Graciotti L, Faronato M, Orlando F, Ricci M. Sonorous waves effect on oedema induced by eccentric contraction in rat skeletal muscle. Eur J Lymphol XVII, n° 50, 2007: 18–20. ISSN 0778-5569.
13. Cau N, Cimolin V, Aspesi V, Galli M, Postiglione F, Todisco A, Tacchini E, Debbi D, Capodaglio P. Preliminary evidence of effectiveness of TECAR in lymphedema. Lymphology. 2019;52(1):35–43.

Whole-Body Vibration

10

Matteo Zago, Cristina Ferrario, Giuseppe Annino, Marco Tarabini, Nicola Cau, Paolo Capodaglio, and Manuela Galli

Key Points

- Whole-body vibration training recently emerged as an alternative exercise modality for the treatment of obesity.
- Interventions longer than 6 weeks can improve cardiac autonomic function and reduce arterial stiffness.
- Interventions of at least 10 weeks lead to reduction in fat mass, improvements in leg strength, and enhanced glucose regulation when added to hypocaloric diet.
- Further research is advised to standardize the application of whole-body vibration training in terms of posology, vibration settings, and exercise modality.

M. Zago (✉) · M. Galli
Dipartimento di Elettronica, Informazione e Bioingegneria, Politecnico di Milano, Milano, Italy
e-mail: matteo2.zago@polimi.it

C. Ferrario
Dipartimento di Elettronica, Informazione e Bioingegneria, Politecnico di Milano, Milano, Italy

Dipartimento di Meccanica, Politecnico di Milano, Milano, Italy

G. Annino
Department of Systems Medicine, Faculty of Medicine and Surgery, Tor Vergata University of Rome, Rome, Italy

Department of Human Sciences and Promotion of the Quality of Life, San Raffaele Roma Open University, Rome, Italy

M. Tarabini
Dipartimento di Meccanica, Politecnico di Milano, Milano, Italy

N. Cau · P. Capodaglio
Research Laboratory in Biomechanics and Rehabilitation, Orthopedic Rehabilitation Unit, IRCCS Istituto Auxologico Italiano, Ospedale San Giuseppe, Piancavallo, Italy

P. Capodaglio (ed.), *Rehabilitation Interventions in the Patient with Obesity*,
https://doi.org/10.1007/978-3-030-32274-8_10

Humans are exposed to whole-body vibration (WBV) in many situations, both at the workplace or in controlled environments for treatment purposes. WBV training (WBVT) usually involves exercising on a vibrating platform; the vibration generates rapid length variations in muscle-tendon complex [1], inducing repetitive eccentric-concentric muscular work and reflexive muscle contractions [2]. In the clinical setting, WBV training is used as a rehabilitative method in a range of chronic diseases, as well as neurological, musculoskeletal, and metabolic conditions [3]. In particular, in the last decade, interventions based on WBV emerged as adjuvant therapies for obese patients [4]. The correct setting of the vibration parameters is crucial, as different literature studies showed that the regular exposure to vibration might have adverse health effect [5]. When the stimulus reaches the human through the hands, workers might develop a range of conditions collectively known as hand-arm vibration syndrome, as well as specific diseases such as the secondary Raynaud's syndrome, carpal tunnel syndrome, and tendinitis [6]. The long-term exposure to WBV increases the risk of low-back pathologies [5], although the low correlation between the measured vibration exposure and the incidence of back pain suggests the importance of the posture in the etiology of the professional disease [7, 8].

Therefore, the aim of this chapter is to present the most actual intervention strategies, strength, and potential limitations of WBV in the treatment of obesity. The main topics presented are the following:

10.1 Physical Principles

The main parameters used to describe the vibration are the amplitude and the frequency. Magnitude, or amplitude, is typically expressed in terms of acceleration (m/s^2 or g) although the motion can be equivalently characterized by the amplitude of the velocity or of the displacement. The other parameter, frequency, defines the number of oscillations completed in a unit of time and is measured in Hertz (Hz).

The mechanical energy of the vibration is transmitted through the human body thanks to compression and rarefaction of tissues and biological fluids (wave propagation) [9]. Different exposure time, amplitude, and frequency of the WBV determine different responses of human body; thus the correct choice of the vibration parameters is fundamental to avoid side effects. The amplitude of the vibration reaching different body parts depends on the magnitude of the vibration at the driving point (the feet in case of WBVT) and on the transmissibility of vibration between the driving point and the body segment [10]. Consequently, the frequency of the vibration should be different from the natural frequencies of the human body to avoid the resonance condition (Fig. 10.1). This phenomenon produces large oscillations of specific body segments and can lead to a harmful state of stress and to different disorders in case of prolonged exposure. In case of vibration frequency matching with the vertical resonance of the head, the mechanical energy might be

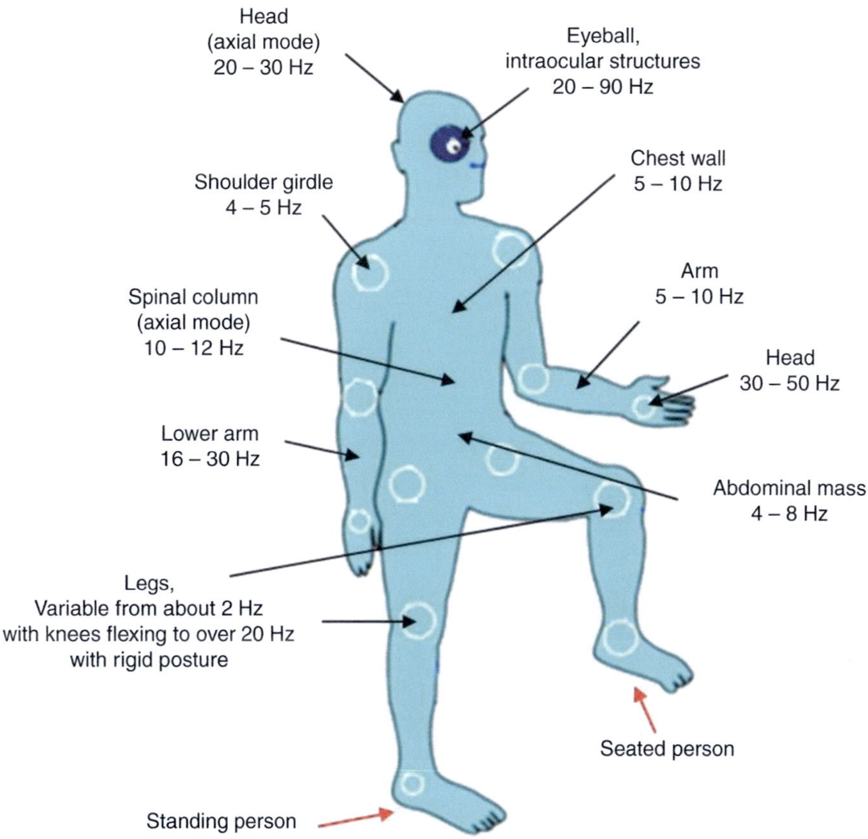

Fig. 10.1 Natural frequencies of human body

harmful for the brain health and thus must be avoided [11]. Two methods that help to reduce the acceleration transmitted to the head are (1) to use a side-alternating whole-body vibrating platform (WBVp) or (2) to instruct the subject to keep his/her knee flexed [2]. Thus, maintaining a straight-legged posture on a WBVp is not only not recommended, but also potentially dangerous.

The vibration is generated by the vibration platform which can provide two different types of stimulus: synchronous and side-alternating vibration (Fig. 10.2). The first refers to a vibration transmitted to both feet synchronously along the same spatial direction (usually vertical). The second type is a displacement alternated between the feet: the right foot goes down while the left one is pushed up (and vice versa).

Another important element that must be controlled is the body posture that subjects should maintain during the vibration treatment. To do this, an indication about the alignment of body segments (posture) is commonly given based on a description of the trunk, knee, and ankle angle.

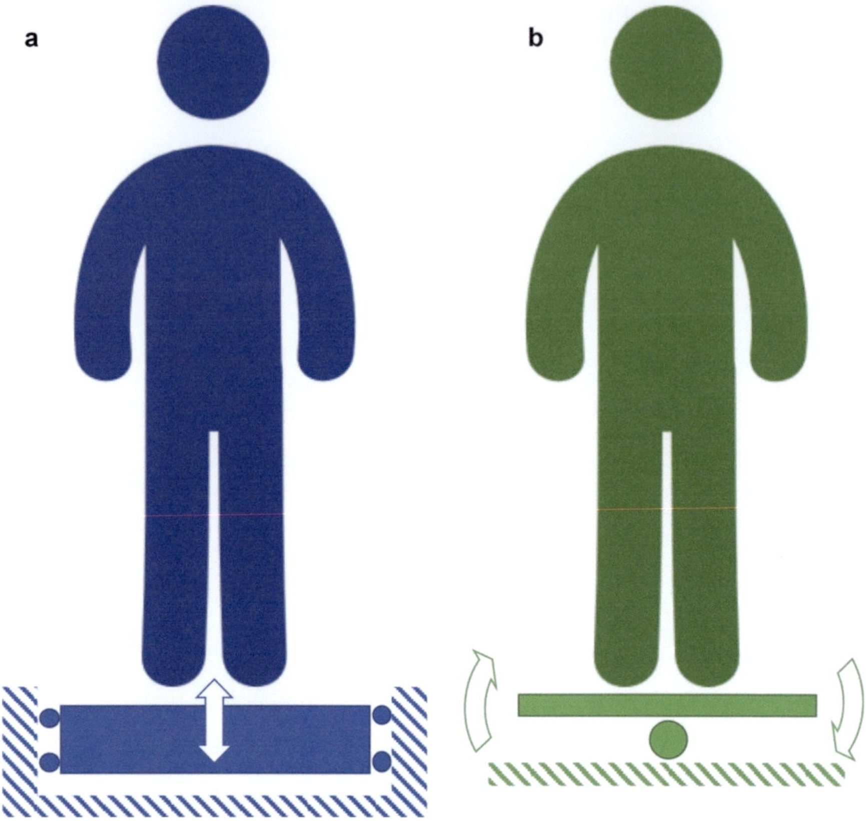

Fig. 10.2 Synchronous (**a**) and side-alternating vibration (**b**)

10.2 WBV as a Therapeutic Intervention

Vibration can provide benefits if correctly used: it can change the concentration of hormones, and prevent muscular atrophy, functional impairment, obesity, cardiovascular diseases, and fragility fractures among the elderly population [12]. Vibration can also be useful to heal osteoporosis in postmenopausal women [13].

The neurological conditions treated with WBV are multiple sclerosis (MS), Parkinson's disease (PD), stroke, cerebral palsy, and spinal cord injury. The studies on patients with MS evaluated that the effects of two different frequency settings (2 and 26 Hz) are in terms of strength [14], balance, gait, mobility, and spasticity [15]. The results obtained showed a greater strength outcome both in acute [14] and chronic [16] treatment with WBV. The chronic exposure to WBV led also to a decrease in spasticity and pain levels in those patients. No significant change was detected in terms of gait, balance, and mobility, and most notably no differences were outlined between the two frequency settings. Considering patients with PD and evaluating the long-term and the acute effect of vibration, improvement was found on balance control, gait [17], motor impairment, and proprioception [18]. The stroke patients treated with WBV showed a balance [19] and strength improvement during the acute exposure [20]. In this last case, no differences were outlined using a chronic exposure in those patients. The vibration treatment was also used on patients with cerebral palsy; motor impairment and spasticity decreased after WBVT, and no effects were reported on gait and mobility [21]. Considering patients affected by spinal cord injury and subjected to a 4-week WBVT, a significant improvement was found in terms of gait speed, cadence, and step length [22].

From a musculoskeletal point of view, also patients with fibromyalgia, low-back pain, osteoarthritis, and surgical treatments of anterior cruciate ligament were treated with WBV. The long-term effects reported on fibromyalgic patients were a reduction of pain and fatigue [23] and an improvement in dynamic balance [24]. Also in patients with low-back pain, a decrease in pain was reported as a long-term effect, although this is in contrast with the majority of the scientific literature on occupational diseases [25]; there was also a slight increase in the lumbar range of motion (ROM) [26]. The effects of WBVT on women with osteoarthritis were a significant increase in the muscle strength and a reduction of pain [27]. Considering anterior cruciate ligament patients, the WBVT resulted in an improvement of balance and proprioception [28].

Patients with cystic fibrosis showed a marked increase in muscle force, power, flexibility [29], and jumping ability and ability to rise up from a chair [30]. The treatment lasted for 6 months and used two frequency settings (12 and 26 Hz). Patients suffering from type 2 diabetes were treated using WBV for 12 weeks with an increase in muscle strength, and a decrease in the systolic blood pressure and in the glucose concentration [31].

The actual effect of vibration could not be mechanistically established since the studies have several limitations: often, the control group was not present, changes were not statistically significant, the vibration parameters were not specified, and the details of the treatment were not explained.

10.3 WBV and Obesity

Obesity is a chronic disease which increases the risk of debilitating and death-leading health problems [32]. Obesity has a detrimental effect on several hormonal, hematic, and functional parameters, and it is also related to cardiovascular complications, due to the hypertriglyceridemia and insulin resistance that lead to impaired fasting glucose, high blood sugar levels, inflammation, and visceral adipose tissue (VAT) accumulation.

In obese patients, even a moderate weight loss (5–10% of body weight) can reduce cardiovascular risk [33]. This is the reason why weight and VAT loss are the primary treatment aims, generally achieved by diets or healthier eating habits, behavioral correction, and/or exercise prescription. However, these therapies often have a low success rate: radical dietary restriction alone may lead to a reduction in muscle mass and a decline in physical fitness [34]. Regular aerobic and resistance training exercises may improve heart rate variability, physical strength, and body composition [35] but most obese people are reluctant to change their sedentary lifestyle due to physical limitations, musculoskeletal discomfort, and lack of self-motivation [36].

To overcome the limitations of the traditional therapies, in the last 20 years, WBV training was introduced. The typical interventions consist of exercises, such as calf-raises and squats at different degrees of knee flexion, performed on a WBV platform. Treatments commonly last from 6 to 12 weeks and generally are administrated three times per week. The vibration frequencies range from 12.5 to 60 Hz; the most common choices are frequencies between 25 and 40 Hz, with an amplitude of 1–2 mm. The duration of the exercises spans from 30 to 60 s with planned work:rest ratio from 1:1 to 1:2.

A large number of outcomes were evaluated to outline if the WBV was effective on obese patients. The results obtained can be divided into three major groups that evaluate body composition, cardiovascular parameters, and hormonal, hematic, and functional parameters [37].

10.3.1 Effects on Body Composition

The first group of parameters evaluated after WBVT includes the body weight (BW), body mass index (BMI), fat mass, waist circumference, lean body mass, bone mineral density, and insulin. When WBVT lasted for at least 10 weeks, a weight reduction was always reported [38]. The amount of weight loss seemed to be related to the intervention settings, but to date the association between these two factors is unclear. Two studies reported that a side-alternating vibration below 16 Hz produced small-to-moderate weight loss [13]. The same effect was also evidenced with a synchronous vibration from 40 to 60 Hz [38]. The amplitude considered in both cases was from 2 to 5 mm. Considering 6 weeks of WBVT with frequencies from 30 to 35 Hz and an amplitude of 2 mm, a larger weight loss was obtained [39]. Not all studies reported a reduction in body weight but even in those cases the WBVT often induced a remodeling of body composition. Reduction of visceral adipose tissue (VAT) [40] and fat mass [39, 40] was observed after 8 or less weeks of WBVT with a daily exposure to vibration from 5.1 to 12.7 m/s^2 [41]. The greatest fat mass loss was at the trunk level: in fact, a reduction of VAT and waist circumferences was reported in several studies [38, 40]. To sum up, there are three main factors that may contribute to fat mass reduction:

- The innervation of white adipose tissue by the central sympathetic nervous system, activated by acute exposure to vibration triggers lipolysis [42].
- Thanks to WBVT, glycemic control is enhanced improving the glucose regulation and the insulin action [43].
- WBVT increased the growth hormone (GH) concentration in obese subjects with the effect of a stimulation of the metabolism [12]; this is an important change for those patients who are characterized by low levels of this hormone.

In postmenopausal obese women, an improved glycemic control is fundamental to avoid insulin resistance. A study of Bellia and collaborators found that the insulin sensitivity increased 35% after 8 weeks of WBVT with static squats. An increase of adiponectin and a decrease of leptin levels were also observed [43].

Another population of obese patients that must be studied is those with type 2 diabetes mellitus. In this case, the WBVT improved the insulin-mediated glucose uptake in the skeletal muscle; this fact seemed to be related to the increase in femoral artery blood flow [44].

An important problem for obese patients, worsening with aging, is that bone mineral density tends to decrease. In particular, in women after menopause this process is enhanced by the decrease of estrogen concentrations, which can lead to osteoporosis. Some studies found that WBVT increased bone density [2] thanks to the shear stresses produced by vibration on the plasma membranes of highly sensitive cells like bone-lining cells and resident osteocytes and osteoblasts [45].

10.3.2 Cardiovascular Outcomes of WBV

In the second group were considered variations in systemic arterial stiffness, blood pressure (BP), sympathovagal balance, heart rate (HR), and blood flow velocity. Many studies examined the effect of WBVT on the previously mentioned adverse cardiovascular outcomes related with obesity and exacerbated by aging, menopause, and diabetes. Many studies found that a WBVT lasting for at least 6 weeks could reduce the sympathovagal balance [46] and central/peripheral arterial stiffness [4, 39] in obese women. The same results were found in men only in one paper [44].

An important improvement for the health of obese women is represented by the reduction of sympathovagal balance, associated to a lower cardiovascular risk and a greater longevity [39]. The measure of sympathovagal balance consists of the ratio between the low-frequency (LF) and the high-frequency (HF) power of heart rate variability spectrum: LF/HF ratio or R-R duration. WBVT leads to a reduction of the sympathovagal balance because vibration generates an increase of LF and a decrease of HF and thus the ratio of LF/HF decreases. This result was not achieved using traditional exercise such as resistance or aerobic training in postmenopausal women [47].

In the latter population, a 6-week vibration training also had beneficial effects on aortic stiffness leading to a reduction of the aortic systolic BP of 8–10 mmHg [48]. Many studies stated that an effect of the WBVT is the lower systemic, aortic, and leg arterial stiffness in terms of brachial-ankle, carotid-femoral, and femoral-ankle pulse wave velocity (PWV), respectively, found out in different studies [39, 48]. This is an important result because a reduction of the aortic systolic and diastolic BP from 5 to 10 mmHg corresponds to a decrement of 30–40% in the risk of death due to stroke and other cardiovascular complications [49]. It must be noticed that these hemodynamic effects of WBVT were not obtained simply using traditional resistance training in obese women [50]; this fact outlines the benefits that can be obtained using the vibration instead of traditional training and dietary program.

Another effect obtained after 6 weeks of WBVT is the increase of a nonprotein amino acid, L-citrulline, in hypertensive postmenopausal women [48], and the conversion of L-citrulline into L-arginine, which is the substrate for endothelial production of nitric oxide (NOx) [51].

The benefits that vibration produces at a cardiovascular level are related to different factors:

- WBVT acts on an inhibitor of cardiovagal activity, increasing the angiotensin II [52], and on the local production of vasodilatory substances, including NOx. The effect of NOx is a reduction of systolic BP and AIx, and thus the vascular tone of small arteries is reduced [53].
- The mechanical oscillation of vibration produces rapid variations in the length of the muscle-tendon complex [1]; these contractions act as an active muscle pump increasing the stroke volume, probably increasing venous return and preload [54].
- During WBVT, there is also an increase of the total peripheral resistance to blood flow. As a reaction to maintain a necessary level of cardiac output, more capillaries are opened resulting in more efficient gas and material metabolism between the blood and muscle fibers [11]. The increase in leg muscle blood flow contributes to improving the muscle mass in elderly [55].
- Another factor enhancing the blood flow is the friction forces applied by the vibration on the endothelial cells [2]. If there is a weekly repetition, this acute vascular effect is probably the cause of the improvements in arterial stiffness and wave reflection [56].

10.3.3 Functional and Hormonal Effects of WBVT

Obese individuals are very sensitive to fatigue and this can hinder the amount of daily motor activity. An effective strategy to improve this condition is to increase the muscle strength with low-intensity exercise that helps patients in preventing muscle dysfunction, vascular complications, and physical disability [57]. To do that, the WBVT is a good solution: choosing the correct training protocols, this innovative treatment produced similar positive effects on muscle strength [38] in both young and elderly subjects, and improvements in sit-to-stand and sit-and-reach functional tests [58]. Also an increase in GH hormone was reported in different studies (Table 10.1) as an acute

Table 10.1 Studies that reported an increase of GH and the parameters used

Authors and year	External load	Frequency (hz)	Wbvp	Subjects	Gh peak
Giunta et al. 2013 [59]	Yes	30	Sync	7	1.3 ± 0.6 ng/ml
Giunta et al. 2012 [60]	Yes	35	Sync	7	5.1 ± 1.9 ng/ml
Kvorning et al. 2006 [61]	Yes	20–25	SA	10	1.17 ± 0.81 μIU/ml
Bosco et al. 2000 [62]	Yes	26	Sync	14	28.6 ± 29.6 ng/ml
Di Giminiani et al. 2014 [63]	No	40	Sync	10	NA
Elmantaser et al. 2012 [64]	No	22	SA	10	0.52 ± 0.06 μg/l

WBVp whole-body vibration platform, *Sync* synchronous, *SA* side alternating

effect of WBVT using different frequencies and different WBVp. From a comparison of these studies it seems that the variation in GH is independent of the addition of an external load, the frequency of vibration, and the WBVp used.

It seems that WBVT improves the efficiency of agonist/antagonist muscles and the synchronization of motor units. This implies a simultaneous contraction of more fibers, thus producing a greater force [1]. This leads also to an improvement in balance control: in obese patients a better single leg balance [58] and a decreased fall rate [65] are found. With respect to simple static and dynamic exercises, if an opportune vibration is added to these, what is obtained is a significant increase in oxygen uptake and caloric output [2, 40]. Actually, the energy consumption thanks to vibration is modest: 4.5 mL/min/kg when the WBVT consisted of a stimulus with frequency of 26 Hz and amplitude of 3 mm [2]. Thus, the increase of oxygen uptake could be explained considering the higher metabolism due to hormonal and cardiovascular changes [11, 12], increase of lean mass, and muscle activation [66] as a consequence of the WBVT.

10.4 Side Effects and Limitations of Vibration Treatment

The most critical aspect emerging from the actual body of literature is that too often the vibration parameters, such as frequency, amplitude, and duration, and the exercise training (type of exercises, volume, and intensity) are not chosen in a safe manner [46]. Considering the ISO 2631-1:1997 regulation, the vibration can be divided into "tolerable" and "dangerous" for the health of people depending on the vibration magnitude and exposure time. The ISO 2631-1:1997 defines the exposure action value and limit value of 0.5 and 1 m/s^2 for workers that are exposed to a continuous WBV for 8 h/day; the maximum tolerable acceleration increases if the exposure decreases, but to date there are no clear indications about the levels that will surely lead to adverse health effects [67].

Another dangerous side effect is the possible damage that vibration transmitted to the head of patients can cause to brain, suggested in some literature studies. Even if the values considered safe are often not respected, the majority of studies reported that the WBVT did not cause on patients side effects or unfavorable symptoms [57, 58, 68, 69]. Few studies report sporadic side effects accused by patients that underwent WBVT, such as mild knee pain [70], lower leg phlebitis [40], and back pain after 2 weeks of treatment [43].

An attempt to define a safety level for vibration for medical application was proposed by Muir and collaborators, who claimed that a WBVT can be considered reasonably safe if it has a maximum exposure of 15 min/day, with frequencies between 30 and 50 Hz and an acceleration of 2.25–7.98 g [71].

Very few studies explicitly reported the vibration parameters, the exercise types used for the WBVT, whether or not the patients were standing freely on the platform or were holding a support, and if footwear were used [72]. All these factors can play a role in the outcome, and their effects are still under investigation, especially in the long term.

Lastly, potential biases as sex or ethnical specificities can play a relevant part in the outcomes such as insulin and GH hormone concentration, systolic BP and AIx, and hemodynamic effects [73].

10.5 Conclusion

In light of the reported results, we can conclude that WBVT is a promising useful intervention therapy in the management of obese patients. Relevant effects were found as follows: (1) cardiac autonomic function, following a WBVT lasting for at least 6 weeks [46, 74]; (2) significant body weight loss after 10 or more weeks [38–40, 44], as well as improvements of leg strength [38, 46, 57, 75]; (3) in addition to hypocaloric diet, there was also an enhancement of insulin sensitivity and glucose regulation [43]; and (4) combined with dietary restrictions, WBVT can be as effective as aerobic exercise in decreasing the BMI [40, 76] and improving the muscle strength [58, 74].

As a first step in a weight loss program, WBVT can be prescribed without other exercises, because it implies low levels of joint stress and self-motivation [43, 54]. Although obese patients are very sensitive to fatigue, they can tolerate this treatment as passive vibration does not imply voluntary action and requires a lower contribution of central command [77] compared to traditional exercises.

References

1. Cardinale M, Bosco C The use of vibration as an exercise intervention. Exerc Sport Sci Rev. 2003;31:3–7. [Internet] [cited 2019 Mar 16]. Available from: http://www.ncbi.nlm.nih.gov/pubmed/12562163.
2. Rittweger J. Vibration as an exercise modality: how it may work, and what its potential might be. Eur J Appl Physiol 2010 108:877–904. [Internet]. Springer [cited 2019 Mar 16] Available from: http://www.ncbi.nlm.nih.gov/pubmed/20012646.
3. Chanou K, Gerodimos V, Karatrantou K, Jamurtas A. Whole-body vibration and rehabilitation of chronic diseases: a review of the literature 187–200. 2012;187–200. Available from: http://www.jssm.org/vol11/n2/1/v11n2-1text.php.
4. Figueroa A, Kalfon R, Wong A. Whole-body vibration training decreases ankle systolic blood pressure and leg arterial stiffness in obese postmenopausal women with high blood pressure. Menopause. 2015 22:423–427. [cited 2019 Mar 16] [Internet] Available from http://www.ncbi.nlm.nih.gov/pubmed/25225715.
5. Krajnak K. Health effects associated with occupational exposure to hand-arm or whole body vibration. J Toxicol Environ Health B Crit Rev; 2018 21:320–334. [cited 2019 Jul 2] [Internet]. NIH Public Access Available from http://www.ncbi.nlm.nih.gov/pubmed/30583715.
6. Bovenzi M Exposure-response relationship in the hand-arm vibration syndrome: an overview of current epidemiology research. Int Arch Occup Environ Health . 1998 71:509–519. [Internet] [cited 2019 Jul 2] Available from http://www.ncbi.nlm.nih.gov/pubmed/9860158.
7. Tarabini M, Valsecchi M, Saggin B, Scaccabarozzi D. Whole-body vibration exposure in sport: four relevant cases. Ergonomics; 2015 58:1143–1150. [cited 2019 Jul 2] [Internet]. Cham: Springer International Publishing Available from http://www.ncbi.nlm.nih.gov/pubmed/25267689.

8. Tarabini M, Valsecchi M. Whole-body vibration in extreme sports. Extrem Sport Med. 2017:389–95. [cited 2019 Jul 2] [Internet]. Cham: Springer International Publishing. https://doi.org/10.1007/978-3-319-28265-7_30.
9. Griffin MJ. Handbook of human vibration: Academic Press; 1990.
10. Goggins KA, Tarabini M, Lievers WB, Eger TR Biomechanical response of the human foot when standing in a natural position while exposed to vertical vibration from 10–200 Hz. Ergonomics 2019 62:644–656. [Internet] [cited 2019 Jul 2] Available from: http://www.ncbi.nlm.nih.gov/pubmed/30560711.
11. Mester J, Kleinöder H, Yue Z. Vibration training: benefits and risks. J Biomech; 2006; 39:1056–1065. [cited 2019 Mar 17] Elsevier [Internet] Available from: https://www.sciencedirect.com/science/article/pii/S0021929005001041?via%3Dihub.
12. Rigamonti AE, Giunta M, Compri E, Patrizi A, Agosti F, Sartorio A, et al. Growth hormone-releasing effects of whole body vibration alone or combined with squatting plus external load in severely obese female subjects. Obes Facts Karger Publishers; 2012 5:567–574. [cited 2019 Mar 22] [Internet] Available from: http://www.ncbi.nlm.nih.gov/pubmed/22922806.
13. Zaki ME. Effects of whole body vibration and resistance training on bone mineral density and anthropometry in obese postmenopausal women. J Osteoporos; 2014 2014:702589. Hindawi Publishing Corporation [cited 2019 Mar 17] [Internet] Available from: http://www.ncbi.nlm.nih.gov/pubmed/25136473.
14. Jackson KJ, Merriman HL, Vanderburgh PM, Brahler CJ. Acute effects of whole-body vibration on lower extremity muscle performance in persons with multiple sclerosis. J Neurol Phys Ther 2008 32:171–176. [Internet] [cited 2019 Jun 24] Available from: http://www.ncbi.nlm.nih.gov/pubmed/19265758.
15. Broekmans T, Roelants M, Alders G, Feys P, Thijs H, Eijnde B. Exploring the effects of a 20-week whole-body vibration training programme on leg muscle performance and function in persons with multiple sclerosis. J Rehabil Med. 2010;42:866–72. [Internet]. [cited 2019 Jun 24]. https://doi.org/10.2340/16501977-0609.
16. Schyns F, Paul L, Finlay K, Ferguson C, Noble E. Vibration therapy in multiple sclerosis: a pilot study exploring its effects on tone, muscle force, sensation and functional performance. Clin Rehabil 2009 23:771–781. https://doi.org/10.1177/0269215508101758. [Internet] [cited 2019 Jun 24].
17. Ebersbach G, Edler D, Kaufhold O, Wissel J. Whole body vibration versus conventional physiotherapy to improve balance and gait in Parkinson's disease. Arch Phys Med Rehabil. 2008;89:399–403.. [Internet]. [cited 2019 Jun 24] Available from: http://www.ncbi.nlm.nih.gov/pubmed/18295614.
18. Haas CT, Turbanski S, Kessler K, Schmidtbleicher D The effects of random whole-body-vibration on motor symptoms in Parkinson's disease. NeuroRehabilitation 2006;21:29–36. [Internet]. [cited 2019 Jun 24] Available from: http://www.ncbi.nlm.nih.gov/pubmed/16720935.
19. van Nes IJW, Latour H, Schils F, Meijer R, van Kuijk A, Geurts ACH. Long-term effects of 6-week whole-body vibration on balance recovery and activities of daily living in the postacute phase of stroke. Stroke 2006 37:2331–2335. [cited 2019 Jun 24]; [Internet]. Available from http://www.ncbi.nlm.nih.gov/pubmed/16902175.
20. Tihanyi TK, Horváth M, Fazekas G, Hortobágyi T, Tihanyi J. One session of whole body vibration increases voluntary muscle strength transiently in patients with stroke. Clin Rehabil. 2007;21:782–93.. [Internet]. [cited 2019 Jun 24] Available from: http://www.ncbi.nlm.nih.gov/pubmed/17875558.
21. Ahlborg L, Andersson C, Julin P Whole-body vibration training compared with resistance training: effect on spasticity, muscle strength and motor performance in adults with cerebral palsy. J Rehabil Med 2006 ;38:302–308. [Internet] [cited 2019 Jun 24] Available from: http://www.ncbi.nlm.nih.gov/pubmed/16931460.
22. Ness LL, Field-Fote EC. Whole-body vibration improves walking function in individuals with spinal cord injury: a pilot study. Gait Posture; 2009 30:436–440. [cited 2019 Jun 24] [Internet]. NIH Public Access Available from: http://www.ncbi.nlm.nih.gov/pubmed/19648013.

23. Alentorn-Geli E, Moras G, Padilla J, Fernández-Solà J, Bennett RM, Lázaro-Haro C, et al. Effect of acute and chronic whole-body vibration exercise on serum insulin-like growth factor–1 levels in women with fibromyalgia. J Altern Complement Med 2009 15:573–578. [Internet]. [cited 2019 Jun 24] Available from http://www.ncbi.nlm.nih.gov/pubmed/19425819.
24. Gusi N, Parraca JA, Olivares PR, Leal A, Adsuar JC Tilt vibratory exercise and the dynamic balance in fibromyalgia: a randomized controlled trial. Arthritis Care Res (Hoboken) 2010 62:1072–1078. [Internet] [cited 2019 Jun 24];Available from: http://www.ncbi.nlm.nih.gov/pubmed/20235191.
25. Bovenzi M, Schust M, Mauro M An overview of low back pain and occupational exposures to whole-body vibration and mechanical shocks. Med Lav 2017 108:419–433. [Internet] [cited 2019 Jul 2]; Available from: http://www.ncbi.nlm.nih.gov/pubmed/29240039.
26. Rittweger J, Just K, Kautzsch K, Reeg P, Felsenberg D. Treatment of chronic lower back pain with lumbar extension and whole-body vibration exercise a randomized controlled trial. Spine (Phila Pa 1976) 27:1829–1834. [Internet]. [cited 2019 Jun 24]; Available from: www.galileo2000.de.
27. Trans T, Aaboe J, Henriksen M, Christensen R, Bliddal H, Lund H Effect of whole body vibration exercise on muscle strength and proprioception in females with knee osteoarthritis. Knee 2009 16:256–261. [Internet] [cited 2019 Jun 24] Available from: http://www.ncbi.nlm.nih.gov/pubmed/19147365.
28. Moezy A, Olyaei G, Hadian M, Razi M, Faghihzadeh S A comparative study of whole body vibration training and conventional training on knee proprioception and postural stability after anterior cruciate ligament reconstruction. Br J Sports Med 2008; 42:373–385. [Internet]. [cited 2019 Jun 24]; Available from: http://www.ncbi.nlm.nih.gov/pubmed/18182623.
29. Rietschel E, van Koningsbruggen S, Fricke O, Semler O, Schoenau E. Whole body vibration: a new therapeutic approach to improve muscle function in cystic fibrosis? Int J Rehabil Res 2008 31:253–256. [Internet]. [cited 2019 Jun 24]; Available from: http://www.ncbi.nlm.nih.gov/pubmed/18708849.
30. Roth J, Wust M, Rawer R, Schnabel D, Armbrecht G, Beller G, et al. Whole body vibration in cystic fibrosis – a pilot study. J Musculoskelet Neuronal Interact 2008 8:179–187. [Internet]. [cited 2019 Jun 24] Available from: http://www.ncbi.nlm.nih.gov/pubmed/18622087.
31. Baum K, Votteler T, Schiab J. Efficiency of vibration exercise for glycemic control in type 2 diabetes patients. Int J Med Sci ; 2007 4:159–163. [Internet]. Ivyspring International Publisher [cited 2019 Jun 24]. Available from: http://www.ncbi.nlm.nih.gov/pubmed/17554399
32. Hales CM, Fryar CD, Carroll MD, Freedman DS, Ogden CL. Trends in Obesity and Severe Obesity Prevalence in US Youth and Adults by Sex and Age, 2007-2008 to 2015-2016. JAMA;319:1723. [Internet]. American Medical Association; 2018 [cited 2019 Jun 20]. https://doi.org/10.1001/jama.2018.3060
33. Yumuk V, Tsigos C, Fried M, Schindler K, Busetto L, Micic D, et al. European guidelines for obesity management in adults. Obes Facts. 2015 8:402–424. [cited 2019 Jun 20] Karger Publishers; [Internet] Available from: http://www.ncbi.nlm.nih.gov/pubmed/26641646.
34. Janssen I, Ross R Effects of sex on the change in visceral, subcutaneous adipose tissue and skeletal muscle in response to weight loss. Int J Obes Relat Metab Disord 1999 23:1035–1046. [Internet]. [cited 2019 Jun 20]; Available from: http://www.ncbi.nlm.nih.gov/pubmed/10557024.
35. Gerage A, Forjaz CL, Nascimento M, Januário RS, Polito M, Cyrino E. Cardiovascular adaptations to resistance training in elderly postmenopausal women. Int J Sports Med ; 2013 34:806–813. [Internet]. © Georg Thieme Verlag KG [cited 2019 Jun 20]. https://doi.org/10.1055/s-0032-1331185
36. Guérin E, Fortier MS. Situational motivation and perceived intensity: their interaction in predicting changes in positive affect from physical activity. J Obes 2012;2012:1–7. [Internet]. Hindawi; [cited 2019 Jun 20]. Available from: http://www.hindawi.com/journals/jobe/2012/269320/

37. Zago M, Capodaglio P, Ferrario C, Tarabini M, Galli M. Whole-body vibration training in obese subjects: a systematic review. PLoS One 2018 13:e0202866. [cited 2019 Mar 24]; [Internet]. Rogan S, editor. https://doi.org/10.1371/journal.pone.0202866
38. Milanese C, Piscitelli F, Zenti MG, Moghetti P, Sandri M, Zancanaro C. Ten-week whole-body vibration training improves body composition and muscle strength in obese women. Int J Med Sci 2013 10:307–311. [cited 2019 Mar 17]; [Internet]. Available from: http://www.medsci.org/v10p0307.htm.
39. Miyaki A, Maeda S, Choi Y, Akazawa N, Tanabe Y, So R, et al. The addition of whole-body vibration to a lifestyle modification on arterial stiffness in overweight and obese women. Artery Res 2012;6:85–91. . No longer published by Elsevier. [cited 2019 Mar 22] [Internet]. Available from: https://www.sciencedirect.com/science/article/pii/S187293121200021X?via%3Dihub.
40. Vissers D, Verrijken A, Mertens I, Van Gils C, Van De Sompel A, Truijen S, et al. Effect of long-term whole body vibration training on visceral adipose tissue: a preliminary report. Obes Facts; 2010 3:93–100. [cited 2019 Mar 22]; Karger Publishers [Internet]. Available from: http://www.ncbi.nlm.nih.gov/pubmed/20484941.
41. Wilms B, Frick J, Ernst B, Mueller R, Wirth B, Schultes B. Whole body vibration added to endurance training in obese women - a pilot study. Int J Sports Med. 2012;33:740–3. [cited 2019 Mar 17] [Internet]. © Georg Thieme Verlag KG. https://doi.org/10.1055/s-0032-1306284.
42. Kvorning T, Bagger M, Caserotti P, Madsen K. Effects of vibration and resistance training on neuromuscular and hormonal measures. Eur J Appl Physiol 2006;96:615–625. [cited 2019 Mar 22] [Internet]. Springer. https://doi.org/10.1007/s00421-006-0139-3
43. Bellia A, Sallì M, Lombardo M, D'Adamo M, Guglielmi V, Tirabasso C, et al. Effects of whole body vibration plus diet on insulin-resistance in middle-aged obese subjects. Int J Sports Med. 2013;35:511–6. https://doi.org/10.1055/s-0033-1354358.. [Internet]. © Georg Thieme Verlag KG; [cited 2019 Mar 22].
44. Sañudo B, Alfonso-Rosa R, del Pozo-Cruz B, del Pozo-Cruz J, Galiano D, Figueroa A. Whole body vibration training improves leg blood flow and adiposity in patients with type 2 diabetes mellitus. Eur J Appl Physiol 2013; 113:2245–2252. https://doi.org/10.1007/s00421-013-2654-3 [cited 2019 Mar 22]; [Internet]. Springer, Berlin, Heidelberg.
45. Rubin C, Turner AS, Mallinckrodt C, Jerome C, McLeod K, Bain S. Mechanical strain, induced noninvasively in the high-frequency domain, is anabolic to cancellous bone, but not cortical bone. Bone 2002 30:445–452. [Internet]. [cited 2019 mar 23]; Available from: http://www.ncbi.nlm.nih.gov/pubmed/11882457.
46. Severino G, Sanchez-Gonzalez M, Walters-Edwards M, Nordvall M, Chernykh O, Adames J, et al. Whole-body vibration training improves heart rate variability and body fat percentage in obese Hispanic postmenopausal women. J Aging Phys Act 2017 25:395–401. [cited 2019 Mar 17]; [Internet]. Human Kinetics, Champaign, Illinois, USA. https://doi.org/10.1123/japa.2016-0087
47. Ryan AS, Pratley RE, Elahi D, Goldberg AP. Resistive training increases fat-free mass and maintains RMR despite weight loss in postmenopausal women. J Appl Physiol 1995 79:818–823. [Internet]. [cited 2019 Mar 23]; Available from: http://www.ncbi.nlm.nih.gov/pubmed/8567523.
48. Figueroa A, Alvarez-Alvarado S, Ormsbee MJ, Madzima TA, Campbell JC, Wong A. Impact of l-citrulline supplementation and whole-body vibration training on arterial stiffness and leg muscle function in obese postmenopausal women with high blood pressure. Exp Gerontol 2015; 63:35–40. .[cited 2019 Mar 22]; [Internet]. Pergamon; Available from: https://www.sciencedirect.com/science/article/pii/S0531556515000595?via%3Dihub.
49. Vlachopoulos C, Aznaouridis K, O'Rourke MF, Safar ME, Baou K, Stefanadis C. Prediction of cardiovascular events and all-cause mortality with central haemodynamics: a systematic review and meta-analysis. Eur Heart J 2010 ;31:1865–1871. https://doi.org/10.1093/eurheartj/ehq024. [cited 2019 Mar 23] [Internet]. Narnia

50. Beck DT, Martin JS, Casey DP, Braith RW. Exercise training reduces peripheral arterial stiffness and myocardial oxygen demand in young prehypertensive subjects. Am J Hypertens 2013 ;26:1093–1102. [cited 2019 Mar 23] [Internet]. Narnia. https://doi.org/10.1093/ajh/hpt080
51. Schwedhelm E, Maas R, Freese R, Jung D, Lukacs Z, Jambrecina A, et al. Pharmacokinetic and pharmacodynamic properties of oral L-citrulline and L-arginine: impact on nitric oxide metabolism. Br J Clin Pharmacol; 2008 ; 65:51–59. [cited 2019 Mar 23]; [Internet]. John Wiley & Sons, Ltd (10.1111) Available from: https://doi.org/10.1111/j.1365-2125.2007.02990.x
52. Townend JN, Al-Ani M, West JN, Littler WA, Coote JH. Modulation of cardiac autonomic control in humans by angiotensin II. Hypertens (Dallas, Tex 1979). 1995;25:1270–5.. [Internet] [cited 2019 Mar 23] Available from: http://www.ncbi.nlm.nih.gov/pubmed/7768573.
53. Kelly RP, Millasseau SC, Ritter JM, Chowienczyk PJ Vasoactive drugs influence aortic augmentation index independently of pulse-wave velocity in healthy men. Hypertens (Dallas, Tex 1979) 2001;37:1429–1433. [cited 2019 Mar 23] [Internet]. Available from: http://www.ncbi.nlm.nih.gov/pubmed/11408390.
54. Dipla K, Kousoula D, Zafeiridis A, Karatrantou K, Nikolaidis MG, Kyparos A, et al. Exaggerated haemodynamic and neural responses to involuntary contractions induced by whole-body vibration in normotensive obese *versus* lean women. Exp Physiol 2016 ;101:717–730. https://doi.org/10.1113/EP085556 [cited 2019 Mar 23] [Internet]. John Wiley & Sons, Ltd (10.1111).
55. Dillon EL, Casperson SL, Durham WJ, Randolph KM, Urban RJ, Volpi E, et al. Muscle protein metabolism responds similarly to exogenous amino acids in healthy younger and older adults during NO-induced hyperemia. Am J Physiol Integr Comp Physiol; 2011 ;301:R1408–R1417. American Physiological Society Bethesda, MD [Internet]. [cited 2019 Mar 23]. https://doi.org/10.1152/ajpregu.00211.2011
56. Figueroa A, Gil R, Wong A, Hooshmand S, Park SY, Vicil F, et al. Whole-body vibration training reduces arterial stiffness, blood pressure and sympathovagal balance in young overweight/obese women. Hypertens Res ; 2012 ;35:667–672. [cited 2019 Mar 17] [Internet]. Nature Publishing Group. https://doi.org/10.1038/hr.2012.15
57. Alvarez-Alvarado S, Jaime SJ, Ormsbee MJ, Campbell JC, Post J, Pacilio J, et al. Benefits of whole-body vibration training on arterial function and muscle strength in young overweight/obese women. Hypertens Res 2017; 40:487–492. [cited 2019 Mar 17]; [Internet]. Nature Publishing Group; Available from: http://www.nature.com/articles/hr2016178.
58. So R, Eto M, Tsujimoto T, Tanaka K. Acceleration training for improving physical fitness and weight loss in obese women. Obes Res Clin Pract; 2014;8:e238–e248. [cited 2019 Mar 17] [Internet]. Elsevier Available from: https://www.sciencedirect.com/science/article/pii/S1871403X13000276?via%3Dihub.
59. Giunta M, Rigamonti A, Agosti F, Patrizi A, Compri E, Cardinale M, et al. Combination of external load and whole body vibration potentiates the GH-releasing effect of squatting in healthy females. Horm Metab Res. 2013 ;45:611–616. [Internet] [cited 2019 Jun 26]. https://doi.org/10.1055/s-0033-1341464
60. Giunta M, Cardinale M, Agosti F, Patrizi A, Compri E, Rigamonti AE, et al. Growth hormone-releasing effects of whole body vibration alone or combined with squatting plus external load in severely obese female subjects. Obes Facts 2012; 5:567–574. [cited 2019 Jun 26]; [Internet]. Available from: http://www.ncbi.nlm.nih.gov/pubmed/22922806.
61. Kvorning T, Bagger M, Caserotti P, Madsen K Effects of vibration and resistance training on neuromuscular and hormonal measures. Eur J Appl Physiol 2006 96:615–625. [cited 2019 Jun 26]; [Internet]. Available from: http://www.ncbi.nlm.nih.gov/pubmed/16482475..
62. Bosco C, Iacovelli M, Tsarpela O, Cardinale M, Bonifazi M, Tihanyi J, et al. Hormonal responses to whole-body vibration in men. Eur J Appl Physiol 2000 ;81:449–454. [cited 2019 Jun 26] [Internet]. Available from: http://www.ncbi.nlm.nih.gov/pubmed/10774867.
63. Di Giminiani R, Fabiani L, Baldini G, Cardelli G, Giovannelli A, Tihanyi J. Hormonal and neuromuscular responses to mechanical vibration applied to upper extremity muscles. PLoS One 2014;9:e111521. [cited 2019 Jun 26]; Public Library of Science; [Internet]. Alemany M, editor. https://doi.org/10.1371/journal.pone.0111521
64. Elmantaser M, McMillan M, Smith K, Khanna S, Chantler D, Panarelli M, et al. A comparison of the effect of two types of vibration exercise on the endocrine and musculoskeletal system. J

Musculoskelet Neuronal Interact 2012 12:144–154. [cited 2019 Jun 26]; [Internet]. Available from: http://www.ncbi.nlm.nih.gov/pubmed/22947546.
65. Yang FF, Munoz J, Han L, Yang FF. Effects of vibration training in reducing risk of slip-related falls among young adults with obesity. J Biomech 2017;57:87–93. Elsevier; [Internet]. [cited 2019 Mar 17] Available from: https://www.sciencedirect.com/science/article/pii/S0021929017301859?via%3Dihub.
66. Vissers D, Baeyens J-P, Truijen S, Ides K, Vercruysse C-C, Gaal L Van. The effect of whole body vibration short-term exercises on respiratory gas exchange in overweight and obese women. Phys Sportsmed; 2009;37:88–94. [cited 2019 Mar 23]; [Internet]. Taylor & Francis. https://doi.org/10.3810/psm.2009.10.1733
67. ISO 2631-1:1997 – Mechanical vibration and shock – Evaluation of human exposure to whole-body vibration – Part 1: General requirements [Internet]. [cited 2019 Mar 17]. Available from: https://www.iso.org/standard/7612.html
68. Adsuar JC, Pozo-Cruz D, Parraca, Corzo, Olivares, Gusi Y. Vibratory exercise training effects on weight in sedentary women with fibromyalgia. [cited 2019 Mar 22]; Available from: http://cdeporte.rediris.es/revista/revista50/artefecto368.pdf
69. Wong A, Alvarez-Alvarado S, Jaime SJ, Kinsey AW, Spicer MT, Madzima TA, et al. Combined whole-body vibration training and l -citrulline supplementation improves pressure wave reflection in obese postmenopausal women. Appl Physiol Nutr Metab; 2016;41:292–297. [cited 2019 Mar 17] [Internet]. NRC Research Press. https://doi.org/10.1139/apnm-2015-0465
70. Song G-EE, Kim K, Lee DJ-J, Joo N-SS. Whole body vibration effects on body composition in the postmenopausal Korean obese women: Pilot study. Korean J Fam Med; 2011;32:399–405. [cited 2019 Mar 23] The Korean Academy of Family Medicine [Internet]. https://doi.org/10.4082/kjfm.2011.32.7.399
71. Muir J, Kiel DP, Rubin CT. Safety and severity of accelerations delivered from whole body vibration exercise devices to standing adults. J Sci Med Sport 2013;16:526–531. [cited 2019 Mar 23] Sports Medicine Australia; [Internet]. Available from: https://linkinghub.elsevier.com/retrieve/pii/S1440244013000248
72. Rauch F, Sievanen H, Boonen S, Cardinale M, Degens H, Felsenberg D, et al. Reporting whole-body vibration intervention studies: recommendations of the International Society of Musculoskeletal and Neuronal Interactions. J Musculoskelet Neuronal Interact 2010;10:193–198. [cited 2019 Mar 17] [Internet]. Available from: http://www.ncbi.nlm.nih.gov/pubmed/20811143.
73. Ives SJ, McDaniel J, Witman MAH, Richardson RS. Passive limb movement: evidence of mechanoreflex sex specificity. Am J Physiol Circ Physiol. 2013;304:H154–H161. [cited 2019 Mar 23] American Physiological Society Bethesda, MD; [Internet]. https://doi.org/10.1152/ajpheart.00532.2012
74. Wong A, Alvarez-Alvarado S, Kinsey AW, Figueroa A. Whole-body vibration exercise therapy improves cardiac autonomic function and blood pressure in obese pre- and stage 1 hypertensive postmenopausal women. J Altern Complement Med; 2016; 22:970–976. [cited 2019 Mar 17]; Mary Ann Liebert, Inc. 140 Huguenot Street, 3rd Floor New Rochelle, NY 10801 USA [Internet]. https://doi.org/10.1089/acm.2016.0124
75. Figueroa A, Kalfon R, Madzima TA, Wong A. Effects of whole-body vibration exercise training on aortic wave reflection and muscle strength in postmenopausal women with prehypertension and hypertension. J Hum Hypertens; 2014;28:118–122. [cited 2019 Mar 17]; Nature Publishing Group [Internet]. Available from: http://www.nature.com/articles/jhh201359.
76. Nam S, Sunoo S, Park H, Moon H. The effects of long-term whole-body vibration and aerobic exercise on body composition and bone mineral density in obese middle-aged women. J Exerc Nutr Biochem . 2016;20:19–27. [cited 2019 Jun 28] [Internet] Available from: http://jenb.or.kr/_common/do.php?a=full&bidx=532&aidx=6604.
77. Ogoh S, Fisher JP, Dawson EA, White MJ, Secher NH, Raven PB. Autonomic nervous system influence on arterial baroreflex control of heart rate during exercise in humans. J Physiol; 2005;566:599–611. [cited 2019 Jun 28] [Internet]. John Wiley & Sons, Ltd (10.1111). https://doi.org/10.1113/jphysiol.2005.084541

11 Whole-Body Cryotherapy: Possible Application in Obesity and Diabesity

Giovanni Lombardi, Ewa Ziemann, and Giuseppe Banfi

Key Points

- Cryotherapies are based on the exposure to extremely cold air in special devices.
- Cold effectively counteracts pain and inflammation through the activation of the sympathetic nervous system.
- Whole-body cryotherapy has a proven efficacy in several inflammatory conditions.
- Low-grade inflammation can be counteracted by cryotherapy and even better if associated with physical activity.

11.1 Introduction

Cold treatment is a popular therapy used by anyone in order to relieve or prevent pain and swelling after trauma, inflammatory conditions or any other condition from which pain originates. However, the application of cold is often driven by an

G. Lombardi (✉)
Laboratory of Experimental Biochemistry & Molecular Biology, IRCCS Istituto Ortopedico Galeazzi, Milano, Italy

Department of Athletics, Strength and Conditioning, Poznan University of Physical Education, Poznan, Poland
e-mail: giovanni.lombardi@grupposandonato.it; lombardi@awf.poznan.pl

E. Ziemann
Department of Athletics, Strength and Conditioning, Poznan University of Physical Education, Poznan, Poland

G. Banfi
Laboratory of Experimental Biochemistry & Molecular Biology, IRCCS Istituto Ortopedico Galeazzi, Milano, Italy

Vita-Salute San Raffaele University, Milano, Italy

P. Capodaglio (ed.), *Rehabilitation Interventions in the Patient with Obesity*,
https://doi.org/10.1007/978-3-030-32274-8_11

"intrinsic knowledge" and only seldom based on a scientific conscience. A 10-year-old survey to Irish emergency physicians, interviewed about the therapeutic use of cold, clearly confirms this shared feeling: 73% of respondents declared to "prescribe" cold application frequently while 7% had never suggested its use. But, more interestingly, 30% of the respondents doubt about the benefits of cold application and its use is mainly driven by experience (47%) and common sense (27%) while only 17% declared to base its application to a precise scientific reasoning [1].

The knowledge about the beneficial effects of cold on bodily functions has a long history and was common to several cultures. Egyptians discovered the invigorating benefits of submerging the body in cold water and Roman soldiers were used to take a quick dip in icy-cold rivers after battles, with recovery purposes. Hippocrates (460–370 BC), the father of the Western medicine, proved that icy-cold water (drunk or used for bathing) had efficacy in multiple medical conditions; he often prescribed ice-cold water as the perfect treatment for relieving pain, oedema and inflammation [2, 3].

Currently, local, partial and whole-body cold therapies (cryotherapies) are used as aids to relieve pain associated to several acute and chronic pathological conditions as well as in case of injuries, trauma and overuse [4, 5]. Besides the wide variety of local cold therapies, the concept of whole-body cryotherapy (WBC), and subsequently of partial-body cryotherapy (PBC), was born about 40 years ago based on the personal observations of Prof. Toshiro Yamauchi. In his clinics, where he treated rheumatologic patients, he noted that those rheumatoid arthritis patients who spent a period on mountain localities, where they conjugated cold exposure and physical activities, during winter, experienced improved clinical outcomes compared to those who remained at home. Thereafter, Yamauchi started treating these patients with cold air exposures, in specially designed cryochambers, opening the season of the clinical use of whole-body cryotherapy [6, 7]. Nowadays, the available cold therapy treatments, referable as both WBC and PBC, are based on the exposure to extremely cold air (either atmospheric air or liquid nitrogen vapours), with the temperature generally ranging between −110 °C and −160 °C, in special chambers [8]. Other cold-based practices have also developed in contemporary times, especially in northern countries, e.g. winter swimming: this activity relies on regularly bathing in ice-cold water, during the winter season, based on the belief that it reduces the frequency of sickness and improves the ability to address with daily stresses [3, 9–11].

Besides its application in pathology, cold exposure has become widely popular among sportsmen who use it as a recovery-enhancing practice [12]. Maybe as a consequence of the great media publicity, especially coming from its use by famous sportsmen, the use of cryotherapy has grown exponentially in the last few years as well as the number of scientific studies aimed at highlighting its efficacy. However, as often happens in the case of such popular treatments, the claimed effectiveness is not always sustained by scientific evidences [13].

11.2 Whole- and Partial-Body Cryotherapies: Technical Features of the Devices

Since the conceptualization of the cryotherapy, several PBC and WBC technologies have been developed and several devices are currently commercialized. Although often confused and defined interchangeably, PBC and WBC differ in several aspects and need to be named differently. Indeed, while in WBC the subject moves within a chamber and the entire body is exposed to cold, in PBC the subject enters into a "tank" with the head placed outside. The WBC devices are greater in size and the subject is more or less free to move within the chamber; on the contrary, the PBC devices are smaller (even transportable) and the subject cannot move within [14]. The moderate-sized mobile devices used for PBC allow its application on the field with sports teams, while WBC is more often used to treat pathological conditions in medical contexts. Also the cooling concepts are different among the different devices: PBC is cooled with liquid nitrogen that is inlet from the bottom of the tank and, generally, the working temperature declared by the producer is the one measured at the inlet, despite the natural gradient generated within the tank. The chambers for WBC are, instead, similar to a refrigerator since the cooling agent (liquid nitrogen) runs within the wall of the chamber, where it cools the atmospheric air, and, hence, the body comes in contact with cold air only [8].

Subjective feelings of patients exposed to cryotherapy indicate that the temperature felt into a nitrogen chamber (PBC) is noticeably colder compared to that felt into a cold-air chambers. This cold is felt particularly strong at the level of the lower extremities. There are, however, no scientific reports confirming this greater range of change in temperature in these conditions.

11.2.1 Partial-Body Cryotherapy

PBC treatment is performed in a cryosauna that is an open tank with a raising platform which allows the positioning of head and neck of the subject outside the device. Cold is generated by spraying nitrogen vapours within the tank and the treatment depends upon the direct contact between the patients and the cold nitrogen vapours. The patient's head must be out of the tank to prevent breathing nitrogen, and the associated risk of asphyxia, which is an important safety problem [8]. This was probably the first kind of extreme cold technology for the body, first developed by Yamauchi and presented in 1979 at the European Congress of Rheumatology which was subsequently improved by Fricke in Germany and Zagrobelny in Poland, between 1980 and 1990. Compared to the cryochambers, the cryosauna devices have some advantages: limited costs of the device and maintenance, despite the large consumption of liquid nitrogen (est. 20 k–30 k €/year); limited space needed and limited logistics issues; possibility to move the device allowing the use of PBC during itinerant sports events (e.g. Tour de France, Vuelta d'España and European Basketball Championship). On the contrary, important safety issues are related to handling and storage of liquid nitrogen and, hence, a professional technical assistance is always needed [8].

A main concern is related to the exposure temperature that ranges, according to the manufacturer indications, between −110 °C and −195 °C, which is a rather wide range, and the consequent difficulty to precisely set the treatment temperature. This is intrinsically due to the cold source: the nitrogen is stored in a liquid form and vaporized at temperatures above −195 °C; the temperature rapidly rises depending on the length of the pipes (from the reservoir to the cabin inlet). When the nitrogen is sprayed into the cryosauna a gradient is generated from the nozzle to the opposite portions of the tank (along both the horizontal and the vertical directions) and it is further accentuated when a warm body (e.g., the subject) is within the tank [8]. As elegantly demonstrated by Savic et al., in an empty cryosauna, the temperature increased from <−150 °C, next to the nozzle, to −60 °C, in the centre of the cabin; after 3 min of exposure, the temperature next to a manikin, placed into the tank, was not homogeneous: −100 °C at the top and −140 °C at the bottom of the cabin with differences between the front and the back of the manikin, too. In the presence of a human participant the recorded mean temperatures were comprised between −20 °C, at the chest, and −40 °C, at the shank, due to the participant's boundary layer consequent to convection [15].

11.2.2 Whole-Body Cryotherapy Devices

WBC is performed into cryochambers in which the subject is entirely exposed to the cold air. Traditionally, these chambers are divided into two or three compartments kept at different temperatures, generally −10 °C, −60 °C and −110 °C to −160 °C, in order to allow a more comfortable adaptation to cold, and are large enough to accommodate three or more subjects. Various cooling systems are available for the WBC devices but in all cases a direct visual contact (window or camera) between the operator, who is always present during the treatment, and the subject within the chamber, is required.

Compared to PBC devices, those for WBC are much more expensive since their costs range between 80 k € and 350 k € (compared to 45 k–60 k € of PBC) and also the maintenance costs are higher. The power supply can also represent a problem since, generally, the WBC devices require a 380 V line. Moreover, the WBC technology is not truly mobile, considering that WBC might be installed within a dedicated room or, eventually, within a container [8]. However, the market is now offering novel WBC devices with physical features resembling those of the cryosauna devices since they are designed as single-place chambers but maintaining the technical features of a WBC device.

Besides the disadvantages about costs, management (including electricity consumption) and logistics of WBC devices, a significant number of evidences have demonstrated that WBC confers benefits in most domains. Moreover, as explained in the next sections, WBC induces greater skin temperature and core temperature variations than PBC [8]. Authors speculated that, since a cryochamber contains a bigger volume of cold air than a cryosauna, the temperature is more constant in the former than in the latter. This is also sustained by the fact that a cryochamber is equipped with several nozzles located at different heights [15]. WBC devices enable the treatment of several patients at the same time, and this could be important in the clinical implementation of the treatment. WBC is also considered safer than PBC since, generally, the subject does not come in contact with the nitrogen vapours. The third limitation is given by the heterogeneity of the temperature during exposure that is greater in PBC devices than in WBC. However, the real difference in the temperature of exposure within the two devices is not clear also considering that there is no standardized method of assessing these temperatures [8].

11.3 Molecular Mechanisms of the Response to Cold

Although still not completely clear, the mechanisms leading to pain and inflammatory symptom alleviation seem to be related to the direct effects of cold on the molecular mechanisms involved in analgesia, inflammation and oxidative stress [16–21]. According to Guillot et al., after cold stimulation several molecular pathways are affected [22]. The first, and possibly the main, target of the cold stimulus is the sympathetic branch of the autonomic nervous system [23]: cold activates the thermosensitive receptors of the afferent nerves to the central nervous system (CNS) and efferent sympathetic nerve terminals are induced to release acetylcholine (ACh) and noradrenaline (NA). These neurotransmitters act on α7nAChR and β2-adrenergic receptors, respectively, and induce intracellular pathways that converge on nuclear factor κB (NF-κB) [21, 23–25]. The inhibition of this key inflammatory hub affects the expression of several downstream effectors involved in inflammation and oxidative stress as interleukin (IL)-1β [26, 27], IL-6 [28], tumor necrosis factor (TNF)α [27], IL-10 [29], inducible nitric oxide synthase (iNOS) and myeloperoxidase (MPO) [27, 30], superoxide dismutase (SOD) [31], glutathione peroxidase (GPx) [32], and intracellular adhesion molecule 1 (ICAM-1) [33]. By acting on α-adrenoreceptors expressed on vascular wall, NA also induces vasoconstriction [34] which is further sustained by the decreased angiogenesis determined by the cold-induced NF-κB-dependent downregulation of vascular endothelial growth factor (VEGF) [35]. The cold-dependent effects on NF-κB are mainly explicated at the macrophage levels even though all the cells of the body are responsive in this sense [22]. The cold stimulus acts also directly on the enzymatic activities, limiting the action of collagenases [36] and matrix metalloproteinases (MMPs) [37, 38], and on the mediators of pain, like prostaglandin E2 (PGE2) [29, 39]. Cold is also able to limit the release of histamine from mast cells. A painful stimulus causes the release of neuropeptides from sensory nerve endings that bind their cognate receptors expressed on mast cells that are induced at releasing histamine. Histamine, in turn, acts on nerve endings throughout a positive feedback to further induce the release of the neuropeptides. Hence, cold limits the painful sensation through this additional way [40].

Because of these molecular events, cold explicates analgesic, anti-inflammatory, anti-oedema, and anti-bleeding effects. The analgesic effects are due to cold-induced gate control activation, increased nociceptor excitability threshold, reduced nerve conduction rate, and decreased muscle spasm rate and strength. Cold stimulus directly reduces nerve conduction and the sympathetic system stimulation, the release of NA from peripheral nerve endings and brainstem nuclei and the vasoconstriction during and after the cold exposure have an impact on pain and joint and/or muscle soreness [17]. Circulating NA reaches the spinal cord via the posterior spinal arteries supplying, for example the *substantia gelatinosa*, where pain afferent neurons from skin end. A cold-induced increase in NA may therefore be involved in the mechanisms that lower pain at the spinal level [41]. Parallel, the slowed down enzymatic activity, the reduced synthesis and release of pro-inflammatory mediators, and the slowed down cell metabolism, all account for the anti-inflammatory effect [19, 42, 43]. Moreover, the cold exposure decreases the oxidative stress and/or increases the antioxidant buffering capacity [20, 42, 44, 45]. Finally, the cold-induced vasoconstriction and the decreased vascular permeability limit oedema and bleeding [2].

11.4 Evidences for WBC Effectiveness in Pathological Conditions

11.4.1 Indications and Contraindications

Based on their proved anti-inflammatory effects, WBC and PBC have been successfully applied to symptomatically treat rheumatic and inflammatory diseases such as RA [28, 46], fibromyalgia [4] and ankylosing spondylitis [47]. Currently, the entire spectrum of inflammatory, autoinflammatory, immune-mediated and autoimmune diseases can be effectively and safely treated with cryotherapy with the aim to reduce the symptoms of inflammation. However, the broadest application has been in sports medicine, surely for its effectiveness in limiting, but also preventing, exercise-induced muscle damages and muscle soreness as well as improving recovery from trauma, but also due to the media hype coming from the use of cryotherapy by famous sportsmen [13].

Recently, WBC and PBC have also been used in psychiatry, to improve mental well-being, in depression and anxiety syndromes [48], a research topic borrowed from previous investigations in winter swimmers, demonstrating a decrease in tension and fatigue and an improvement in mood, memory and well-being [9]. Improvement of sleep quality has also been reported [8]. Current indications for WBC are summarized in Table 11.1.

Table 11.1 Indications and pathophysiological response to whole-body cryotherapy

Indications (according to ref. [13])	Effects (according to ref. [8])
Pathological conditions	
Degenerative articular pain	*Molecular*
Back pain from degenerative disc disease or arthritis	↓ TNFα (RA)
Cervical pain from muscle stiffness, inflammation or degenerative disc disease	↓ Catalase (MS)
	↑ Uric acid (MS)
Skeletal muscle inflammation	↑ TAS (MS)
Joint, tendinous or muscle overload	↑ SOD (MS)
Psoriasis and psoriatic arthritis	*Clinical*
Myositis and fibromyositis	↓ Inflammation (RA)
Chronic polyarthritis	↓ Pain (RA, FM, AS, LBP)
Autoimmune diseases (RA, MS, SEL)	↓ Fatigue (RA, FM, MS)
Painful osteoporosis	↓ Disease score activity (RA, FM, AS)
Paresis and spastic contractures	↓ Morning stiffness (RA)
Fibromyalgia	↓ Disability index (LBP)
Cellulitis	↓ Depressive-anxiety symptoms (ADS)
Atopic dermatitis	↑ Walking (RA)
Anxious-depressive syndrome	↑ Physician's global assessment (RA)
Sleep disturbances	↑ Quality of life (RA, FM)
	↑ Functional score index (AS)
	↑ Spinal mobility parameters (AS)
	↑ Functional abilities (MS)
	↑ General well-being (SPS, PJD)
	↑ Mood (SS, PJD)

Table 11.1 (continued)

Indications (according to ref. [13])	Effects (according to ref. [8])
Sports medicine	
Muscle injuries, painful or fatigue syndromes Skeletal muscle overload Acute and overload tendinopathies Post-exercise recovery Power and resistance Exercise-induced muscle damage and delayed-onset muscle soreness Soft-tissue injuries	*Molecular* ↓ TNFα (RA) ↓ IL-1α and IL-1β (limited post-exercise increase) ↓ IL-2 ↓ IL-8 ↓ CRP (limited post-exercise increase) ↓ sICAM ↓ PGE2 ↓ Lactate production ↓ Lipid peroxidation products ↓ Markers of muscle damage ↓ GPx ↓ TBARS ↑ IL-1ra ↑ IL-10 ↑ IL-6 ↑ Catecholamines ↑ TAS *Clinical* ↓ Muscle damage ↓ Pain ↑ Muscle strength ↑ Maximal voluntary contraction ↑ Well-being ↑ Workout power ↑ Autonomic response ↑ Sleep quality

TNFα tumour necrosis factor α, *RA* rheumatoid arthritis, *MS* multiple sclerosis, *SEL* systemic erythematosus lupus, *TAS* total antioxidant status, *SOD* superoxide dismutase, *FM* fibromyalgia, *AS* ankylosing spondylitis, *LBP* low-back pain, *ADS* anxiety-depressive syndrome, *SPS* spinal pain syndrome, *PJD* peripheral joint diseases, *IL* interleukin, *CRP* C-reactive protein, *sICAM* soluble intracellular adhesion molecule, *PGE2* prostaglandin E2, *GPx* glutathione peroxidase, *TBARS* thiobarbituric acid-reactive substances, *IL-1ra* interleukin-1 receptor antagonist

As better described below, recent researches have shown positive effects of WBC on metabolic profile, low-to-moderate chronic inflammation and related diseases (e.g., obesity, insulin resistance, type 2 diabetes). Being cheap and easily accessible, WBC could be intended as an adjuvant method in the treatment of several dysmetabolic conditions, such as overweight or obesity.

As a medical treatment, it must be performed in specialized centres based on specific medical indications. Contraindications to the treatment are known, although some of them are just precautionary, since evidence are not always available, and they include: cryoglobulinaemia, cold intolerance, Raynaud's disease, hypothyroidism, acute respiratory system disorders, cardiovascular diseases (unstable angina pectoris, NYHA stage III and IV cardiac failure), purulent-gangrenous cutaneous lesions, sympathetic nervous system neuropathies, local blood flow disorders, cachexia and hypothermia. Obviously, claustrophobia and other conditions hindering the cooperation with patients, during the treatment, must be also considered. When appropriately performed, WBC is safe even for lung [49] and heart functions [50] and, contrarily to what was previously described [51], both single and multiple WBC sessions slightly reduce systolic and diastolic pressures (unpublished data).

A specific warning for PBC only is the possible risk of asphyxia associated with the unwanted inhalation of liquid nitrogen vapours during the treatment.

11.4.2 Evidences in Inflammatory Diseases

WBC effectiveness has been demonstrated in several conditions and diseases. In RA WBC at −110 °C had effects greater than WBC at −60 °C or local cold on the disease activity score (DAS), visual analogue scale (VAS) for pain [46] and swollen joint count, regardless of steroid treatment [28]. Although WBC was unable to elicit a measurable humoral response (e.g., inflammatory markers), but on histamine [40], it clearly improved several qualitative functional parameters more than the traditional physical therapies [22, 52]. Similarly, based on our and other groups' studies, compared to analgesia/kinesiotherapy alone, the association with WBC had strong positive effects on pain, fatigue and indexes of physical and mental health (SF36) in a wide cohort of fibromyalgic patients [4] and on disease activity indexes, pain and spine mobility in ankylosing spondylitis patients [47]. Thanks to its antihistamine activity, WBC had also 8-week-lasting effects on mild-to-moderate atopic dermatitis in terms of itch, quality of sleep (<30%), disease activity and skin damages (<19%) [53]. Anti-inflammatory effects of WBC are due to immune system activation whose pattern mimics exercise. Indeed, a single WBC session is sufficient to mobilize white blood cells and to increase IL-6 [19, 20]. IL-6, for long time considered to be pro-inflammatory, actually exerts both pro- and anti-inflammatory functions depending on the expression profile and the persistence in circulation: liver-derived chronically (even moderate) elevated levels sustain inflammation (as in sedentary and obesity); skeletal muscle-derived contraction-associated pulsating increases (even very high) exert anti-inflammatory effects (as in exercise) [54]; hence it is described as a myokine. Furthermore, WBC-dependent cytokine expression profile is precisely timed: IL-10 (anti-inflammatory) increases already after 5 WBC, while IL-1β (pro-inflammatory) starts to decrease after around 10 sessions. At 20 sessions this effect remains for the following 2 weeks [19]. WBC improved muscle damage (creatine kinase, CK) and cytokine profile (IL-6, IL-1β, IL-10) in healthy and physically active young men who underwent a muscle damage-inducing eccentric exercise protocol [55]. WBC also limits oxidative stress, which is intimately linked to inflammation [8, 56]. In multiple sclerosis (MS), an immune-mediated disease featured by an imbalanced oxidative stress, WBC, associated to kinesiotherapy, improved total antioxidant status (TAS) [31, 43] and erythrocyte superoxide dismutase (eSOD) and, in males, it lowered circulating and pro-oxidant species to levels comparable to those of healthy subjects [31]. WBC also increased serum uric acid [31, 57], an important endogenous antioxidant (up to 1 month post-treatment), and reduced disability (up to 3 months) [57]. Overall, published data record more or less significant shifts in immunological indicators; however, it is yet to be determined how long these changes are maintained.

Although, sometimes, with either no or only little measurable effects on biochemical markers of disease, WBC always improves both functional indexes and feeling (e.g., pain, fatigue). This means that it modulates other, mainly unknown, homeostatic functions: for example, we and others have reported that WBC decreases the stress hormone cortisol [58, 59] and improves sleep quality in stressful periods [60]. WBC also slightly lowers erythrocytes and haemoglobin, at least in active subjects, by enhancing the rate of intravascular haemolysis [61, 62], an effect that is completely abolished after 30 sessions thanks to a slight increase in erythropoietin [62].

WBC positively affects bone metabolism, too: in professional rugby players, WBC combined with training, but not training alone, induced circulating osteoprotegerin (OPG) while left unchanged the receptor activator of NF-κB (RANK) and its ligand (RANKL), key factors for osteoclast differentiation (the bone resorbing cells). Since OPG antagonizes RANKL, the raised OPG:RANKL ratio induced by WBC indicates a greater bone formation potential. Actually, RANKL is an immune-derived modulator of bone metabolism: this is another anti-inflammatory effect of WBC [63].

11.4.3 Evidences in Metabolic Diseases: Perspectives for the Treatment of Obesity and Related Conditions

Recently, positive effects of WBC on the systemic metabolic profile [42, 55, 64] and on the metabolism of tissues involved in energy use and storage (skeletal muscle [65], adipose tissue [65, 66], bone [63]) have been shown. It is important to underline that the evidences in this field are still limited and, only very recently, researchers have started to investigate this potential effect of WBC. However, by borrowing the results obtained in studies on the metabolic effects of WBC in healthy subjects, along with the limited number of studies involving subjects affected by dysmetabolic conditions (e.g. obesity), it is possible to argue its potential effectiveness in these conditions.

WBC dose-dependently affected the metabolic profile, in active males: 5 sessions were ineffective; 10 sessions reduced triglycerides (TG) by a third; 20 sessions decreased TG (from 108.0 ± 50.0 to 69.4 ± 27.2 mg/dL), total cholesterol (TC, from 172.6 ± 44.5 to 151.8 ± 53.8 mg/dL) and LDL cholesterol (from 97.7 ± 48.3 to 72.8 ± 52.0 mg/dL), and improved HDL cholesterol (from 53.2 ± 16.5 to 63.1 ± 27.4 mg/dL) and non-esterified fatty acids (NEFA, from 0.64 ± 0.4 to 0.79 ± 0.3 mmol/L), and their relative ratios, but not glycaemia [64]. HDL, LDL and TG were also improved in obese adults by combining a 6-month aerobic exercise program and 20 WBC sessions at the start and at the end of the protocol [42]. Being lipids, the main source of energy, as well as the main thermogenic substrate, it is conceivable that the WBC-induced intense cold stimulus has an effect on lipid metabolism [13].

In physically active young males, who performed a 30-min step-up/ step-down exercise, blood TC and LDL decreased in those who underwent twice-daily sessions of WBC over 5 consecutive days (43% and 52%, respectively) while it increased in those who passively recovered. Similar improvements were recorded for TC and TG [55]. Importantly, the same group of researchers showed that WBC positively affected the obesity-associated low-grade inflammation but the size of this effect was dependent upon the muscle mass and the cardiorespiratory fitness (CF) [66]. Chronic low-grade inflammation (also named metabolic inflammation) is defined as a chronic inflammatory state driven by the chronically elevated liver- and white adipose tissue (WAT)-derived IL-6 that keeps the phlogistic process turned on [67, 68]. The trigger is represented by the accumulation of lipids into the WAT that attracts the macrophages. Activated macrophages release cytokines that determine a shift of the entire WAT towards a pro-inflammatory phenotype characterized by the increased secretion of pro-inflammatory mediators (IL-6, TNFα, plasminogen activator inhibitor 1 (PAI1), leptin, macrophage chemoattractant protein 1 (MCP1), IL-18, resistin, visfatin) and the inhibition of the anti-inflammatory species (adiponectin). This immune activation, together with the hyperglycaemia-dependent hyperinsulinaemia and hypercortisolism, causes, in turn, the establishment of a vicious cycle that feeds the inflammation and its deleterious effects. Indeed, for instance, chronically elevated TNFα impairs the ability of insulin to stimulate the translocation of the insulin-dependent glucose transporter 4 (GLUT4) to the cell membrane and, consequently, further reduces the already impaired glucose uptake into muscle cells. Also IL-6, when chronically elevated, fails in stimulating the GLUT4 translocation to the plasma membrane. Chronic low-grade inflammation, other than being linked to metabolic syndrome (insulin resistance, type 2 diabetes, cardiovascular disease, atherosclerosis and fatty liver disease) and to aging and lifestyle factors (smoking, obesity, dietary patterns, cognitive decline and cachexia), is also an independent and consistent predictor of all-cause mortality [69].

Recent findings support the concept that WBC somehow mimics exercise and it can thus be applied as an adjuvant to exercise interventions in obesity and dysmetabolic conditions [13]. In obese subjects, who underwent to ten sessions of WBC over 2 weeks, the drop of chronically elevated IL-6, TNFα and adipokines (resistin, visfatin) was greater in subjects with a low CF (LCF, i.e., those with the a worse metabolic phenotype) than in those with a high CF (HCF). IL-10, instead, was similarly increased [66]. In another study, LCF and HCF middle-aged obese men (BMI >30 kg/m^2), exposed to ten consecutive sessions of WBC over 2 weeks, displayed a similar decrease in CRP but a different response in terms of circulating irisin concentration. This myokine, that is induced by exercise, stimulates WAT browning and is linked to an enhanced thermogenic capacity ([70, 54]), was slightly increased in both groups within 24 h after the first session of WBC but, more interestingly, the magnitude of the increase was greater in LCF than in HCF subjects [65]. These results match with the observation of Lee and colleagues who described the rise of irisin and the decrease of fibroblast growth factor 21 (FGF21) in response to cold-water immersion that was interpreted as a sign of non-shivering thermogenesis [71]. Very recently we have confirmed that WBC is also able to decrease circulating

FGF21 in a cohort of female volleyball players [72]. Both WAT and brown adipose tissues (BAT) are activated during cold exposure and, particularly, BAT is "consumed" during exposure to cold, contributing to energy metabolism [13].

In our recent research involving 45 healthy male students from a military academy who were exposed to 30 consecutive WBC sessions, we confirmed the positive changes in lipid profile (decrease in TC and increase in HDL) and, moreover, we found a decrease in ApoB:ApoA-I ratio, constituents of LDL and HDL, respectively. These changes, initiated after the 20th WBC session, were further pushed at the 30th session and were kept for a month after the last session. These findings confirm the metabolic benefits resulting from a prolonged exposure to cryogenic temperatures and support the postulate of using WBC as an intervention to improve lipid metabolism and to prevent cardiovascular diseases [73].

Redox balance is known to be linked to inflammatory response and, hence, to metabolic inflammation [69]. As described above, WBC is effective in counteracting the production of pro-oxidant species and in increasing the amount of antioxidant compounds. In a cohort of healthy subjects (24 males and 22 females) those who were exposed to ten consecutive WBC sessions displayed increased plasma levels of uric acid, SOD and total antioxidants compared to both baseline and those subjects who were not submitted to WBC [31].

Taken together, the available evidences support the hypothesis about the beneficial effect of WBC on lipid metabolism and on the inflammatory phenotype of the adipose tissue and, hence, as a possible approach in the treatment of dysmetabolic conditions such as obesity, insulin resistance and metabolic syndrome.

11.5 Conclusion: Current Limitation and Future Perspectives

Despite the increasing interest around the metabolic effects of WBC, no studies have gone deeper into the investigation of its effects on the functionality of pancreatic islets, insulin sensitivity and metabolic syndrome as well as on the hormonal axis connecting the different tissues involved in the whole-body management of energy. Inflammation is the key feature of all the dysmetabolic conditions [54, 74] and WBC has proven anti-inflammatory exercise-mimicking effects; hence it is conceivable that patients affected by dysmetabolic conditions, such as obesity and glucose intolerance, could benefit from the treatment alone or even better in association with physical activity interventions.

However, despite these putative beneficial effects, several issues still limit a wide clinical application of WBC. Besides the limited availability of WBC devices, differently from PBC devices that, despite the above-mentioned issues, are more diffused (and advertised), the main limitation is represented by the lack of any protocol customization. In other terms, besides the differences in the working temperature of cryochambers (generally ranging from −110 °C to −140 °C) and the theories about the most effective number of sessions [18, 20, 62, 64], the majority of protocols contemplate 3-min-long exposures (30 s in a pre-chamber and 2 min 30 s-to-3 min in a cryochamber) without considering the body composition and, therefore, the cooling potential of each subject. Indeed, it is well established that body composition (i.e., fat mass) is the main variable affecting the decrease in body (skin and core) temperature. Consequently, the decrease in temperature obtained in obese subjects is smaller compared to that gained in normal-weighted persons [75]. In addition, body composition is constitutively different between men and women [76] and it changes with age, too [76].

In conclusion, the clinical application of WBC as an adjuvant in the treatment of obesity and related co-morbidities is desirable but, at the same time, a great effort in the determination of the optimal treatment regimen is needed.

References

1. Collins NC. Is ice right? Does cryotherapy improve outcome for acute soft tissue injury? Emerg Med J. 2008;25(2):65–8. https://doi.org/10.1136/emj.2007.051664.
2. Demoulin C, Vanderthommen M. Cryotherapy in rheumatic diseases. Joint Bone Spine. 2012;79(2):117–8. https://doi.org/10.1016/j.jbspin.2011.09.016.
3. Dugue B, Leppanen E. Adaptation related to cytokines in man: effects of regular swimming in ice-cold water. Clin Physiol. 2000;20(2):114–21.
4. Bettoni L, Bonomi FG, Zani V, Manisco L, Indelicato A, Lanteri P, Banfi G, Lombardi G. Effects of 15 consecutive cryotherapy sessions on the clinical output of fibromyalgic patients. Clin Rheumatol. 2013;32(9):1337–45. https://doi.org/10.1007/s10067-013-2280-9.
5. Jastrzabek R, Straburzynska-Lupa A, Rutkowski R, Romanowski W. Effects of different local cryotherapies on systemic levels of TNF-alpha, IL-6, and clinical parameters in active rheumatoid arthritis. Rheumatol Int. 2013;33(8):2053–60. https://doi.org/10.1007/s00296-013-2692-5.
6. Yamauchi T, Kim S, Nogami S, Kawano AD. Extreme cold treatment (−150°C) on the whole body in rheumatoid arthritis. Rev Rheumatol. 1981;48(Suppl):P1054.
7. Yamauchi T, Nogami S, Miura K. Various application of the extreme cryotherapy and strenuous exercise program. Physiother Rehabil. 1981;5:35–9.
8. Bouzigon R, Grappe F, Ravier G, Dugue B. Whole-body and partial-body cryostimulation/cryotherapy: current technologies and practical applications. J Therm Biol. 2016;61:67–81.
9. Huttunen P, Kokko L, Ylijukuri V. Winter swimming improves general well-being. Int J Circumpolar Health. 2004;63(2):140–4.
10. Lombardi G, Ricci C, Banfi G. Effect of winter swimming on haematological parameters. Biochem Med. 2011;21(1):71–8.
11. Lubkowska A, Dolegowska B, Szygula Z, Bryczkowska I, Stanczyk-Dunaj M, Salata D, Budkowska M. Winter-swimming as a building-up body resistance factor inducing adaptive changes in the oxidant/antioxidant status. Scand J Clin Lab Invest. 2013;73(4):315–25. https://doi.org/10.3109/00365513.2013.773594.
12. Furmanek MP, Slomka K, Juras G. The effects of cryotherapy on proprioception system. Biomed Res Int. 2014;2014:696397. https://doi.org/10.1155/2014/696397.
13. Lombardi G, Ziemann E, Banfi G. Whole-body cryotherapy in athletes: from therapy to stimulation. An updated review of the literature. Front Physiol. 2017;8:258. https://doi.org/10.3389/fphys.2017.00258.
14. Hausswirth C, Schaal K, Le Meur Y, Bieuzen F, Filliard JR, Volondat M, Louis J. Parasympathetic activity and blood catecholamine responses following a single partial-body cryostimulation and a whole-body cryostimulation. PLoS One. 2013;8(8):e72658. https://doi.org/10.1371/journal.pone.0072658.
15. Savic M, Fonda B, Sarabon N. Actual temperature during and thermal response after whole-body cryotherapy in cryo-cabin. J Therm Biol. 2013;38:186–91.

16. Hausswirth C, Louis J, Bieuzen F, Pournot H, Fournier J, Filliard JR, Brisswalter J. Effects of whole-body cryotherapy vs. far-infrared vs. passive modalities on recovery from exercise-induced muscle damage in highly-trained runners. PLoS One. 2011;6(12):e27749. https://doi.org/10.1371/journal.pone.0027749.
17. Leppaluoto J, Westerlund T, Huttunen P, Oksa J, Smolander J, Dugue B, Mikkelsson M. Effects of long-term whole-body cold exposures on plasma concentrations of ACTH, beta-endorphin, cortisol, catecholamines and cytokines in healthy females. Scand J Clin Lab Invest. 2008;68(2):145–53. https://doi.org/10.1080/00365510701516350.
18. Lubkowska A, Dolegowska B, Szygula Z. Whole-body cryostimulation—potential beneficial treatment for improving antioxidant capacity in healthy men—significance of the number of sessions. PLoS One. 2012;7(10):e46352. https://doi.org/10.1371/journal.pone.0046352.
19. Lubkowska A, Szygula Z, Chlubek D, Banfi G. The effect of prolonged whole-body cryostimulation treatment with different amounts of sessions on chosen pro- and anti-inflammatory cytokines levels in healthy men. Scand J Clin Lab Invest. 2011;71(5):419–25. https://doi.org/10.3109/00365513.2011.580859.
20. Lubkowska A, Szygula Z, Klimek AJ, Torii M. Do sessions of cryostimulation have influence on white blood cell count, level of IL6 and total oxidative and antioxidative status in healthy men? Eur J Appl Physiol. 2010;109(1):67–72. https://doi.org/10.1007/s00421-009-1207-2.
21. Pournot H, Bieuzen F, Louis J, Mounier R, Fillard JR, Barbiche E, Hausswirth C. Time-course of changes in inflammatory response after whole-body cryotherapy multi exposures following severe exercise. PLoS One. 2011;6(7):e22748. https://doi.org/10.1371/journal.pone.0022748.
22. Guillot X, Tordi N, Mourot L, Demougeot C, Dugue B, Prati C, Wendling D. Cryotherapy in inflammatory rheumatic diseases: a systematic review. Exp Rev Clin Immunol. 2014;10(2):281–94. https://doi.org/10.1586/1744666X.2014.870036.
23. Mourot L, Cluzeau C, Regnard J. Hyperbaric gaseous cryotherapy: effects on skin temperature and systemic vasoconstriction. Arch Phys Med Rehabil. 2007;88(10):1339–43. https://doi.org/10.1016/j.apmr.2007.06.771.
24. Pavlov VA, Tracey KJ. The cholinergic anti-inflammatory pathway. Brain Behav Immun. 2005;19(6):493–9. https://doi.org/10.1016/j.bbi.2005.03.015.
25. Tracey KJ. Reflex control of immunity. Nat Rev Immunol. 2009;9(6):418–28. https://doi.org/10.1038/nri2566.
26. Hildebrand F, van Griensven M, Giannoudis P, Luerig A, Harwood P, Harms O, Fehr M, Krettek C, Pape HC. Effects of hypothermia and re-warming on the inflammatory response in a murine multiple hit model of trauma. Cytokine. 2005;31(5):382–93. https://doi.org/10.1016/j.cyto.2005.06.008.
27. Zhang H, Zhou M, Zhang J, Mei Y, Sun S, Tong E. Therapeutic effect of post-ischemic hypothermia duration on cerebral ischemic injury. Neurol Res. 2008;30(4):332–6. https://doi.org/10.1179/174313208X300279.
28. Straub RH, Pongratz G, Hirvonen H, Pohjolainen T, Mikkelsson M, Leirisalo-Repo M. Acute cold stress in rheumatoid arthritis inadequately activates stress responses and induces an increase of interleukin 6. Ann Rheum Dis. 2009;68(4):572–8. https://doi.org/10.1136/ard.2008.089458.
29. Banfi G, Melegati G, Barassi A, Dogliotti G, d'Eril GM, Dugue B, Corsi MM. Effects of whole-body cryotherapy on serum mediators of inflammation and serum muscle enzymes in athletes. J Therm Biol. 2009;34(2):55–9. https://doi.org/10.1016/j.jtherbio.2008.10.003.
30. Kang J, Albadawi H, Casey PJ, Abbruzzese TA, Patel VI, Yoo HJ, Cambria RP, Watkins MT. The effects of systemic hypothermia on a murine model of thoracic aortic ischemia reperfusion. J Vasc Surg. 2010;52(2):435–43. https://doi.org/10.1016/j.jvs.2010.03.021.
31. Miller E, Markiewicz L, Saluk J, Majsterek I. Effect of short-term cryostimulation on antioxidative status and its clinical applications in humans. Eur J Appl Physiol. 2012;112(5):1645–52. https://doi.org/10.1007/s00421-011-2122-x.
32. Zhang H, Zhang JJ, Mei YW, Sun SG, Tong ET. Effects of immediate and delayed mild hypothermia on endogenous antioxidant enzymes and energy metabolites following global cerebral ischemia. Chin Med J. 2011;124(17):2764–6.

33. Cao J, Xu J, Li W, Liu J. Influence of selective brain cooling on the expression of ICAM-1 mRNA and infiltration of PMNLs and monocytes/macrophages in rats suffering from global brain ischemia/reperfusion injury. Biosci Trends. 2008;2(6):241–4.
34. Shepherd JT, Rusch NJ, Vanhoutte PM. Effect of cold on the blood vessel wall. Gen Pharmacol. 1983;14(1):61–4.
35. Coassin M, Duncan KG, Bailey KR, Singh A, Schwartz DM. Hypothermia reduces secretion of vascular endothelial growth factor by cultured retinal pigment epithelial cells. Br J Ophtalmol. 2010;94(12):1678–83. https://doi.org/10.1136/bjo.2009.168864.
36. Harris ED Jr, McCroskery PA. The influence of temperature and fibril stability on degradation of cartilage collagen by rheumatoid synovial collagenase. New Eng J Med. 1974;290(1):1–6. https://doi.org/10.1056/NEJM197401032900101.
37. Suehiro E, Fujisawa H, Akimura T, Ishihara H, Kajiwara K, Kato S, Fujii M, Yamashita S, Maekawa T, Suzuki M. Increased matrix metalloproteinase-9 in blood in association with activation of interleukin-6 after traumatic brain injury: influence of hypothermic therapy. J Neurotrauma. 2004;21(12):1706–11. https://doi.org/10.1089/neu.2004.21.1706.
38. Truettner JS, Alonso OF, Dietrich WD. Influence of therapeutic hypothermia on matrix metalloproteinase activity after traumatic brain injury in rats. J Cereb Blood Flow Metab. 2005;25(11):1505–16. https://doi.org/10.1038/sj.jcbfm.9600150.
39. Stalman A, Berglund L, Dungnerc E, Arner P, Fellander-Tsai L. Temperature-sensitive release of prostaglandin E(2) and diminished energy requirements in synovial tissue with postoperative cryotherapy: a prospective randomized study after knee arthroscopy. J Bone Joint Surg Am. 2011;93(21):1961–8. https://doi.org/10.2106/JBJS.J.01790.
40. Wojtecka-Lukasik E, Ksiezopolska-Orlowska K, Gaszewska E, Krasowicz-Towalska O, Rzodkiewicz P, Maslinska D, Szukiewicz D, Maslinski S. Cryotherapy decreases histamine levels in the blood of patients with rheumatoid arthritis. Inflamm Res. 2010;59(Suppl 2):S253–5. https://doi.org/10.1007/s00011-009-0144-1.
41. Pertovaara A, Kalmari J. Comparison of the visceral antinociceptive effects of spinally administered MPV-2426 (fadolmidine) and clonidine in the rat. Anesthesiology. 2003;98(1):189–94.
42. Lubkowska A, Dudzinska W, Bryczkowska I, Dolegowska B. Body composition, lipid profile, Adipokine concentration, and antioxidant capacity changes during interventions to treat overweight with exercise Programme and whole-body cryostimulation. Oxidative Med Cell Longev. 2015;2015:803197. https://doi.org/10.1155/2015/803197.
43. Miller E, Mrowicka M, Malinowska K, Zolynski K, Kedziora J. Effects of the whole-body cryotherapy on a total antioxidative status and activities of some antioxidative enzymes in blood of patients with multiple sclerosis-preliminary study. J Med Investig. 2010;57(1–2):168–73.
44. Dugue B, Smolander J, Westerlund T, Oksa J, Nieminen R, Moilanen E, Mikkelsson M. Acute and long-term effects of winter swimming and whole-body cryotherapy on plasma antioxidative capacity in healthy women. Scand J Clin Lab Invest. 2005;65(5):395–402. https://doi.org/10.1080/00365510510025728.
45. Lubkowska A, Dolegowska B, Szygula Z, Klimek A. Activity of selected enzymes in erythrocytes and level of plasma antioxidants in response to single whole-body cryostimulation in humans. Scand J Clin Lab Invest. 2009;69(3):387–94. https://doi.org/10.1080/00365510802699246.
46. Hirvonen HE, Mikkelsson MK, Kautiainen H, Pohjolainen TH, Leirisalo-Repo M. Effectiveness of different cryotherapies on pain and disease activity in active rheumatoid arthritis. A randomised single blinded controlled trial. Clin Exp Rheumatol. 2006;24(3):295–301.
47. Stanek A, Cholewka A, Gadula J, Drzazga Z, Sieron A, Sieron-Stoltny K. Can whole-body cryotherapy with subsequent kinesiotherapy procedures in closed type cryogenic chamber improve BASDAI, BASFI, and some spine mobility parameters and decrease pain intensity in patients with ankylosing spondylitis? Biomed Res Int. 2015;2015:404259. https://doi.org/10.1155/2015/404259.
48. Rymaszewska J, Ramsey D, Chladzinska-Kiejna S. Whole-body cryotherapy as adjunct treatment of depressive and anxiety disorders. Arch Immunol Ther Exp. 2008;56(1):63–8. https://doi.org/10.1007/s00005-008-0006-5.

49. Smolander J, Westerlund T, Uusitalo A, Dugue B, Oksa J, Mikkelsson M. Lung function after acute and repeated exposures to extremely cold air (−110 degrees C) during whole-body cryotherapy. Clin Physiol Funct Imaging. 2006;26(4):232–4. https://doi.org/10.1111/j.1475-097X.2006.00675.x.
50. Banfi G, Melegati G, Barassi A, d'Eril GM. Effects of the whole-body cryotherapy on NTproBNP, hsCRP and troponin I in athletes. J Sci Med Sport. 2009;12(6):609–10. https://doi.org/10.1016/j.jsams.2008.06.004.
51. Lubkowska A, Szygula Z. Changes in blood pressure with compensatory heart rate decrease and in the level of aerobic capacity in response to repeated whole-body cryostimulation in normotensive, young and physically active men. Int J Occup Med Environ Health. 2010;23(4):367–75. https://doi.org/10.2478/v10001-010-0037-0.
52. Gizinska M, Rutkowski R, Romanowski W, Lewandowski J, Straburzynska-Lupa A. Effects of whole-body cryotherapy in comparison with other physical modalities used with kinesitherapy in rheumatoid arthritis. Biomed Res Int. 2015;2015:409174. https://doi.org/10.1155/2015/409174.
53. Klimenko T, Ahvenainen S, Karvonen SL. Whole-body cryotherapy in atopic dermatitis. Arch Dermatol. 2008;144(6):806–8. https://doi.org/10.1001/archderm.144.6.806.
54. Lombardi G, Sanchis-Gomar F, Perego S, Sansoni V, Banfi G. Implications of exercise-induced adipo-myokines in bone metabolism. Endocrine. 2016;54(2):284–305.
55. Ziemann E, Olek RA, Grzywacz T, Kaczor JJ, Antosiewicz J, Skrobot W, Kujach S, Laskowski R. Whole-body cryostimulation as an effective way of reducing exercise-induced inflammation and blood cholesterol in young men. Eur Cytokine Net. 2014;25(1):14–23. https://doi.org/10.1684/ecn.2014.0349.
56. Banfi G, Lombardi G, Colombini A, Melegati G. Whole-body cryotherapy in athletes. Sports Med. 2010;40(6):509–17. https://doi.org/10.2165/11531940-000000000-00000.
57. Miller E, Saluk J, Morel A, Wachowicz B. Long-term effects of whole body cryostimulation on uric acid concentration in plasma of secondary progressive multiple sclerosis patients. Scand J Clin Lab Invest. 2013;73(8):635–40. https://doi.org/10.3109/00365513.2013.841986.
58. Grasso D, Lanteri P, Di Bernardo C, Mauri C, Porcelli S, Colombini A, Zani V, Bonomi FG, Melegati G, Banfi G, Lombardi G. Salivary steroid hormones response to whole-body cryotherapy in elite rugby players. J Biol Regul Homeost Agents. 2014;28(2):291–300.
59. Wozniak A, Mila-Kierzenkowska C, Szpinda M, Chwalbinska-Moneta J, Augustynska B, Jurecka A. Whole-body cryostimulation and oxidative stress in rowers: the preliminary results. Arch Med Sci. 2013;9(2):303–8. https://doi.org/10.5114/aoms.2012.30835.
60. Schaal K, Y LEM, Louis J, Filliard JR, Hellard P, Casazza G, Hausswirth C. Whole-body Cryostimulation limits overreaching in elite synchronized swimmers. Med Sci Sports Exerc. 2015;47(7):1416–25. https://doi.org/10.1249/MSS.0000000000000546.
61. Lombardi G, Lanteri P, Porcelli S, Mauri C, Colombini A, Grasso D, Bonomi FG, Zani V, Melegati G, Banfi G. Hematological profile and martial status in rugby players during whole body cryostimulation. PLoS One. 2013;8(2):e55803.
62. Szygula Z, Lubkowska A, Giemza C, Skrzek A, Bryczkowska I, Dolegowska B. Hematological parameters, and hematopoietic growth factors: EPO and IL-3 in response to whole-body cryostimulation (WBC) in military academy students. PLoS One. 2014;9(4):e93096. https://doi.org/10.1371/journal.pone.0093096.
63. Galliera E, Dogliotti G, Melegati G, Corsi Romanelli MM, Cabitza P, Banfi G. Bone remodelling biomarkers after whole body cryotherapy (WBC) in elite rugby players. Injury. 2012;44(8):1117–21. https://doi.org/10.1016/j.injury.2012.08.057.
64. Lubkowska A, Banfi G, Dolegowska B, d'Eril GV, Luczak J, Barassi A. Changes in lipid profile in response to three different protocols of whole-body cryostimulation treatments. Cryobiology. 2010;61(1):22–6. https://doi.org/10.1016/j.cryobiol.2010.03.010.
65. Dulian K, Laskowski R, Grzywacz T, Kujach S, Flis DJ, Smaruj M, Ziemann E. The whole body cryostimulation modifies irisin concentration and reduces inflammation in middle aged, obese men. Cryobiology. 2015;71(3):398–404. https://doi.org/10.1016/j.cryobiol.2015.10.143.
66. Ziemann E, Olek RA, Grzywacz T, Antosiewicz J, Kujach S, Luszczyk M, Smaruj M, Sledziewska E, Laskowski R. Whole-body cryostimulation as an effective method of reduc-

ing low-grade inflammation in obese men. J Physiol Sci. 2013;63(5):333–43. https://doi.org/10.1007/s12576-013-0269-4.
67. Lombardi G. Exercise-dependent modulation of bone metabolism and bone endocrine function: new findings and therapeutic perspectives. J Sci Sport Exerc. 2019;1:20–8. https://doi.org/10.1007/s42978-019-0010-y.
68. Lombardi G, Ziemann E, Banfi G. Physical activity and bone health: what is the role of immune system? A narrative review of the third way. Front Endocrinol. 2019;10:60. https://doi.org/10.3389/fendo.2019.00060.
69. Khandekar MJ, Cohen P, Spiegelman BM. Molecular mechanisms of cancer development in obesity. Nat Rev Cancer. 2011;11(12):886–95. https://doi.org/10.1038/nrc3174.
70. Boström P, Wu J, Jedrychowski MP, Korde A, Ye L, Lo JC, Rasbach KA, Boström EA, Choi JH, Long JZ, Kajimura S, Zingaretti MC, Vind BF, Tu H, Cinti S, Højlund K, Gygi SP, Spiegelman BM. A PGC1-a-dependent myokine that drives brown-fat-like development of white fat and thermogenesis. Nature 2012;481(7382):463–8. https://doi.org/10.1038/nature10777.
71. Lee P, Linderman JD, Smith S, Brychta RJ, Wang J, Idelson C, Perron RM, Werner CD, Phan GQ, Kammula US, Kebebew E, Pacak K, Chen KY, Celi FS. Irisin and FGF21 are cold-induced endocrine activators of brown fat function in humans. Cell Metab. 2014;19(2):302–9. https://doi.org/10.1016/j.cmet.2013.12.017.
72. Jaworska J, Micielska K, Kozłowska M, Wnorowski K, Skrobecki J, Radzimin L, Babin A, Rodziewicz E, Lombardi G, Ziemann E. A 2-week specific volleyball training supported by the whole body cryostimulation protocol induced an increase of growth factors and counteracted deterioration of physical performance. Front Physiol. 2018;9(1711) https://doi.org/10.3389/fphys.2018.01711.
73. Lubkowska A, Bryczkowska I, Szygula Z, Giemza C, Skrzek A, Rotter I, Lombardi G, Banfi G. The effect of repeated whole-body cryostimulation on the HSP-70 and lipid metabolisms in healthy subjects. Physiol Res. 2019;68(3):419–29.
74. Lombardi G, Perego S, Luzi L, Banfi G. A four-season molecule: osteocalcin. Updates in its physiological roles. Endocrine. 2015;48:394–404.
75. Cholewka A, Stanek A, Sieron A, Drzazga Z. Thermography study of skin response due to whole-body cryotherapy. Skin Res Technol. 2012;18(2):180–7. https://doi.org/10.1111/j.1600-0846.2011.00550.x.
76. Hammond LE, Cuttell S, Nunley P, Meyler J. Anthropometric characteristics and sex influence magnitude of skin cooling following exposure to whole body cryotherapy. Biomed Res Int. 2014;2014:628724. https://doi.org/10.1155/2014/628724.

Virtual Reality

12

Giuseppe Riva, Clelia Malighetti, Alice Chirico, Daniele Di Lernia, Fabrizia Mantovani, and Antonios Dakanalis

Key Points

- Virtual reality (VR) technology is an integrated experiential platform able to engage obese individuals in mastering physical activity, diet, and self-regulatory strategies—targeting both emotions and experience of the body.
- It provides a safe environment for learner experimentation, real-time personalized behavioral weight management tasks, and strategies.
- It is able to target negative emotions and body image dissatisfaction that play a critical role in the onset and maintenance of this disorder.
- It has the potential of improving treatment adherence, addressing a critical issue to achieve successful weight loss and weight maintenance.

G. Riva (✉)
Applied Technology for Neuro-Psychology Lab, IRCSS Istituto Auxologico Italiano, Milan, Italy

Department of Psychology, Università Cattolica del Sacro Cuore, Milan, Italy
e-mail: giuseppe.riva@unicatt.it

C. Malighetti · A. Chirico · D. Di Lernia
Department of Psychology, Università Cattolica del Sacro Cuore, Milan, Italy
e-mail: Clelia.malighetti@unicatt.it; alice.chirico@unicatt.it; daniele.dilernia@unicatt.it

F. Mantovani
CESCOM, Università Milano—Bicocca, Milan, Italy
e-mail: Fabrizia.mantovani@unimib.it

A. Dakanalis
Department of Medicine and Surgery, Università degli Studi di Milano Bicocca, Milan, Italy

Department of Brain and Behavioral Sciences, University of Pavia, Pavia, Italy
e-mail: Antonios.dakanalis@unimib.it

P. Capodaglio (ed.), *Rehabilitation Interventions in the Patient with Obesity*,
https://doi.org/10.1007/978-3-030-32274-8_12

12.1 Introduction

The evolution of technology is providing new tools and methods for health care [1]. Between them, an emerging trend is the use of virtual reality (VR) [2–4].

Computer scientists define VR as a set of fancy technologies used to create a simulated environment [5]: an interactive 3D visualization system (a computer, a game console, or a smartphone) supported by one or more position trackers and head-mounted display. The trackers sense the movements of the user and report them to the visualization system which updates the images for display in real time.

However, psychology and neuroscience define VR as [6] "an advanced form of human-computer interface that allows the user to interact with and become immersed in a computer-generated environment in a naturalistic fashion" (p. 82). In fact, from a cognitive viewpoint, VR is mainly a *subjective experience* that makes the user believe that he/she is there, that the experience is real [7]. Why? As underlined recently [8, 9], VR shares with our brain the same basic mechanism: embodied simulations. According to neuroscience our brain, to effectively regulate and control the body in the world, creates an embodied simulation of the body in the world used to represent and predict actions, concepts, and emotions. VR works in a similar way: the VR experience tries to predict the sensory consequences of the individual's movements providing to him/her the same scene he/she will see in the real world. This transforms VR into an experiential technology that is able to target at the same time both the body and the mind.

As underlined by two different meta-reviews [7, 8] discussing 48 different systematic reviews and meta-analyses, VR is a powerful clinical tool for behavioral health, able to provide assessment and effective treatment options for different mental health problems. Specifically, VR compares favorably to existing treatments in anxiety disorders, eating and weight disorders, and pain management, with long-term effects that generalize to the real world. Moreover, they show the potential of VR as an assessment tool with practical applications that range from social and cognitive deficits to addiction. Finally, they suggest a clinical potential in the treatment of psychosis and in the pediatric field.

In this chapter we focus our analysis to the field of obesity, discussing the potential of VR to achieve successful weight loss and weight maintenance [10–13]. In particular we discuss three different applications of VR in this field: exergames, emotion regulation, and multisensory integration.

12.2 VR for Exergames

The term "exergames," the fusion of the words "exercise" and "gaming," indicates video games that provide also a form of exercise. As explained by Rizzo and colleagues [13]: "The core concept of exergaming rests on the idea of using vigorous body activity as the input for interacting with engaging digital game content with the hope of supplanting the sedentary activity that typifies traditional game interaction that relies on keyboards, gamepads, and joysticks." (p. 259).

By creating engaging digital gaming interacted via body movements, the motivation to participate in calorie-burning cardiovascular exercise activities is increased. In particular, the three factors influencing motivation and compliance [14]—feedback, challenge, and rewards—are all supported by virtual reality experiences.

Feedback is a critical part of physical exercise because it offers informative and evaluative feedback on skill development and progress, allowing the perceptions of competence and the identification of possible errors or shortcomings. Typically feedbacks can be visual, auditory, or sensory, but in VR their integration and multiple use are possible: for example, a progress bar with the remaining time and tasks, physical indications in the player avatar (stumbling, showing a slower pace, etc.), a sound to indicate the amount of exercise left, and other avatars (e.g., the virtual coach) commenting on the performance.

According to the theory of "flow" introduced by Csikszentmihalyi [15, 16] an optimal match between skill and challenge is critical to achieve an intrinsically motivating experience. In this view, the ability of the exergame to assess the skill of the user and to provide a level of challenge matched to it is required to guarantee compliance and motivation. VR facilitates this process. Using VR it is possible to develop exergames in which subjects experience themselves as competent and efficacious [5, 17]. Specifically, the VR experience can offer different difficulty levels—from easy tasks to very difficult ones—offering a controlled setting in which the individual is able to develop new skills through trials and errors. Using this approach, the level of challenge can be balanced to the skill of the user so that failures can support perceived relatedness and competence without reducing perceived competence [14].

The final component for the success of exergames is reward. It is well known that external rewards support behavior as long as the rewards are present, but intrinsically motivated activity is more likely to produce long-term change [18]. Again, VR supports the provision of effective reward, by allowing two different types of reward [14]: controlling rewards that are task and performance contingent and autonomy-supportive rewards that are verbal and task noncontingent. In particular, it allows the use of embodiment as a form of autonomy-supportive reward through specific poses and ballets that can be replicated and shared by users. Differently by non-VR videogames, the use of embodied avatars with normal body size has the potential to increase the effectiveness of exergames among overweight children as demonstrated by a recent study [19].

These principles have been used in different successful exergames [20–23]. For example, Astrojumper is an immersive virtual reality exergame used to engage children and adults in rigorous, full-body exercise [20]. The overall goal of this exergames is relatively easy: users fly through an immersive, stereoscopic outer space environment in first-person perspective and they have to avoid or grab the different virtual planets that are speeding toward them. As the authors explain [20]: "To make sure that Astrojumper would be playable for users at all levels of physical fitness, Astrojumper begins very slowly, providing all users with a warm-up phase. After this phase is complete, planets will begin to gradually come out at a slightly faster rate. If the player is successfully able to avoid these planets, the speed will continue to increase. If the player starts to collide with the planets, their speed will reduce. This back-and-forth adjustment finds a speed where the player can successfully avoid almost all of the planets, and will continuously update throughout the game." (p. 87).

The achieved results support this approach. A study involving 30 subjects (10 participants were children and 20 were adults) demonstrated that Astrojumper is an effective way to provide a workout, motivating both children and adults to exercise through immersive VR [20].

Up to now the most significant barrier to the wide use of VR exergames is cost [22]. However, the appearance of cheaper stand-alone VR devices (see Table 12.1) associated to successful commercial VR exergames like Beat Saber or Dance Central may improve the use of this approach in the prevention and treatment of obesity.

12.3 VR for Emotion Regulation

Stress and negative emotions have been shown to be critical factors in inducing overeating as a form of maladaptive coping in some patients with obesity. According to the theory of emotional eating [24], eating is used as a strategy to regulate or escape negative emotions and it is related to both obesity and binge eating disorders. Specifically, Macht identified five classes of emotion-induced changes of eating [24]: (1) emotional control of food choice, (2) emotional suppression of food intake, (3) impairment of cognitive eating controls, (4) eating to regulate emotions, and (5) emotion-congruent modulation of eating. Different studies suggest the ability of VR to address many of them.

First, using VR is possible to modulate food craving, the intense desire to consume a specific food (selective hunger). According to Jansen [25] once eating behavior has been established, exposure to specific food cues—i.e., cues systematically associated with food intake such as the presence of high-calorie food—induces a conditioned response (hyperinsulinemia), which thus activates a hypoglycemic compensatory response. This biochemical response is experienced as food craving and may lead to an eating episode. However, by exposing participants to these cues, cue exposure therapy is designed to progressively break the mental links that typically precede using. For example, in cue exposure therapy (CET), an obese individual may be exposed to a chocolate cake or any other high-calorie food. Initially, the exposure to the cue prompts the brain to "expect" consumption. However, frequent exposure to different cues—without eating—reduces the likelihood of a cue-induced eating in the future by desensitizing the brain's reaction.

VR is perfect for CET. On one side, as demonstrated by Gorini and colleagues [26], real food and virtual food induced a comparable emotional reaction in patients that is higher than the one elicited by photos of the same food. More, unlike exposure to photographs, in vivo exposure, and guided imagination, VR offers a good ecological validity, and also a fair internal validity, while allowing strict control over the variables. This is true also for social interactions in VR. As demonstrated by Balzarotti and colleagues [27], VR avatars are recognized as intentional agents and users adjust their emotion nonverbal behavior according to the behavior of the

Table 12.1 Commercial VR devices

	PC based			Mobile based			Console based	Stand-alone		
System	Oculus Rift	HTC Vive/ Vive Pro	Microsoft Mixed Reality	Samsung Gear VR	Google Cardboard	Google Daydream	Playstation VR	Oculus Go	Oculus Quest	Mirage Solo
Cost	399 US$	499/799 US$	249/449 US$	99 US$	10–50 US$	69–149 US$	299 US$	199 US$	399 US$	299 US$
Hardware requirements	High-end PC (>1000 US$)	High-end PC (>1000 US$)	Mid-level PC (>600 US$)	High-end Samsung phone (>600 US$)	Middle/ high-end Android phone or iPhone (>299 US$)	High-end Android phone (>499 US$)	PS4 (299 US$) or PS4 Pro (399 US$)	None (Internal Snapdragon 821 processor)	None (Internal Snapdragon 835 processor)	None (Internal Snapdragon 835 processor)
Resolution	2160 × 1200	2160 × 1200/2880 × 1660	2880 × 1440	2560 × 1440	Depends on the phone (minimum 1024 × 768)	Depends on the phone (minimum 1920 × 1080)	1920 × 1080	2560 × 1440	2560 × 1440	2560 × 1440
Refresh rate	90 Hz	90 Hz	90 Hz	60 Hz	60 Hz	90 Hz minimum	120 Hz	72 Hz	72 Hz	75 Hz
Field of view	110°	110°	100/110°	101°	From 70°	96°	100°	90°	100°	100°
Body tracking	Medium/ high: Head tracking (rotation) and positional tracking (forward/ backward)	High: Head tracking (rotation) and volumetric tracking (full room size—15 ft × 15 ft—movement)	Medium/ high: Head tracking (rotation) and positional tracking (forward/ backward)	Medium: Head tracking (rotation)	Medium: Head tracking (rotation)	Medium: Head tracking (rotation)	Medium/ high: Head tracking (rotation) and positional tracking (forward/ backward)	Medium: Head tracking (rotation)	Medium/ high: Head tracking (rotation) and positional tracking (forward/ backward)	Medium/ high: Head tracking (rotation) and positional tracking (forward/ backward)

(continued)

Table 12.1 (continued)

	PC based			Mobile based			Console based	Stand-alone		
User interaction with VR	High (using a joystick or controllers)	High (using controllers)	High (using a joystick or controllers)	Medium (using gaze, a built-in pad, or joystick)	Low (using gaze or a button)	Medium (using gaze or joystick)	High (using a joystick or controllers)	Medium (using gaze, a built-in pad, or joystick)	High (using a joystick or controllers)	Medium (using gaze, a built-in pad, or joystick)
Software availability	Oculus Store	Steam Store	Microsoft Store	Oculus Store	Google Play or IOS Store	Google Play	Playstation Store	Oculus Store	Oculus Store	Google Play

avatar. On the other side, several studies support the ability of food-related VR environments to induce food craving [28, 29].

Their results [30] suggest that craving experienced in VR environments incorporating cues and contexts related to binging behavior was consistent with trait and state craving assessed (with questionnaires) outside the VR environments. In addition, participants with the highest scores on trait and state craving also experienced craving when exposed to food in VR. Finally, scores on questionnaires assessing trait and state craving were able to predict the average craving experienced in VR.

These results provide a clear rationale for the use of VR-CET with eating-disordered patients. And different studies are providing an experimental support to this claim.

A first study assessed the efficacy of CET based on VR (VR-CET) as a second-level treatment in patients with bulimia nervosa (BN) and binge eating disorders [31]. With this objective in mind, 64 patients diagnosed with BN or BED, according to DSM-5 who were treatment resistant (that is, their binges persisted after CBT), were randomly assigned to one of the two booster session conditions: a VR-CET booster sessions group, and a CBT booster sessions group (the control group).

Booster sessions consisted of six 60-min sessions held twice weekly over a period of 3 weeks. Over the six sessions, participants in the experimental group were exposed to different VR environments related to binge behavior, according to a previously constructed hierarchy. During exposure, patients faced high-risk situations and handled the virtual foods using a computer mouse. Exposure ended after a significant reduction in the level of anxiety, or after 60 min. Participants in the control group received six CBT booster sessions to improve treatment outcome.

A significant interaction between group (VR-CET vs. CBT) and time (before and after booster sessions) was expected, showing the maintenance of the number of binges and purges before and after booster sessions in the control group (CBT) and a reduction in the experimental group (VR-CET).

After the six booster sessions, patients in both CBT and VR-CET conditions presented improvement. However, participants in the VR-CET group showed significantly higher reductions in binges, purges, bulimia symptoms (assessed with the Bulimia scale of the Eating Disorders Inventory-3; EDI-3), craving for food (assessed with the Food Craving Questionnaire-State/Trait; FCQ-S/T), and anxiety (State and Trait Anxiety Inventory, STAI) than patients in the CBT group. A follow-up study showed that the VR-CET group maintained the obtained results also after 6 months [32]. Moreover the obtained reductions were greater after VR-CET, regarding binge and purge episodes, as well as the decrease of self-reported tendency to engage in overeating episodes.

In sum, these results support the use of VR-CET as an effective way for reducing food craving and related behaviors in eating- and weight-disordered individuals.

Second, VR can also be used to improve emotion regulation. In a different study Manzoni and colleagues [33] evaluated the efficacy of a 3-week relaxation protocol enhanced by VR in reducing emotional eating in a sample of 60 female inpatients with obesity who report emotional eating. To reach this goal they used a three-arm exploratory randomized controlled trial with 3 months of follow-up. The intervention included 12 individual relaxation training sessions provided traditionally (imagination condition) or supported by virtual reality (virtual reality condition). Control participants received only standard hospital-based care. Their data show that VR-enhanced relaxation training was effective in reducing emotional eating episodes and depressive and anxiety symptoms, and in improving perceived self-efficacy for eating control at 3-month follow-up after discharge. The virtual reality condition proved better than the imagination condition in the reduction of emotional eating. Weight decreased in subjects in all three conditions without significant differences between them, probably due to the common treatment all inpatients received. In conclusion, VR-enhanced relaxation training is a useful tool for reducing emotional eating episodes and thereby reducing weight and obesity.

12.4 VR for Improving Multisensory Integration

In our culture most women are dissatisfied with their body: one adolescent girl out of two reports body dissatisfaction [34]. And recent studies highlighted that socio-cultural pressure to be thin is central to the development of negative feelings about the body, which are recognized as critical risk factor for the emergence of overweight and obesity [35–37].

A first longitudinal study [37] used data from a prospective study of 496 adolescent girls who completed a baseline assessment at age 11–15 years and four annual follow-ups to test whether behavioral and psychological risk factors predict the onset of obesity during adolescence and to compare the predictive power of these factors with that of parental obesity. Contrary to hypotheses, elevated intake of high-fat foods, binge eating, and exercise did not predict obesity onset. Instead the most important predictor was elevated dietary restraint scores associated to maladaptive compensatory behaviors for weight control, such as vomiting or laxative abuse.

Moreover, a second study [35] tried to identify 10-year longitudinal predictors of overweight incidence during the transition from adolescence to young adulthood using a population-based cohort ($N = 2134$). At 10-year follow-up, 51% of young adults were overweight (26% increase from baseline). Among females and males, higher levels of body dissatisfaction, weight concerns, unhealthy weight control behaviors (e.g., fasting, purging), dieting, binge eating, weight-related teasing, and parental weight-related concerns and behaviors during adolescence and/or increases in these factors over the study period predicted the incidence of overweight at 10-year follow-up.

Finally, a third longitudinal study [36] explored whether weight-based teasing in adolescence predicts adverse eating and weight-related outcomes 15 years later. The results are quite clear: weight-based teasing in adolescence predicted higher BMI and obesity 15 years later. For women, these longitudinal associations occurred across peer- and family-based teasing sources, but for men, only peer-based teasing predicted higher BMI.

For this reason, the "objectification theory" suggests a significant role of culture and society in the etiology of eating and weight disorders. Introduced by Fredrickson and Roberts [38], this theory suggests that our culture imposes a specific self-evaluation model—self-objectification—defining women's behavioral and emotional responses [39–41]. At its simplest, the objectification theory holds that [1] there exists an objectified societal ideal of beauty (within a particular culture) that is [2] transmitted via a variety of sociocultural channels. This ideal is then [3] internalized by individuals, so that [4] satisfaction (or dissatisfaction) with appearance will be a function of the extent to which individuals do (or do not) meet the ideal prescription [42].

The internalization of an observer's perspective on one's own body is labeled as "self-objectification" [43, 44] and reduces a woman's worth to her perception of her body's semblance to cultural standards of attractiveness [45].

Even if self-objectification can be a critical risk factor for the development of obesity and overweight through its link with teasing, body image dissatisfaction, and unhealthy weight control behaviors the objectification theory is still not able to answer two critical questions [46]: Why do not all the individuals experiencing self-objectification develop EDs? What is the role of the body experience in the etiology of obesity?

Here we will embrace an emerging field of neuroscience—the multisensory integration of bodily representations and signals [47, 48]—to answer the above questions.

Multisensory body integration is a critical cognitive and perceptual process, allowing the individual to protect and extend his/her boundaries at both the homeostatic and psychological levels [49, 50]. To achieve this goal the brain integrates sensory data arriving from real-time multiple sensory modalities and internal bodily information with predictions made using the stored information about the body from conceptual, perceptual, and episodic memory. In this view the emotional [51], motor [52], proprioceptive [53], and interoceptive [54] deficits reported by many authors in individuals with obesity may reflect a broader impairment in multisensory body integration [55]. Specifically it can affect the individual's abilities [47, 48]: (a) to identify the relevant interoceptive signals that predict potential pleasant (or aversive) consequences and (b) to modify/correct the autobiographical allocentric (observer view) memories of body-related events (self-objectified memories).

The first effect of an impaired multisensory body integration is a prospective aversive body state [56]. This situation makes it difficult for obese individuals to obtain and regulate a sense of self and could contribute to the problems with body image and self-disturbances.

The second effect of an impaired multisensory body integration is that obese patients may be locked to an allocentric disembodied negative memory of the body that is not updated even after a demanding diet and a significant weight loss [57, 58]. Therefore, successful dieting attempts are not able to improve body dissatisfaction and subjects may either start more radical dieting attempts or, at the opposite end, engage in "disinhibited" eating behaviors [44].

VR allows to target an impaired multisensory body integration through two different strategies—"reference frame shifting" [59, 60] and "body swapping" [61, 62]—that can be integrated within a classical cognitive-behavioral training (CBT) for obesity.

The first method, "reference frame shifting" [59, 60], structures the individual's bodily self-consciousness (see Table 12.2) through the focus and reorganization of its contents [60, 63].

Table 12.2 The VR body image rescripting protocol (adapted from Riva, 2011)

Phase 1: Interview	During a clinical interview the patient is asked to relive the contents of the allocentric negative body image and the situation/s in which it was created and/or reinforced (e.g., being teased by my boyfriend at home) in as much detail as possible. The meaning of the experience for the patient was also elicited.
Phase 2: Development of the VR scene	The clinician reproduces the setting of the identified situation (e.g., the corridor of the classroom where my boyfriend teased me) using the VR development toolkit.
Phase 3: Egocentric experience of the VR scene	The patient is asked to re-experience the event in VR from a first-person perspective (the patient does not see his/her body in the scene) expressing and discussing his/her feelings. The patient is then asked what was needed to happen to change the feelings in a positive direction. The main cognitive techniques used in this phase, if needed, are: *Countering*: Once a list of distorted perceptions and cognitions is developed, the process of countering these thoughts and beliefs begins. *Label shifting*: The patient first tries to identify the kinds of negative words she uses to interpret situations in her life, such as bad, terrible, obese, inferior, and hateful. The situations in which these labels are used are then listed. The patient and therapist replace each emotional label with two or more descriptive words.
Phase 4: Allocentric experience of the VR scene	The patient is asked to re-experience the event in VR from a third-person perspective (the patient sees his/her body in the scene) intervening both to calm and reassuring his/her virtual avatar and to counter any negative evaluation. The therapist follows the Socratic approach. For example: "What would need to happen for you to feel better? How does it look through the eyes of a third person? Is there anything you as a third person like to do? How do the other people respond?" The main cognitive techniques used in this phase, if needed, are: *Alternative interpretation*: The patient learns to stop and consider other interpretations of a situation before proceeding to the decision-making stage. *Deactivating the illness belief:* The therapist first helps the client list her beliefs concerning weight and eating.

To achieve it, the subject re-experiences in VR a negative situation related to the body (e.g., teasing) both in first person and in third person (e.g., seeing and supporting his/her avatar in the VR world) integrating the therapeutic methods used by Butters and Cash [64] and Wooley and Wooley [65]. Specifically, the VR situations are used in the same way as guided imagery [66] is used in the cognitive and visual/motorial approach. In general, the therapist asks the patient to give detailed descriptions of the virtual experience and of the feelings associated with it. Furthermore, the patient is taught how to cope with them [66].using different techniques (see Table 12.2).

This approach has been successfully used in different randomized trials with obese patients [67, 68] allowing both to update the contents of their body memory and to improve the clinical outcomes over traditional CBT.

In the second—"body swapping" [61, 62]—VR is used to induce the illusory feeling of ownership of a virtual body with a different shape and/or size. Since the publication by Botvinick and Cohen [69] revealing that it is simple to generate in people the illusion that a rubber hand is part of their body (rubber hand illusion—RHI), there has been increasing research interest in the study of bodily illusions.

Specifically, this term refers to controlled illusory generation of unusual bodily feelings, such as the feeling of ownership over a rubber hand that affects the experience of a body part or the entire body (i.e., a body-swap illusion).

More recently, an increasing body of pioneered research conducted by Riva team [70, 71] revealed that the embodiment in a virtual body that substitutes the own body in virtual reality with visuo-tactile stimulation (body-swap illusion) alters body percept (i.e., participants are significantly fatter or thinner than they really are) suggesting, among others, that virtual reality is more than a way of placing people in a simulated world (i.e., manipulating their sense of place).

A first study [70] has showed that the body-swap illusion is able to induce an update of the negative stored representation of the body. In particular, it has been found that after embodying a virtual body with a skinny belly there was an update of the "remembered body," with women reporting a significant (post-illusion) decrease in their body-size distortion. Consistent with this perspective, Preston and Ehrsson [72] induced an illusory ownership over a slimmer mannequin by synchronously stroking the mannequin body and the corresponding part of the participants' body. It has been found that that the illusory ownership over a slimmer body decreases significantly participants' perceived body size but also increases significantly participants' body satisfaction.

Support for the use of bodily illusions to alter the dysfunctional experience of the body in obesity comes from a recent published study [71]. Serino and colleagues showed that a (virtual reality) body-swap illusion, which generates the (converse) illusion that a fat person is thin, was able to increase body satisfaction and reduce body-size distortion in a non-operable super-super-obese patient (i.e., with body mass index >60 kg/m^2). In addition to the improvement in the bodily experience, the illusion was able to increase patient's motivation to maintain healthy eating behaviors. While no studies to date have directly exploited the capability of the bodily illusions in obese treatment, the evidence deriving from the extant experimental studies for a (a) direct link between perceptual (described as an inability to accurately estimate body size) and affective (described as subjective body dissatisfaction) body-image components and (b) a positive affective response with the body illusion-modulated severe obesity [71] may suggest clinical applications for these methods.

12.5 Conclusions

Most clinicians and patients consider obesity just as a problem of energy input and expenditure: more energy input than expenditure. However, the clinical practice and epidemiological data clearly show that obesity is more complex than expected by this simple equation.

In this chapter we underlined significant potential of VR in this process by discussing three different applications of VR: exergames, emotion regulation, and multisensory integration.

The term "exergames," the fusion of the words "exercise" and "gaming," indicates digital experiences that provide also a form of exercise able to increase the motivation to participate in calorie-burning cardiovascular activities. In particular,

VR is able to support the three factors influencing motivation and compliance [14]—feedback, challenge, and rewards—with different studies supporting its clinical efficacy. Up to now the most significant barrier to the wide use of VR exergames is cost [22]. However, the appearance of cheaper stand-alone VR devices (see Table 12.1) associated to successful commercial VR exergames may improve the use of this approach in the prevention and treatment of obesity.

Stress and negative emotions have been shown to be critical factors in inducing overeating as a form of maladaptive coping in some patients with obesity. Different studies suggest the ability of VR to address many of them.

First, using VR is possible to modulate food craving, the intense desire to consume a specific food (selective hunger) and related behaviors in eating- and weight-disordered individuals. Moreover, VR-enhanced relaxation training is a useful tool for reducing emotional eating episodes and thereby reducing weight and obesity.

Other critical risk factors for the emergence of overweight and obesity are that sociocultural pressure to be thin is central and the development of negative feelings about the body, in particular self-objectification [35–37]. When these factors are associated to an impaired multisensory body integration they produce a paradoxical situation [57, 58]: obese patients may be locked to an allocentric disembodied negative memory of the body that is not updated even after a demanding diet and a significant weight loss. Therefore, successful dieting attempts are not able to improve body dissatisfaction and subjects may either start more radical dieting attempts or, at the opposite end, engage in "disinhibited" eating behaviors [44]. VR is able to correct an impaired multisensory body integration through two different strategies—"reference frame shifting" [59, 60] and "body swapping" [61, 62]—that can be integrated within a classical cognitive-behavioral training (CBT) for obesity. If the first strategy is already backed by different randomized controlled trials with obese patients [67, 68], no randomized studies to date have directly exploited the capability of the bodily illusions in obese treatment. However, the evidence deriving from different basic research studies and the result of a case study [71] may suggest clinical applications for this method, too.

In conclusion, the available clinical data suggest the added value of VR as part of an integrated obesity treatment targeting both the physical and the psychological side of the problem. Longer follow-up data and multicentric trials are required to investigate the possible effects of the behavioral, emotional, and body image changes on the long-term maintenance of the weight loss.

References

1. Riva G, Vatalaro F, Davide F, Alcañiz M, editors. Ambient intelligence: the evolution of technology, communication and cognition towards the future of human-computer interaction. Amsterdam: IOS Press; 2004. Online: http://www.emergingcommunication.com/volume6.html.
2. Satava RM, Jones SB. Medical applications of virtual reality. In: Stanney KM, editor. Handbook of virtual environments: design, implementation, and applications. Mahwah, NJ: Lawrence Erlbaum Associates, Inc.; 2002. p. 368–91.

3. Riva G, Gamberini L. Virtual reality in telemedicine. Telemed J e-Health. 2004;6(3):327–40.
4. Riva G, Gaggioli A. Virtual clinical therapy. Lect Notes Comput Sci. 2008;4650:90–107.
5. Riva G, Botella C, Baños R, Mantovani F, García-Palacios A, Quero S, et al. Presence-inducing media for mental health applications. In: Lombard M, Biocca F, Freeman J, Ijsselsteijn W, Schaevitz RJ, editors. Immersed in media. New York: Springer International Publishing; 2015. p. 283–332.
6. Schultheis MT, Rizzo AA. The application of virtual reality technology in rehabilitation. Rehabil Psychol. 2001;46(3):296–311.
7. Riva G, Baños RM, Botella C, Mantovani F, Gaggioli A. Transforming experience: the potential of augmented reality and virtual reality for enhancing personal and clinical change. Front Psychiatry. 2016;7:164.
8. Riva G, Wiederhold BK, Mantovani F. Neuroscience of virtual reality: from virtual exposure to embodied medicine. Cyberpsychol Behav Soc Netw. 2019;22(1):82–96.
9. Riva G, Wiederhold BK, Chirico A, Di Lernia D, Mantovani F, Brain GA. Virtual reality: what do they have in common and how to exploit their potential. Annu Rev Cyberther Telemed. 2018;16:3–7.
10. Riva G. Letter to the editor: virtual reality in the treatment of eating and weight disorders. Psychol Med. 2017;47(14):2567–8.
11. Gutierrez-Maldonado J, Wiederhold BK, Riva G. Future directions: how virtual reality can further improve the assessment and treatment of eating disorders and obesity. Cyberpsychol Behav Soc Netw. 2016;19(2):148–53.
12. Riva G, Gutierrez-Maldonado J, Wiederhold BK. Virtual worlds versus real body: virtual reality meets eating and weight disorders. Cyberpsychol Behav Soc Netw. 2016;19(2):63–6.
13. Rizzo AS, Lange B, Suma EA, Bolas M. Virtual reality and interactive digital game technology: new tools to address obesity and diabetes. J Diabetes Sci Technol. 2011;5(2):256–64.
14. Lyons EJ. Cultivating engagement and enjoyment in exergames using feedback, challenge, and rewards. Games Health J. 2015;4(1):12–8.
15. Csikszentmihalyi M. Flow: the psychology of optimal experience. New York: HarperCollins; 1990.
16. Nakamura J, Csikszentmihalyi M. Flow theory and research. In: Lopez SJ, Snyder CR, editors. Handbook of positive psychology. New York: Oxford University Press; 2009. p. 195–206.
17. Botella C, Quero S, Banos RM, Perpina C, Garcia Palacios A, Riva G. Virtual reality and psychotherapy. Stud Health Technol Inform. 2004;99:37–54.
18. Ryan RM, Mims V, Koestner R. Relation of reward contingency and interpersonal context to intrinsic motivation: a review and test using cognitive evaluation theory. J Pers Soc Psychol. 1983;45(4):736.
19. Li BJ, Lwin MO, Jung Y. Wii, myself, and size: the influence of Proteus effect and stereotype threat on overweight Children's exercise motivation and behavior in exergames. Games Health J. 2014;3(1):40–8.
20. Finkelstein S, Nickel A, Lipps Z, Barnes T, Wartell Z, Suma EA. Astrojumper: motivating exercise with an immersive virtual reality exergame. Presence Teleop Virt. 2011;20(1): 78–92.
21. Bolton J, Lambert M, Lirette D, Unsworth B. PaperDude: a virtual reality cycling exergame. In: CHI'14 extended abstracts on human factors in computing systems, Toronto, Ontario, Canada. ACM; 2014. p. 475–8.
22. Farič N, Yorke E, Varnes L, Newby K, Potts HWW, Smith L, et al. Younger adolescents' perceptions of physical activity, exergaming, and virtual reality: qualitative intervention study. JMIR Serious Games. 2019;7(2):e11960.
23. Farrow M, Lutteroth C, Rouse PC, Bilzon JLJ. Virtual-reality exergaming improves performance during high-intensity interval training. Eur J Sport Sci. 2019;19(6):719–27.
24. Macht M. How emotions affect eating: a five-way model. Appetite. 2008;50(1):1–11.
25. Jansen A. A learning model of binge eating: cue reactivity and cue exposure. Behav Res Ther. 1998;36(3):257–72.
26. Gorini A, Griez E, Petrova A, Riva G. Assessment of the emotional responses produced by exposure to real food, virtual food and photographs of food in patients affected by eating

disorders. Ann Gen Psychiatr. 2010;9:30. Online: http://www.annals-general-psychiatry.com/content/9/1/.

27. Balzarotti S, Piccini L, Andreoni G, Ciceri R. "I Know That You Know How I Feel": Behavioral and Physiological Signals Demonstrate Emotional Attunement While Interacting with a Computer Simulating Emotional Intelligence. Journal of Nonverbal Behavior, 2014 38, 283–99.
28. Pla-Sanjuanelo J, Ferrer-Garcia M, Gutierrez-Maldonado J, Riva G, Andreu-Gracia A, Dakanalis A, et al. Identifying specific cues and contexts related to bingeing behavior for the development of effective virtual environments. Appetite. 2015;87:81–9.
29. Pla-Sanjuanelo J, Ferrer-García M, Vilalta-Abella F, Riva G, Dakanalis A, Ribas-Sabaté J, et al. Testing virtual reality-based cue-exposure software: which cue-elicited responses best discriminate between patients with eating disorders and healthy controls? Eat Weight Disord. 2019;24:757–65.
30. Gutierrez-Maldonado J, Ferrer-Garcia M, Dakanalis A, Riva G. Virtual reality: applications to eating disorders. In: Agras SW, Robinson A, editors. The Oxford handbook of eating disorders. 2nd ed. Oxford: Oxford University Press; 2017. p. 146–61.
31. Ferrer-Garcia M, Gutierrez-Maldonado J, Pla-Sanjuanelo J, Vilalta-Abella F, Riva G, Clerici M, et al. A randomised controlled comparison of second-level treatment approaches for treatment-resistant adults with bulimia nervosa and binge eating disorder: assessing the benefits of virtual reality cue exposure therapy. Eur Eat Disord Rev. 2017;25(6):479–90.
32. Ferrer-Garcia M, Pla-Sanjuanelo J, Dakanalis A, Vilalta-Abella F, Riva G, Fernandez-Aranda F, et al. A randomized trial of virtual reality-based Cue exposure second-level therapy and cognitive behavior second-level therapy for bulimia nervosa and binge-eating disorder: outcome at six-month follow-up. Cyberpsychol Behav Soc Netw. 2019;22(1):60–8.
33. Manzoni GM, Pagnini F, Gorini A, Preziosa A, Castelnuovo G, Molinari E, et al. Can relaxation training reduce emotional eating in women with obesity? An exploratory study with 3 months of follow-up. J Am Diet Assoc. 2009;109(8):1427–32.
34. Makinen M, Puukko-Viertomies LR, Lindberg N, Siimes MA, Aalberg V. Body dissatisfaction and body mass in girls and boys transitioning from early to mid-adolescence: additional role of self-esteem and eating habits. BMC Psychiatry. 2012;12:35.
35. Quick V, Wall M, Larson N, Haines J, Neumark-Sztainer D. Personal, behavioral and socio-environmental predictors of overweight incidence in young adults: 10-yr longitudinal findings. Int J Behav Nutr Phys Act. 2013;10:37.
36. Puhl RM, Wall MM, Chen C, Bryn Austin S, Eisenberg ME, Neumark-Sztainer D. Experiences of weight teasing in adolescence and weight-related outcomes in adulthood: a 15-year longitudinal study. Prev Med. 2017;100:173–9.
37. Stice E, Presnell K, Shaw H, Rohde P. Psychological and behavioral risk factors for obesity onset in adolescent girls: a prospective study. J Consult Clin Psychol. 2005;73(2):195–202.
38. Fredrickson BL, Roberts T. Objectification theory: toward understanding women's lived experiences and mental health risks. Psychol Women Q. 1997;21:173–206.
39. Calogero RM, Tantleff-Dunn S, Thompson JK. Self-objectification in women: causes, consequences, and counteractions. Washington, DC: American Psychological Association; 2010.
40. Dakanalis A, Di Mattei VE, Bagliacca EP, Prunas A, Sarno L, Riva G, et al. Disordered eating behaviors among Italian men: objectifying media and sexual orientation differences. Eat Disord. 2012;20(5):356–67.
41. Riva G, Waterworth JA, Murray D, editors. Interacting with presence: HCI and the sense of presence in computer-mediated environments. Berlin: De Gruyter Open; 2014. Online: www.presence-research.com.
42. Tiggemann M. Sociocultural perspectives on human appearance and body image. In: Cash TF, Smolak L, editors. Body image: a handbook of science, practice, and prevention. New York: Guilford; 2011. p. 12–9.
43. Riva G. Medical clinical uses of virtual worlds. In: Grimshaw M, editor. The Oxford handbook of virtuality. New York: Oxford University Press; 2014. p. 649–65.
44. Riva G. Out of my real body: cognitive neuroscience meets eating disorders. Front Hum Neurosci. 2014;8:236.

45. Dakanalis A, Riva G. Mass media, body image and eating disturbances: the underline mechanism through the lens of the objectification theory. In: Latzer J, Merrick J, Stein D, editors. Body image: gender differences, sociocultural influences and health implication. New York: Nova Science; 2013. p. 217–36.
46. Riva G, Dakanalis A. Altered processing and integration of multisensory bodily representations and signals in eating disorders: a possible path toward the understanding of their underlying causes. Front Hum Neurosci. 2018;12:49.
47. Tsakiris M. The multisensory basis of the self: from body to identity to others. Q J Exp Psychol. 2017;70(4):597–609.
48. Talsma D. Predictive coding and multisensory integration: an attentional account of the multisensory mind. Front Integr Neurosci. 2015;9:19.
49. Riva G, Gaudio S. Locked to a wrong body: eating disorders as the outcome of a primary disturbance in multisensory body integration. Conscious Cogn. 2018;59:57–9.
50. Riva G. The neuroscience of body memory: from the self through the space to the others. Cortex. 2018;104:241–60.
51. Shriver LH, Dollar JM, Lawless M, Calkins SD, Keane SP, Shanahan L, et al. Longitudinal associations between emotion regulation and adiposity in late adolescence: indirect effects through eating behaviors. Nutrients. 2019;11(3):517.
52. Fink PW, Shultz SP, D'Hondt E, Lenoir M, Hills AP. Multifractal analysis differentiates postural sway in obese and nonobese children. Mot Control. 2019;23(2):262–71.
53. Gardner RM, Salaz V, Reyes B, Brake SJ. Sensitivity to proprioceptive feedback in obese subjects. Percept Mot Skills. 1983;57(3 Suppl):1111–8.
54. Simmons WK, DeVille DC. Interoceptive contributions to healthy eating and obesity. Curr Opin Psychol. 2017;17:106–12.
55. Scarpina F, Migliorati D, Marzullo P, Mauro A, Scacchi M, Costantini M. Altered multisensory temporal integration in obesity. Sci Rep. 2016;6:28382.
56. Paulus MP, Stein MB. Interoception in anxiety and depression. Brain Struct Funct. 2010;214(5–6):451–63.
57. Riva G. Neuroscience and eating disorders: the allocentric lock hypothesis. Med Hypotheses. 2012;78:254–7.
58. Riva G, Gaudio S, Dakanalis AI. I'm in a virtual body: a locked allocentric memory may impair the experience of the body in both obesity and anorexia nervosa. Eat Weight Disord. 2013;19(1):133–4.
59. Akhtar S, Justice LV, Loveday C, Conway MA. Switching memory perspective. Conscious Cogn. 2017;56(Supplement C):50–7.
60. Riva G. The key to unlocking the virtual body: virtual reality in the treatment of obesity and eating disorders. J Diabetes Sci Technol. 2011;5(2):283–92.
61. Normand JM, Giannopoulos E, Spanlang B, Slater M. Multisensory stimulation can induce an illusion of larger belly size in immersive virtual reality. PLoS One. 2011;6(1):e16128.
62. Gutiérrez-Maldonado J, Wiederhold BK, Riva G. Future directions: how virtual reality can further improve the assessment and treatment of eating disorders and obesity. Cyberpsychol Behav Soc Netw. 2016;19:148–53.
63. Osimo SA, Pizarro R, Spanlang B, Slater M. Conversations between self and self as Sigmund Freud—a virtual body ownership paradigm for self-counselling. Sci Rep. 2015;5:13899.
64. Butters JW, Cash TF. Cognitive-behavioral treatment of women's body image satisfaction: a controlled outcome-study. J Consult Clin Psychol. 1987;55:889–97.
65. Wooley SC, Wooley OW. Intensive out-patient and residential treatment for bulimia. In: Garner DM, Garfinkel PE, editors. Handbook of psychotherapy for anorexia and bulimia. New York: Guilford Press; 1985. p. 120–32.
66. Leuner H. Guided affective imagery: a method of intensive psychotherapy. Am J Psychother. 1969;23:4–21.
67. Cesa GL, Manzoni GM, Bacchetta M, Castelnuovo G, Conti S, Gaggioli A, et al. Virtual reality for enhancing the cognitive behavioral treatment of obesity with binge eating disorder: randomized controlled study with one-year follow-up. J Med Internet Res. 2013;15(6):e113.

68. Manzoni GM, Cesa GL, Bacchetta M, Castelnuovo G, Conti S, Gaggioli A, et al. Virtual reality-enhanced cognitive-behavioral therapy for morbid obesity: a randomized controlled study with 1 year follow-up. Cyberpsychol Behav Soc Netw. 2016;19(2):134–40.
69. Botvinick M, Cohen J. Rubber hands 'feel' touch that eyes see. Nature. 1998;391(6669):756.
70. Serino S, Pedroli E, Keizer A, Triberti S, Dakanalis A, Pallavicini F, et al. Virtual reality body swapping: a tool for modifying the allocentric memory of the body. Cyberpsychol Behav Soc Netw. 2016;19(2):127–33.
71. Serino S, Scarpina F, Keizer A, Pedroli E, Dakanalis A, Castelnuovo G, et al. A novel technique for improving bodily experience in a non-operable super-super obesity case. Front Psychol. 2016;7:837.
72. Preston C, Ehrsson HH. Illusory changes in body size modulate body satisfaction in a way that is related to non-clinical eating disorder psychopathology. PLoS One. 2014;9(1):e85773.

Repetitive Transcranial Magnetic Stimulation

13

Matteo Bigoni, Lorenzo Priano, Alessandro Mauro, and Paolo Capodaglio

Key Points

- rTMS modifies cerebral activity level by means of noninvasive application of magnetic fields.
- Low-frequency (<1 Hz) TMS inhibits cortical excitability, and high-frequency (>5 Hz) TMS enhances cortical excitability by increasing neuronal depolarization.
- Nonmajor side effects have been reported; the most frequently reported event is a short-lasting headache; risk of seizure is not high, but more frequent with high-frequency stimulation; epilepsy and medications that reduce seizure threshold represent relative contraindications to rTMS.
- Based on the similarity between food craving and addiction and neuroimaging studies, treatment of eating disorder related to obesity with rTMS and dTMS has been proposed in the last years.

M. Bigoni (✉)
Neurology and Neurorehabilitation Division, "S. Giuseppe" Hospital, Istituto Auxologico Italiano IRCCS, Piancavallo, Italy
e-mail: m.bigoni@auxologico.it

L. Priano · A. Mauro
Neurology and Neurorehabilitation Division, "S. Giuseppe" Hospital, Istituto Auxologico Italiano IRCCS, Piancavallo, Italy

"R. Levi Montalcini" Neuroscience Department, University of Turin, Turin, Italy
e-mail: lorenzo.priano@unito.it; alessandro.mauro@unito.it

P. Capodaglio
Rehabilitation Unit, Physiotherapy and Research Laboratory in Biomechanics and Rehabilitation, "S. Giuseppe" Hospital, Istituto Auxologico Italiano IRCCS, Piancavallo, Italy
e-mail: p.capodaglio@auxologico.it

P. Capodaglio (ed.), *Rehabilitation Interventions in the Patient with Obesity*, https://doi.org/10.1007/978-3-030-32274-8_13

- There is evidence in favor of a reduction of food craving following high-frequency rTMS treatment on the left dorsolateral-prefrontal cortex.
- In general, the level of evidence of rTMS treatment so far is A for mood disorder and neuropathic pain, and B for stroke patient.

New health technologies are a hot topic for rehabilitation treatments [1]. New high-tech instruments are nowadays available and there is also pressure from patients looking for novel effective approaches. This is the case of the transcranial magnetic stimulation (TMS) techniques and in general of the neuromodulation approach. The key feature of these technologies is the chance to modify the cerebral level of activity by means of noninvasive magnetic field application [2, 3]. TMS is not the only way to perform neuromodulation and the technique itself presents different modalities of application. To decide which one is the best for obese patients, it is important to understand the neurocognitive point of view about obesity. There are at least four different models [4]: the "food addiction" model, the reward hyper-responsivity theory, the opposite reward hypo-responsivity theory, and the lack of inhibitory control theory.

In line with the aim of this book, the main topic that will be discussed here is the applications of noninvasive neuromodulation rTMS techniques in psychological and behavioral disorders associated with obesity. Some stimulation protocols have been proven to be of clinical effectiveness in mood disorders [5]. Moreover, scientific research is now addressing the effects of these treatments on metabolic processes [6, 7].

In this chapter, we discuss the following topics:

- The basic theoretical information about rTMS as a tool that can modify the activity of central nervous system for therapeutic purposes
- The recommendations for a safe use of rTMS
- The indications provided by guidelines to orientate among the different protocols of treatment for obese patients
- The new perspective of research in this field

13.1 Plasticity and Neuromodulation: What Is Stimulated and Why

The greater misunderstanding of the twentieth-century neuroscience was the attribution of static property to central nervous system that is not responding to the simplest empiric observation that can be done by everyone, e.g., the learning ability. This happened even if a lot of information about the functioning of the fundamental element of this system (neuron) was already present. The key concept to understand it is the extraordinary feature of these biological "devices" that works through a dialogue between biochemical and electrical phenomena. On the other hand, the great novelty of the twenty-first-century neuroscience was the introduction of the concept of plasticity that involves the basic functioning of the same system that till some years ago was believed to be unchangeable [8].

Plasticity could be described as the ability of a system to permanently modify its function or structure after a stimulus or an experience as occurring in everyone's daily life. Every single experience can contribute to shaping the activity of nervous system. The fundamental rule of this process is that the more intense and repeated the stimulus is, the more it will be able to induce functional and/or structural changes maintained over time [8]. This gives an immediate idea to the burden that could derive from certain behaviors and eating habits in obese patients.

The potential plasticity is known to act in two different directions [9]:

- *Long-term potentiation effect (LTP)*: This leads to a greater neuronal response after repetitive stimuli typically applied with high frequencies (Figs. 13.1 and 13.2).
- *Long-term depression effect (LTD)*: This gives a reduction in the neuronal response after repetitive stimuli applied with low frequencies (Figs. 13.3 and 13.4).

In the plasticity concept, "long term" indicates a regulation divided into two phases: an early phase (within 90 min) and a late phase (lasting more than few hours, due to protein modifications). In the regulation of these responses both electrical and biochemical neuronal activities physiologically interact at different levels:

- *Synaptic activity*: This is the first level of nervous system modulation with gain or lowering function, as far for the possibility to have an extension or a reduction of the dendritic tree, according, respectively, with *potentiation* or *depression* processes explained above; the main driver of synaptic plasticity seems to be glutamate that activates NMDA channels allowing calcium intake in the postsynaptic neurons.

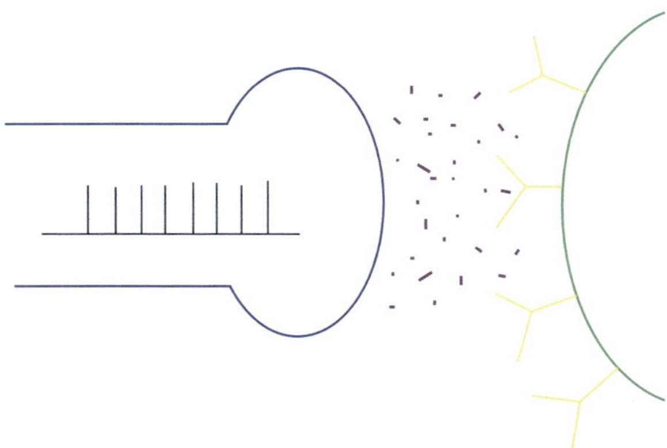

Fig. 13.1 Mechanism of synaptic plasticity where potentiation occurs after a high-frequency stimulation (identified as a sequence of spike in the presynaptic termination) that produces a release of neurotransmitters and an overexpression of postsynaptic receptors

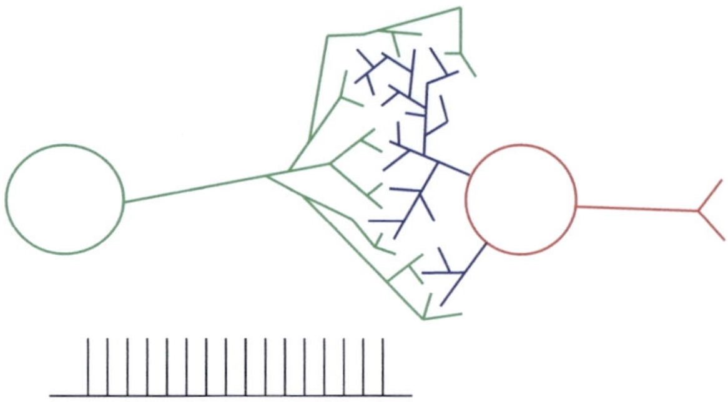

Fig. 13.2 Structural effects of plasticity with widening of the dendritic tree after a high-frequency stimulation

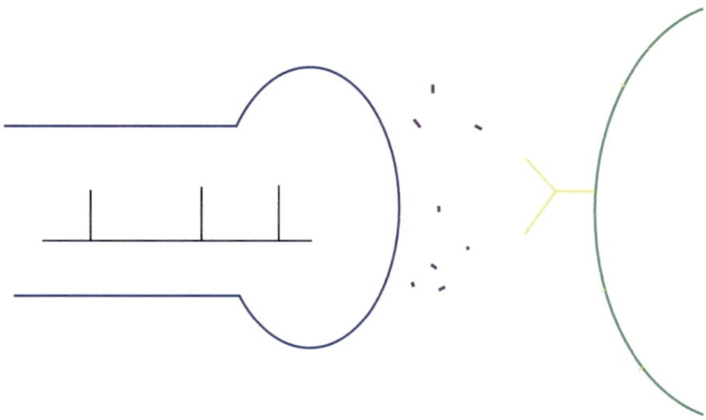

Fig. 13.3 Mechanism of synaptic plasticity where depression occurs after a low-frequency stimulation (identified as a poor sequence of spike in the presynaptic termination) that gives a lowering of the neurotransmitter release and a downregulation of postsynaptic receptors

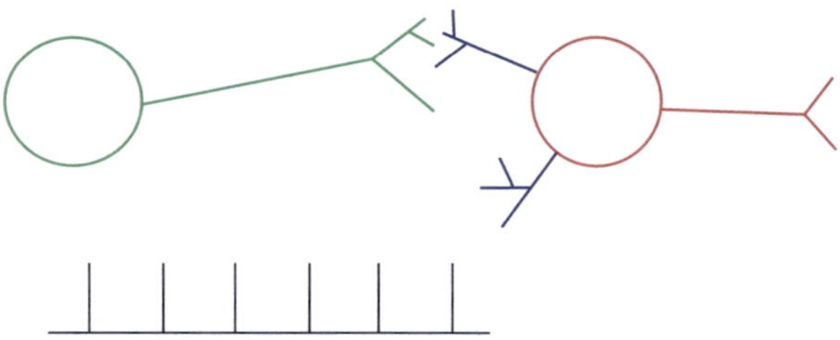

Fig. 13.4 Structural effects of plasticity with reduction of the dendritic tree after a low-frequency stimulation

- *Neuronal differentiation*: It is the second level of structural modulation by means of different growth factors such as the well-known *nerve growth factor* (NGF) and the *brain-derived nerve growth factor* (BDNF) to support the so-called neurogenesis or on the other hand to stimulate apoptotic processes.

– *Neuronal network organization*: This is the last and more wide level of plasticity, by means of changes in the extension of a specific cortical area involved in an as much specific function (these changes were confirmed by TMS cortical mapping studies or functional magnetic resonance studies).

The development of the modern neuromodulation techniques got started with the use of transcranial noninvasive magnetic stimulation in the 80s of the last century, for the assessment of neuron excitability of the central neuronal motor pathways. Applying the same magnetic stimulus in sequences, a potentiation or a depression of the activity of the same motor pathways can be observed.

Such magnetic stimulus is produced by a specific device that can generate a magnetic field obtained with a high-intensity electric current that passes through a metal coil. What is important to remind is that the effect we observe by applying a magnetic stimulus to the patient's scalp is the resultant of the interaction between two physical quantities and the neuronal tissue:

– The electric field, which is not the one that passes through the coil, but a second one, that is generated in the patient's cortex as the result of the neuronal network activation by the magnetic field (perpendicular to it) (Fig. 13.5): The power of the electric field is sufficient to stimulate the axons of the cortical neurons, producing a motor-evoked potential.
– The magnetic field, which is produced within the coil and is perpendicular to the coil itself: Magnetic field is the real one responsible for the plastic phenomena due to the modulation of intercortical neurons (a special neuronal population that connect horizontally cortical neuron in particular of the pyramidal system).

By taking into account all of these information, we acknowledge that only rTMS techniques have both neurostimulation and neuromodulation properties, unlike the widely diffuse transcranial direct current stimulation (TDCS), which has only a neuromodulation effect (due to the low level in current intensity that is not able to activate—and therefore stimulate—axons). According to a difference in impedance between gray matter and white matter, the subcortical structures

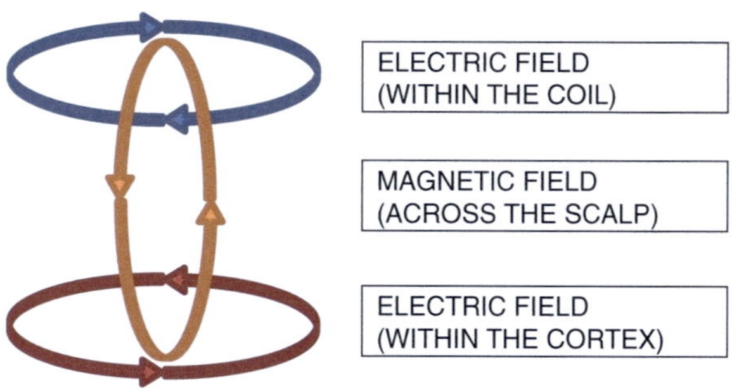

Fig. 13.5 Mechanism of rTMS

(e.g., basal ganglia and thalamus) are not stimulated by rTMS, whose effect is limited to a depth of 1.5 cm [9].

13.1.1 rTMS Techniques, Protocols, and Safety Considerations

There are different types of coils in order to achieve the desired goal (Fig. 13.6): circular coils are used for simple TMS diagnostic studies of motor pathways but are not very focal; eight-shaped coils are more often indicated for rTMS due to their very focal stimulation on cortical area (for rTMS treatment: focal stimulation is considered advantageous); finally, in order to allow a deeper stimulation, a double-cone-shaped coil and an H-shaped coil were developed, which can stimulate at a depth of 4 cm (this is the so-called deep TMS or dTMS), useful to stimulate the insula region [9, 10]. The coils used for rTMS are generally provided with a cooling system because their functioning produces heat.

As for the effects of the different types of stimulation [3]: low-frequency (LF ≤1 Hz) TMS inhibits cortical excitability, whereas high-frequency (HF >5 Hz) TMS enhances cortical excitability by increasing neuronal depolarization. Therefore, different protocols can be defined. The parameters to consider are the following:

- Resting motor threshold (RMT): This is defined as the stimulator intensity output that can evoke a motor potential of 100 μV in the 50% of tests (generally 5/10). It is also accepted to consider the intensity able to generate the muscular twitch in first digital interosseous. LF protocols are performed below RMT, and HF protocols are performed with an intensity higher than RMT.
- Frequency and pattern of stimulation (see Table 13.1): In conventional protocols, the main parameter is the frequency rate; in other patterned protocols every single pulse is replaced by a burst of three pulses at high frequencies (the so-called theta burst stimulation—TBS) and this group of stimuli can be administered at a low-frequency interval in a continuous way (cTBS) or with a higher frequency in an intermittent way (iTBS). Both conventional and patterned can be divided into

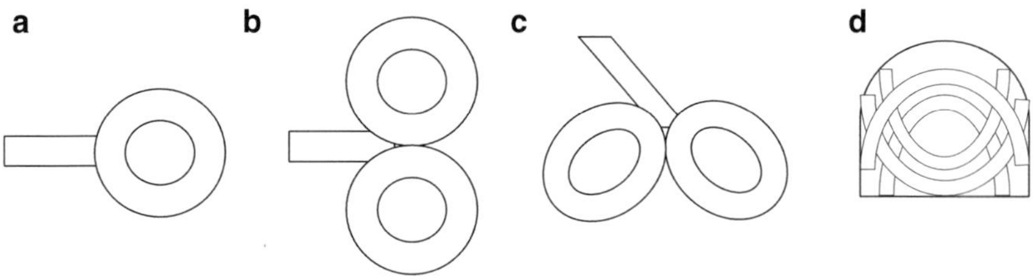

Fig. 13.6 Schematic representation of different types of coil. (**a**) Circular coil (magnetic field has a dimension of few centimeters), (**b**) 8-shaped coil (can produce a focal magnetic field centered in the central point of superimposition of the two rings), (**c**) double-cone coil (also produces a focal magnetic field but at a greater depth than the previous one), (**d**) H coil (it is a helmet with a lot of coils surrounding frontal and lateral parts of the skull: has been indicated by thinner lines)

Table 13.1 Types of rTMS protocols

<table>
<tr><th></th><th>Conventional rTMS</th><th>Patterned (TBS)</th></tr>
<tr><td>Inhibitory effect</td><td>LF = 1 Hz
| | | | | | | | | |</td><td>cTBS (burst run at 1 Hz)
| | | | | | | : 1 Hz
↓ ↘ ↘
||| ||| ||| (3 pulses at 50 Hz)</td></tr>
<tr><td>Activating effect</td><td>HF = 5 Hz – 25 Hz
||||||| ____ |||||||| ____ |||||||</td><td>iTBS (burst run at 5 to 25 Hz)
| | | | ____ | | | | ____ | | | |
↓ ↘ ↘ ↘
||| ||| ||| ||| (3 pulses at 50 Hz)</td></tr>
</table>

inhibitory (applied continuously) and activating protocols (applied in trains of stimuli, see below).

- Train of stimuli: Both conventional and patterned activating protocols are administered in trains of stimuli (between 2 and 5 s) interspersed with pauses that allows cooling of the brain and the coil.
- Number of sessions: Different schemes of treatment have been proposed by different authors, from a single-session treatment to 3–5 sessions per week, repeated for more than 2 weeks.
- Site/sites of stimulation: Depending on the expected effects, it/they can vary and range from one (e.g., left frontal area) to two (e.g., bilateral frontal areas) to a more diffuse stimulation using an H coil, or even associated with peripheral nerve stimulation (the so-called PAS technique) to enhance LTP phenomena.

In 2009, a Consensus Group [3] revised the most important safety considerations:

- *Patient safety*: Avoid overheating (almost every rTMS device includes heat sensors which automatically limit the stimulation, according to the consensus indications). Nonmajor side effects have been reported and the most frequent event is a short-lasting headache. The risk of seizures is not high, but more frequent with HF stimulation. Therefore, epilepsy and medications that reduce seizure threshold represent relative contraindications. Again, when considering patient safety the presence of devices that could interact with magnetic field should be considered. It is recommended to sign an informed consent that excludes relative or absolute contraindications, and those in use for magnetic resonance.
- *Staff safety and training*: Staff who work with magnetic field should refer to guidelines about the correct management of those techniques monitoring electromagnetic exposition and correct training about the use of such medical devices under the supervision of an as well-trained physician. In some countries, neurophysiology technicians undergo a specific training about the management of electric and magnetic field, the technical skill to perform examinations, and the

patients' treatments. It is important, for example, to know the different positions of the possible cerebral target areas, the use of a neuro-navigation system, and the indication about the correct coil positioning (it is known that a simple variation of coil alignment can significantly decrease the treatment effectiveness) parallel to the sagittal plane [11].

13.1.2 rTMS and dTMS

In the past 20 years, the possibility to treat eating disorder and obesity was investigated with the application of different neuromodulation techniques. Among those, rTMS had already shown some evidence about positive effects [12]. In particular, cerebral regions such as the lateral prefrontal cortex (LPCF), striatum, and insula, previously found to be altered in neuroimaging studies [13], are targets of rTMS. These regions are involved in the emotional responses and executive functions, including inhibitory control for food assumption and reward processes. According to McClelland's findings, until 2012 only one study with tDCS had been conducted on people affected by obesity, no studies in patients with binge eating disorder (BED), while different neuromodulation techniques had already been applied to bulimia nervosa and anorexia nervosa as well as to addictions [14]. The overall conclusion was in favor of a reduction of food craving especially with rTMS treatment on the left dorsolateral-prefrontal cortex (DPLFC). Based on these concepts of similarity between food craving and addiction, and the evidence from neuroimaging studies, in the last few years the treatment of eating disorder related to obesity has been proposed [15]. A study investigating the effects of rTMS on metabolic pathways [16] confirmed the positive effect of treating left DPLFC with a high-frequency protocol (HF) in healthy subjects under stress condition, showing a decrease of cortisol level that indicates an influence on the hypothalamic-pituitary-adrenal (HPA) system. A more comprehensive review about neuroimaging techniques in eating disorders [13] confirmed the findings of previous studies supporting the use of neuromodulation techniques in treating obesity. This represents a shift of paradigm in treating obesity: from behavioral to neurocognitive treatments. rTMS should specifically interact with the "food addiction" model or the "lack of inhibitory control" theory with a frontal HF stimulation [4, 17].

Clinical trials specifically designed for obese patients are scanty. A protocol with HF rTMS on left DLPFC for obese women with BED has been proposed [18]. More recently, dTMS was chosen to test the effects of bilateral DLPFC stimulation, with follow-up at 9 weeks and 1 year [7]. This second pilot study showed a significant reduction of food craving and, consequently of body weight and BMI, at 1-year follow-up. Other significant effects observed were a reduction of leptin level and an increase of epinephrine. The protocol included HF, LF, and a sham stimulation for 15 sessions over 5 weeks. Only HF stimulation was able to add benefits to the combined diet and physical activity program. The site of stimulation with an H coil was the PFC and the insula bilaterally. The effect hypothesized by the authors was that HF dTMS could possibly stimulate the dopaminergic pathways, leading to a modulation on behavioral inhibitory control via PFC and the mesolimbic system. The same authors published another paper [6, 7] on the metabolic effects of a single-session treatment in the same patients described above (with HF, LF, and sham stimulations). The main finding was an increase of β-endorphin level. The explanation about the main underlying mechanism of action could be the same as for the longer treatment protocol considered before.

In conclusion, rTMS, and nowadays also dTMS, has a precise rationale and different treatment protocols can provide short- and long-term results. The strength of rTMS relies on its ease of use and the possibility to perform individualized therapy. According to the last guidelines [1], strong evidence of effectiveness exists in different pathologies: level A for mood disorder and neuropathic pain, and level B for motor training in stroke patients and a growing number of evidences in the last very few years. The effects on eating disorder are clear but with respect to obesity further studies should be conducted to define new treatment options addressing the different pathogenic mechanisms of this condition. Another interesting topic is the effectiveness of this treatment alone vs. the effects combined with rehabilitation: according to the 2014 guidelines, the majority of trials showed greater improvement when rTMS was combined with rehabilitative programs performed during the plasticity window provided by LTP mechanism. This is probably the way to define correct neuro-modulation treatments in patients with obesity.

13.1.3 Noninvasive and Invasive Neuromodulation

Noninvasive neuromodulation represents a range of very appealing and different techniques developed in the last 20 years [17, 19–21]. tDCS and its variants have now a widespread diffusion with respect to rTMS, mainly due to reduced costs, ease of use, and transportability. Other noninvasive neuromodulation techniques proposed in the literature are the peripheral noninvasive vagal stimulation and the neuro-biofeedback with functional magnetic resonance. Vivid interest also exists towards invasive neuromodulation techniques such as the invasive vagal nerve stimulation and the deep brain stimulation (DBP). The latter is a consolidated technique in Parkinson's disease. The problems of those latter treatments are the risk of serious side effects of the invasive procedure, high costs, and a still preliminary evidence of effectiveness. It should also be noted, however, that the mechanism of DBS may be different from the other neuromodulation techniques, since it addresses the hyper-responsivity of the food reward system [4].

References

1. Lefaucheur JP, André-Obadia N, Antal A, Ayache SS, Baeken C, Benninger DH, Cantello RM, Cincotta M, de Carvalho M, De Ridder D, Devanne H, Di Lazzaro V, Filipović SR, Hummel FC, Jääskeläinen SK, Kimiskidis VK, Koch G, Langguth B, Nyffeler T, Oliviero A, Padberg F, Poulet E, Rossi S, Rossini PM, Rothwell JC, Schönfeldt-Lecuona C, Siebner HR, Slotema CW, Stagg CJ, Valls-Sole J, Ziemann U, Paulus W, Garcia-Larrea L. Evidence-based guidelines on the therapeutic use of repetitive transcranial magnetic stimulation (rTMS). Clin Neurophysiol. 2014;125(11):2150–206.
2. Klomjai W, Katz R, Lackmy-Vallée A. Basic principles of transcranial magnetic stimulation (TMS) and repetitive TMS (rTMS). Ann Phys Rehabil Med. 2015;58(4):208–13.
3. Rossi S, Hallett M, Rossini PM, Pascual-Leone A, Safety of TMS Consensus Group. Safety, ethical considerations, and application guidelines for the use of transcranial magnetic stimulation in clinical practice and research. Clin Neurophysiol. 2009;120(12):2008–39.
4. Göbel CH, Tronnier VM, Münte TF. Brain stimulation in obesity. Int J Obes. 2017;41(12):1721–7.
5. McClintock SM, Reti IM, Carpenter LL, McDonald WM, Dubin M, Taylor SF, Cook IA, O'Reardon J, Husain MM, Wall C, Krystal AD, Sampson SM, Morales O, Nelson BG, Latoussakis V, George MS, Lisanby SH, National Network of Depression Centers rTMS Task Group, American Psychiatric Association Council on Research Task Force on Novel Biomarkers and Treatments. Consensus recommendations for the clinical application of repetitive transcranial magnetic stimulation (rTMS) in the treatment of depression. J Clin Psychiatry. 2018;79(1):16cs10905.
6. Ferrulli A, Macrì C, Terruzzi I, Ambrogi F, Milani V, Adamo M, Luzi L. High frequency deep transcranial magnetic stimulation acutely increases β-endorphins in obese humans. Endocrine. 2019a;64(1):67–74.
7. Ferrulli A, Macrì C, Terruzzi I, Massarini S, Ambrogi F, Adamo M, Milani V, Luzi L. Weight loss induced by deep transcranial magnetic stimulation in obesity: a randomized, double-blind, sham-controlled study. Diabetes Obes Metab. 2019b;21(8):1849–60.
8. Gulyaeva NV. Molecular mechanisms of neuroplasticity: an expanding universe. Biochemistry (Mosc). 2017;82(3):237–42.
9. Cirillo G, Di Pino G, Capone F, Ranieri F, Florio L, Todisco V, Tedeschi G, Funke K. Di Lazzaro V. Neurobiological after-effects of non-invasive brain stimulation. Brain Stimul. 2017;10(1):1–18.
10. Lu M, Ueno S. Comparison of the induced fields using different coil configurations during deep transcranial magnetic stimulation. PLoS One. 2017;12(6):e0178422.
11. D'Ostilio K, Goetz SM, Hannah R, Ciocca M, Chieffo R, Chen JA, Peterchev AV, Rothwell JC. Effect of coil orientation on strength-duration time constant and I-wave activation with controllable pulse parameter transcranial magnetic stimulation. Clin Neurophysiol. 2016;127(1):675–83.
12. McClelland J, Bozhilova N, Campbell I, Schmidt U. A systematic review of the effects of neuromodulation on eating and body weight: evidence from human and animal studies. Eur Eat Disord Rev. 2013;21(6):436–55.
13. Val-Laillet D, Aarts E, Weber B, Ferrari M, Quaresima V, Stoeckel LE, Alonso-Alonso M, Audette M, Malbert CH, Stice E. Neuroimaging and neuromodulation approaches to study eating behavior and prevent and treat eating disorders and obesity. Neuroimage Clin. 2015;8:1–31.
14. Makani R, Pradhan B, Shah U, Parikh T. Role of repetitive transcranial magnetic stimulation (rTMS) in treatment of addiction and related disorders: a systematic review. Curr Drug Abuse Rev. 2017;10(1):31–43.
15. Rami Bou Khalil, Charline El Hachem, (2014) Potential role of repetitive transcranial magnetic stimulation in obesity. Eating and Weight Disorders - Studies on Anorexia, Bulimia and Obesity 19(3):403–407.

16. C. Baeken, M.A. Vanderhasselt, J. Remue, V. Rossi, J. Schiettecatte, E. Anckaert, R. De Raedt, (2014) One left dorsolateral prefrontal cortical HF-rTMS session attenuates HPA-system sensitivity to critical feedback in healthy females. Neuropsychologia 57:112–121.
17. Lee DJ, Elias GJB, Lozano AM. Neuromodulation for the treatment of eating disorders and obesity. Ther Adv Psychopharmacol. 2018;8(2):73–92.
18. Maranhão MF, Estella NM, Cury ME, Amigo VL, Picasso CM, Berberian A, Campbell I, Schmidt U, Claudino AM. The effects of repetitive transcranial magnetic stimulation in obese females with binge eating disorder: a protocol for a double-blinded, randomized, sham-controlled trial. BMC Psychiatry. 2015;15:194.
19. Jáuregui-Lobera I, Martínez-Quiñones JV. Neuromodulation in eating disorders and obesity: a promising way of treatment? Neuropsychiatr Dis Treat. 2018;14:2817–35.
20. Hall PA, Vincent CM, Burhan AM. Non-invasive brain stimulation for food cravings, consumption, and disorders of eating: a review of methods, findings and controversies. Appetite. 2018;124:78–88.
21. Pleger B. Invasive and non-invasive stimulation of the obese human brain. Front Neurosci. 2018;12:884.

Mobile Technologies 14

Roberto Cattivelli, Anna Guerrini Usubini, Anna Maria Mirto, Camilla Pietrantonio, Nicola Cau, Manuela Galli, Valentina Granese, Giorgia Varallo, Giada Pietrabissa, Gian Mauro Manzoni, Enrico Molinari, and Gianluca Castelnuovo

R. Cattivelli · C. Pietrantonio · V. Granese · G. Varallo · G. M. Manzoni · E. Molinari
G. Castelnuovo (✉)
Psychology Research Laboratory, Istituto Auxologico Italiano IRCCS, Ospedale San Giuseppe, Verbania, Italy

Department of Psychology, Catholic University of Milan, Milan, Italy
e-mail: r.cattivelli@auxologico.it; gm.manzoni@auxologico.it; molinari@auxologico.it; gianluca.castelnuovo@auxologico.it

A. Guerrini Usubini · A. M. Mirto
Psychology Research Laboratory, Istituto Auxologico Italiano IRCCS, Ospedale San Giuseppe, Verbania, Italy

N. Cau
Research Laboratory in Biomechanics and Rehabilitation, Istituto Auxologico Italiano IRCCS, Ospedale San Giuseppe, Verbania, Italy
e-mail: n.cau@auxologico.it

M. Galli
Dipartimento di Elettronica, Informazione e Bioingegneria, Politecnico di Milano, Milan, Italy
e-mail: manuela.galli@polimi.it

G. Pietrabissa
Department of Psychology, Catholic University of Milan, Milan, Italy

Psychology Research Laboratory, Istituto Auxologico Italiano IRCCS, Ospedale San Luca, Milan, Italy

P. Capodaglio (ed.), *Rehabilitation Interventions in the Patient with Obesity*,
https://doi.org/10.1007/978-3-030-32274-8_14

Key Points

- *Broad diffusion of mobile tech and fitness smartphone app for physical activity (PA)*: Thousands of app for smartphone, almost 700 wearables and more than 100 apps directly linked to smartbands and smartwatches.
- *Mobile tech seems to be effective in the promotion of PA*: Wearables and smartphone app for PA are effective to improve PA as midterm outcome compared to PA prescription alone.
- *Five core points of behavioral change techniques (BCT) of mobile app to enhance mobile tech*: (1) Self-monitoring; (2) goal setting with counselor feedback and communication; (3) social support; (4) structured program; and (5) individually tailored program.
- *Guidelines to choose mobile app and wearable devices*: Select apps and wearables that are empirically tested and with an evidence-based cutoff to foster interpretation of results.

Obesity is traditionally defined as a body mass index (BMI) of greater than 30 kg/m^2 and is today considered a public health problem and a global epidemia [1, 2] according to World Health Organization (WHO) that estimates a global incidence of over 700 million individuals [3, 4]. Despite the etiology of obesity being multifactorial, there is a strong consensus in the scientific community that behavioral factors, and in particular poor diet and physical inactivity, are among the main proximal causes linked to obesity [5].

Physical activity (PA) is recommended as an important part of weight management by virtually all public health agencies and scientific organizations including WHO, National Heart, Lung, and Blood Institute (NHLBI) Centers for Disease Control (CDC), American College of Sports Medicine (ACSM), and various medical societies (American Heart Association, American Medical Association, American Academy of Family Physicians) [6, 7]. Guidelines provided by WHO underline that adults aged between 18 and 64 should do at least 150 min of moderate-intensity aerobic physical activity or 75 min of vigorous-intensity physical activity throughout the week or an equivalent combination of moderate- and vigorous-intensity activity [8].

The general physical activity recommendations from the CDC and Prevention for health promotion suggest the consumption of 1000 kcal/week, corresponding approximately to the energy expended in walking 30 min/day [8, 9].

Nevertheless, several studies demonstrated that rehabilitation programs focused on increase of PA have generally only good short-term efficacy [10, 11]. Even the most intensive intervention was ineffective in promoting adherence to exercise in the absence of further incentives to maintain changes in lifestyle (The Newcastle exercise project: a randomized controlled trial of methods to promote physical activity in primary care, Jane Harland, Martin White, Chris Drinkwater, David Chinn, Lorna Farr, Denise Howel).

Behavioral change techniques (BCTs), as goal setting and contingent feedback, seem to be the most effective way to promote healthy lifestyle helping individuals to meet the physical activity recommendations and with mobile technology implementation offer an innovative way to sustain the process of habit changes [12, 13]. Thanks to the large adoption of wearable devices able to measure and store data about PA and to provide contingent feedbacks and reminders, a large-scale health revolution has begun [14–16]. The availability of smartphone applications has contributed to a better understanding of human health by allowing us to assess precious, contingent data for medical and fitness area [14, 16–18] taking advantages of some improvements in app technology (e.g., a built-in camera for heart rate assessment, accelerometers) that have proved useful [19–22] and supported by current reviews of mHealth (healthcare practice supported by mobile devices). Further, the capability of mobile technology to improve access to a large number of people living far from clinical centers, reduce costs, and enhance health outcomes for management of chronic health condition represents the core feature of these apps, connected with their potential and effectiveness for remote monitoring of clinical parameters, such as cardiovascular disease (CVD) risk factors [18], and for implementing behavioral change strategies aimed to promote healthy habits, in particular regarding compliance to therapies, diet, and physical activity. Nevertheless, further investigation is needed to enhance the validity and reliability of existing fitness apps for PA promotion in both contexts [18].

14.1 Role of Mobile Technology to Increase PA: A Perspective

As previously reported, evidences show that the achieved results in long-term habit change are not maintained at 1-year follow-up, with a gradual return to the baseline level of activity [5, 10, 23, 24] in the absence of further incentives to maintain changes in lifestyle. According to the Newcastle exercise project [25], an intervention based on combining exercise plan and behavioral changes will increase physical activity rather than the mere exercise prescription. For these reasons, a promising field of application is represented by implementation of mobile technology and wearable devices with smartphone app, focusing on core aspects of behavioral change such as self-monitoring, for example, using accelerometers to check daily steps, or stimulus control (i.e., with advertising regarding sedentary behavior) and behavioral modification (setting sustainable goals for exercising) [26–28]. In this context, an app-based approach could overcome these challenges associated with traditional approaches, allowing for broader promotion of PA. In clinical and sports setting the use of technological tools such as valid and reliable fitness apps allows professionals to select the optimal assessment protocol for patients or clients and provides a more objective daily measure of physiological signals, but also they support individuals with constant and customized feedback, supporting the whole process of changing lifestyle.

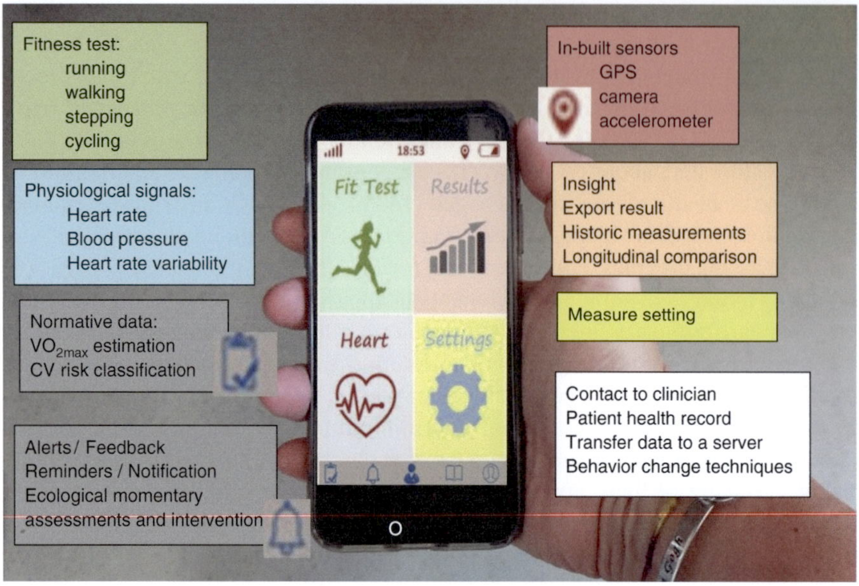

Fig. 14.1 Key factors to be considered when selecting or developing an app for assessing cardio-respiratory fitness

14.2 Efficacy and Cost-Effectiveness of Mobile Technology: Wearables and Smartphone App

In recent years, the field of wearable/mobile technology to enhance and promote PA is growing faster, such as the market of these apps. The main stores for these kind of products, Apple Store and Google Play, count thousands of "Apps," and their diffusion is every day broader [29]. In recent studies [14, 18, 29] focused on accuracy, validity, and reliability, the authors pointed out that, despite the number of the apps, only few are empirically tested [14]. Therefore, the technology seems to be valid and reliable, but further investigations are needed to develop (Fig. 14.1).

14.3 Behavioral Change Technique Components Crucial in Technology-Based Remote Weight-Loss Interventions

In general population only a small portion of individuals meet the required amount of PA [30], so in order to promote the compliance to existing guidelines and general recommendation, it is necessary to establish a starting point, prescribe individualized training programs, and monitor improvements [25, 31]. As mentioned above, BCTs implemented by mobile technologies have to be considered as a potentially determinant factor to foster PA in daily life [32] and therapeutic setting such as the management of obesity [16], and different recent works provide useful guide to select treatments and devices [14, 18]. In this regard, Khaylis et al. [33] provide a conceptualization of the five behavioral and psychological components crucial in technology-based weight-loss interventions that are successful in facilitating PA promotion.

1. Self-monitoring: It is defined as the way in which a person regulates and controls his/her own behavior. Mobile technologies can support this process by providing feedback about food intake and physical activity during daily life. Actually monitors, pedometers, and handheld PDA and other mobile technologies are easy to use and convenient, especially for those who do not have asses to high-speed Internet connections.
2. Counselor feedback and communication: During the period of rehabilitation within weight-loss program, patients and counselor or psychologist stay in contact by using mobile technologies. Participants can share their monitoring about food and exercise, while professionals encourage and sustain the rehabilitation process by providing online feedback and reinforcement using email.
3. Social support: A group treatment represents the preferred format for behavioral weight-loss intervention because it facilitates the social support, one of the most important factors for the promotion of behavioral change. In a group setting chat rooms, online meetings, and forums are useful technologies able to sustain communication, motivation, commonality, and encouragement among participants.
4. Structured program: Behavioral weight-loss interventions are based on a multidimensional approach which includes weekly lessons on nutrition, physical exercises, but also psychological factors such as goal setting, self-regulation strategies, and stimulus control.
5. Individually tailored program: Interventions are customized and individualized for participants in order to facilitate adherence and achievement of goals in terms of weight loss.

In the area of research of application of mobile technologies, only small-sized studies have directly assessed their efficacy for PA [18, 32]. Consequently, further researches are needed in order to improve the effectiveness and the efficacy of the use of mobile technology for the management of obesity.

With wider adoption of electronic health records to measure individual performance, there is a need to explore the use of these valuable tools, not only for identification and assessment of obesity but also for the delivery of obesity interventions.

14.4 Goal Setting Enhanced by Mobile Technology

Through goal setting the patient is supported to express the "representation of the desired outcomes to anchieve and criteria for judging them" [34, 35]. A goal-setting program useful for clinicians in rehabilitation consulting is proposed by Cullen et al. [36] and it is articulated in four specific steps: (1) recognizing a need for change, (2) establishing a goal, (3) adopting a goal-directed activity and self-monitoring it, and (4) finally self-rewarding goal attainment and its full applicability for PA promotion. For an effective goal setting, achievable goals are needed in order to obtain higher performance [35, 37]. Moreover, feedback and internal or external rewards are useful for boosting the motivation for achieving goals with simple tasks. Instead, people are less motivated when difficult assignments are perceived as not achievable [35]. Some recommendations were provided by Strecher et al. [35] for defining goals within BCTs including their implementation in mobile technology: (1) problem analysis and patients' efforts, (2) definition of tasks needed to deal with problems, and (3) provision of contingent feedback. The wearable devices are significantly useful for preventing the interruption of the goal achievement process since they allow data collection, monitoring, encouraging, and feedback delivery [13].

14.5 Self-Monitoring and Wearables

Another clinical strategy developed in the area of behavioral therapy applied to obesity's treatment is self-monitoring [38, 39], a "cornerstone" of behavioral intervention and BCTs [40]. Several processes are involved: self-observation, self-evaluation, and self-reinforcement. Self-monitoring is positively correlated with self-awareness, playing a crucial role in the eating behaviors allowing weight management [41]. In obesity treatment, Baker and Kirschenbaum [42] demonstrated that higher levels of weight control correlate with monitoring over all foods, time, quantity of food eaten, and percentage of fat ingested. New self-monitoring technology applied to weight loss ensures advantages for treatment, allowing individuals to set their own goals, comparing their self-monitoring data, reinforcing their achievements and pointing out higher adherence to self-monitoring and greater weight losses than traditional interventions [43]. Several reviews and meta-analyses reported evidences on eHealth intervention for weight management [20, 44]. A study conducted by Burke [45] compared the use of a personal digital assistant with dietary and exercise software, with and without a feedback message, and a paper diary/record. The results of this study showed that all participants had a significant weight loss, but those who received a personal digital assistant with a feedback message lost more than 5% weight compared to other groups. In conclusion, internet-based weight-loss and maintenance programs seem to be adequate approaches in moderating weight loss in obese patients [46]. Nevertheless, other studies are required to evaluate the efficacy of this new type of interventions.

14.6 NUDGE 2.0: Nudging Provided by Mobile Technology

Thaler and Sunstein's definition of a "nudge" as "any aspect of the choice architecture that alters people's behavior in a predictable way without forbidding any options or significantly changing their economic incentives" (2008) does not provide a precise operational definition of the applied meaning of those terms. The term

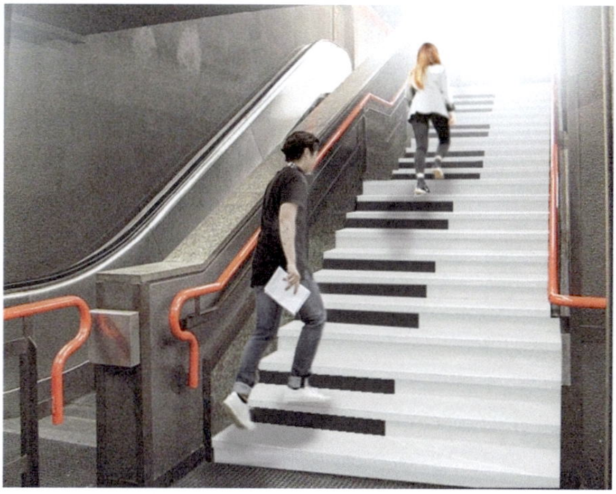

Fig. 14.2 A classical implementation of nudge intervention for physical activity promotion

"choice architecture" is defined as the environment within which people make choices [47, 48]. Hollands et al. [49] systematically review the evidence base for nudge (choice architecture) interventions and propose the following, more precise, operational definition of such interventions: "interventions that involve altering the properties or placement of objects or stimuli within micro-environments with the intention of changing health-related behavior (Fig. 14.2). Such interventions are implemented within the same micro-environment as that in which the target behavior is performed, typically require minimal conscious engagement, can in principle influence the behavior of many people simultaneously, and are not targeted or tailored to specific individuals."

Nudging could be enhanced by mobile technology, smartwatches, and wearables in particular, and could be crucial to promote PA. Some of the most meaningful implementations of nudging regard physical activity but are limited to specific places. Furthermore, merging nudging with smartwatch technology could bring nudge theory to a new level, fostering healthy habits with tailored suggestions, feedback, and advertising directly from the smartwatch display. Many apps for PA already implement basic principles of nudging, for example the vibration advertising for sedentary behaviors, but the future implementations could be crucial to promote more meaningful change. Some pioneering studies already show promising data [50] but we need more empirical works to deepen the feasibility and cost-effectiveness of the nudge procedure (Fig. 14.3).

14.7 Guidelines to Choose the Right Devices for the Scope

With over than 400 different wearable devices in the market to choose the right one could be difficult, in particular if there are specific aims to fulfill. So some recent articles analyze scientific literature providing useful guidelines to select the most useful for both individuals and groups. A work of the 2019 [18] pointed out the

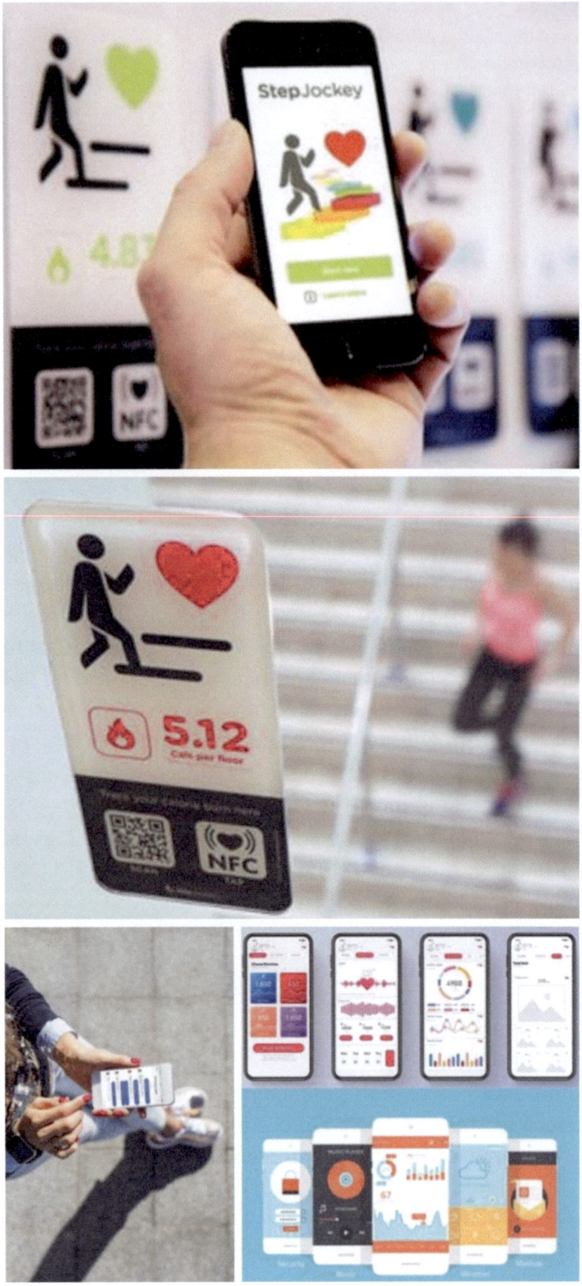

Fig. 14.3 Nudge implementation with smartphone app

importance to take into consideration only devices with adequate empirical support that fit the specific aims of the projects, for example rehabilitation, sport, and healthy habits, and with at least medium-quality smartphone app. Accordingly, Henriksen and colleagues [14] after screening over 500 wearables and smartphone apps suggest to choose only devices with higher count of empirical paper published and with support to develop custom application suited for the specific aims of the research or rehab program.

From the technical point of view, the characteristics of the sensors present inside the smartwatches must be considered. These must meet high standards and ensure the reliability of the measurement and data collection at appropriate sampling rate (for example, provide the heart rate beat per beat and not its average per minute). This mode of acquisition and saving data entails the need for a high storage capacity that complicates data management and the size of the device itself. In most devices, the data is presented in aggregate form (number of steps, HR, calories, etc.) that derives from the processing of the "raw" data through the use of calculation algorithms. We can therefore state that the goodness parameter of the device is directly linked to the level of reliability and optimization of the algorithm used to generate these derived parameters. However, in medical applications, it is good to start from a certain data and therefore the raw data must be of excellent quality. Systems of this type, as already mentioned, are developed for sports use and the measured parameters are dependent activities (it is important to have the GPS data in outdoor activities, while it is less so if the activity is carried out within a gym). In a rehabilitation perspective, for example, it is important to define specific tasks and activities within which to provide significant data precisely for that activity and not for others. In choosing the device, it is important to evaluate the available software development kit (SDK) to define new aggregate parameters and the application programming interface (API) to manage the interface with the software in the smartwatch or inside the smartphone (Figs. 14.4 and 14.5).

14.8 Brief Conclusion

At the state of literature wearable devices and app for PA are well established and show promising findings, highlighting the positive impact of wearable devices on the compliance of patients and adherence to PA programs provided by professionals in the context of promoting healthy lifestyle, as long as the choice of sensors and app is oriented toward the device well studied and validated by research. Today the consumer market of wearable devices and smartphone app is rapidly changing, but only few devices and apps are sufficiently tested for research and rehabilitation [14]. Further studies with larger samples and deepening different aspects of mobile technologies are needed in order to provide more detailed considerations.

Brand	
SDK support	Device count
API support	Article count
Apple Health support	Validation Study count
Google Fit support	Clinical Trials, org count
Device	
Sensors	Battery life
Validation	Robustness
Previous usage	Water resistance
Price	Connectivity
Availability	Usability
Phone environment	Easy to data access
Affiliated app features	Privacy
Look and feel	Security

Fig. 14.4 Characteristics to consider when choosing brand or device. *API* application programming interface, *SDK* software development kit (Adapted from Herisksen et al. [14])

Feature	Apple	FitBit	Garmin	Mio	Misfit	Polar	PulseOn	Samsung	TomTom	Withings	Xiaomi
Supported platform											
Android		✓	✓		✓	✓	✓	✓	✓	✓	✓
iPhone	✓		✓		✓	✓	✓	✓	✓	✓	✓
Windows phone		✓	✓		✓						
Integration											
Automatic syncronization to Apple Health	✓			✓	✓					✓	✓
Automatic synchronization to Google Fit				✓	✓					✓	✓
Private cloud storage		✓	✓		✓	✓		✓	✓	✓	
Cloud storage API [a]	✓	✓	✓		✓	✓		✓	✓	✓	
Developed SDK [b]	✓	✓	✓		✓			✓			
Watch system											
Android Wear					✓	✓					✓
watchOS (Apple)	✓										
Custom		✓	✓				✓	✓	✓	✓	

Fig. 14.5 Comparison between eight brands of wearable devices (Adapted from Henriksen et al. [14])

References

1. Lifshitz F, Lifshitz JZ. Globesity: the root causes of the obesity epidemic in the USA and now worldwide. Pediatr Endocrinol Rev. 2014;12(1):17–34.
2. Pietrabissa G, Manzoni GM, Corti S, Vegliante N, Molinari E, Castelnuovo G. Addressing motivation in globesity treatment: a new challenge for clinical psychology. Front Psychol. 2012;3:317.
3. Davin SA, Taylor NM. Comprehensive review of obesity and psychological considerations for treatment. Psychol Health Med. 2009;14(6):716–25.
4. WHO. Definition and diagnosis of diabetes mellitus and intermediate hyperglycemia. Geneva: WHO; 2006.
5. Haslam DW, James WP. Obesity. Lancet. 2005;366(9492):1197–209.
6. Donnelly JE, Blair SN, Jakicic JM, Manore MM, Rankin JW, Smith BK, et al. American College of Sports Medicine position stand. Appropriate physical activity intervention strategies for weight loss and prevention of weight regain for adults. Med Sci Sports Exerc. 2009;41(2):459–71.
7. Garber CE, Blissmer B, Deschenes MR, Franklin BA, Lamonte MJ, Lee IM, et al. American College of Sports Medicine position stand. Quantity and quality of exercise for developing and maintaining cardiorespiratory, musculoskeletal, and neuromotor fitness in apparently healthy adults: guidance for prescribing exercise. Med Sci Sports Exerc. 2011;43(7):1334–59.
8. Haskell WL, Lee IM, Pate RR, Powell KE, Blair SN, Franklin BA, et al. Physical activity and public health: updated recommendation for adults from the American College of Sports Medicine and the American Heart Association. Med Sci Sports Exerc. 2007;39(8):1423–34.
9. Pate RR, Pratt M, Blair SN, Haskell WL, Macera CA, Bouchard C, et al. Physical activity and public health. A recommendation from the Centers for Disease Control and Prevention and the American College of Sports Medicine. JAMA. 1995;273(5):402–7.
10. Foreyt JP, Poston WS. What is the role of cognitive-behavior therapy in patient management? Obes Res. 1998;6(Suppl 1):18S–22S.
11. Foreyt JP, Poston WS. The challenge of diet, exercise and lifestyle modification in the management of the obese diabetic patient. Int J Obes Relat Metab Disord. 1999;23(Suppl 7):S5–11.
12. Howlett N, Trivedi D, Troop NA, Chater AM. What are the most effective behaviour change techniques to promote physical activity and/or reduce sedentary behaviour in inactive adults? A systematic review protocol. BMJ Open. 2015;5(8):e008573.
13. Yang CH, Maher JP, Conroy DE. Implementation of behavior change techniques in mobile applications for physical activity. Am J Prev Med. 2015;48(4):452–5.
14. Henriksen A, Haugen Mikalsen M, Woldaregay AZ, Muzny M, Hartvigsen G, Hopstock LA, et al. Using fitness trackers and Smartwatches to measure physical activity in research: analysis of consumer wrist-worn Wearables. J Med Internet Res. 2018;20(3):e110.
15. Moulos I, Maramis C, Mourouzis A, Maglaveras N. Designing the user interfaces of a behavior modification intervention for obesity & eating disorders prevention. Stud Health Technol Inform. 2015;210:647–51.
16. Schüll ND. Wearable technology and the design of self-care. BioSocieties. 2016;11(3):317–33.
17. Duncan M, Murawski B, Short CE, Rebar AL, Schoeppe S, Alley S, et al. Activity trackers implement different behavior change techniques for activity, sleep, and sedentary behaviors. Interact J Med Res. 2017;6(2):e13.
18. Muntaner-Mas A, Martinez-Nicolas A, Lavie CJ, Blair SN, Ross R, Arena R, et al. A systematic review of fitness apps and their potential clinical and sports utility for objective and remote assessment of cardiorespiratory fitness. Sports Med. 2019;49(4):587–600.
19. Castelnuovo G, Pietrabissa G, Manzoni GM, Corti S, Ceccarini M, Borrello M, et al. Chronic care management of globesity: promoting healthier lifestyles in traditional and mHealth based settings. Front Psychol. 2015;6:1557.
20. Castelnuovo G, Zoppis I, Santoro E, Ceccarini M, Pietrabissa G, Manzoni GM, et al. Managing chronic pathologies with a stepped mHealth-based approach in clinical psychology and medicine. Front Psychol. 2015;6:407.

21. Estabrooks PA, Nelson CC, Xu S, King D, Bayliss EA, Gaglio B, et al. The frequency and behavioral outcomes of goal choices in the self-management of diabetes. Diabetes Educ. 2005;31(3):391–400.
22. Martínez-Pérez B, de la Torre-Díez I, López-Coronado M. Experiences and results of applying tools for assessing the quality of a mHealth app named Heartkeeper. J Med Syst. 2015;39(11):303.
23. Howlett N, Trivedi D, Troop NA, Chater AM. Are physical activity interventions for healthy inactive adults effective in promoting behavior change and maintenance, and which behavior change techniques are effective? A systematic review and meta-analysis. Transl Behav Med. 2019;9(1):147–57.
24. Janevic MR, McLaughlin SJ, Connell CM. Overestimation of physical activity among a nationally representative sample of underactive individuals with diabetes. Med Care. 2012;50(5):441–5.
25. Shaw K, O'Rourke P, Del Mar C, Kenardy J. Psychological interventions for overweight or obesity. Cochrane Database Syst Rev. 2005;2:CD003818.
26. Foster GD, Makris AP, Bailer BA. Behavioral treatment of obesity. Am J Clin Nutr. 2005;82(1 Suppl):230S–5S.
27. Swencionis C, Rendell SL. The psychology of obesity. Abdom Imaging. 2012;37:733.
28. Wing RR. Behavioral weight control. In: Wadden TA, Stunkard AJ, editors. Handbook of obesity treatment. New York: Guilford Press; 2002. p. 301–16.
29. Henriksen A, Hopstock LA, Hartvigsen G, Grimsgaard S. Using cloud-based physical activity Data from Google fit and apple Healthkit to expand recording of physical activity Data in a population study. Stud Health Technol Inform. 2017;245:108–12.
30. Unick JL, Gaussoin SA, Hill JO, Jakicic JM, Bond DS, Hellgren M, et al. Objectively assessed physical activity and weight loss maintenance among individuals enrolled in a lifestyle intervention. Obesity (Silver Spring). 2017;25(11):1903–9.
31. Spring B, Gotsis M, Paiva A, Spruijt-Metz D. Healthy apps: mobile devices for continuous monitoring and intervention. IEEE Pulse. 2013;4(6):34–40.
32. Direito A, Dale LP, Shields E, Dobson R, Whittaker R, Maddison R. Do physical activity and dietary smartphone applications incorporate evidence-based behaviour change techniques? BMC Public Health. 2014;14:646.
33. Khaylis A, Yiaslas T, Bergstrom J, Gore-Felton C. A review of efficacious technology-based weight-loss interventions: five key components. Telemed J E Health. 2010;16(9):931–8.
34. Cullen KW, Baranowsky T, Smith SP. Using goal setting as a strategy for dietary behavior change. J Am Diet Assoc. 2001;101(5):562–6.
35. Strecher VJ, Seijts GH, Kok GJ, Latham GP, Glasgow R, DeVellis B, et al. Goal setting as a strategy for health behavior change. Health Educ Q. 1995;22(2):190–200.
36. Cullen KW, Thompson DI, Scott AR, Lara-Smalling A, Watson KB, Konzelmann K. The impact of goal attainment on behavioral and mediating variables among low income women participating in an Expanded Food and Nutrition Education Program intervention study. Appetite. 2010;55(2):305–10.
37. Latham GP. Self-regulation through goal setting. Organ Behav Human Decis Processes. 1991;50(2):212–47.
38. Kirschenbaum DS. Self-regulation of sport performance. Med Sci Sports Exerc. 1987;19(5 Suppl):S106–13.
39. Kirschenbaum DS, Kelly KP, Germann JN. Efficacy of a screening procedure to identify potentially disruptive participants in an immersion program for the treatment of adolescent obesity. Obes Facts. 2009;2(2):110–5.
40. Kirschenbaum DS, Stalonas PM, Zastowny TR, Tomarken AJ. Behavioral treatment of adult obesity: attentional controls and a 2-year follow-up. Behav Res Ther. 1985;23(6):675–82.
41. Sperduto WA, Thompson HS, O'Brien RM. The effect of target behavior monitoring on weight loss and completion rate in a behavior modification program for weight reduction. Addict Behav. 1986;11(3):337–40.
42. Baker RC, Kirschenbaum DS. Self-monitoring may be necessary for successful weight control. Behav Ther. 1993;24(3):377–94.

43. Ross KM, Wing RR. Impact of newer self-monitoring technology and brief phone-based intervention on weight loss: a randomized pilot study. Obesity (Silver Spring). 2016;24(8):1653–9.
44. Cattivelli R, Castelnuovo G, Musetti A, Varallo G, Spatola CAM, Riboni FV, et al. ACTonHEALTH study protocol: promoting psychological flexibility with activity tracker and mHealth tools to foster healthful lifestyle for obesity and other chronic health conditions. Trials. 2018;19(1):659.
45. Burke LE. Experiences of self monitoring: successes and struggles during treatment of weight loss. Qual Health Res. 2009;19:815.
46. Neve MJ, Collins CE, Morgan PJ. Dropout, nonusage attrition, and pretreatment predictors of nonusage attrition in a commercial web-based weight loss program. J Med Internet Res. 2010;12(4):e69.
47. Leonard, T. C., Richard H. Thaler, Cass R. Sunstein (2008). Nudge: improving decisions about health, wealth, and happiness.
48. Marteau TM, Ogilvie D, Roland M, Suhrcke M, Kelly MP. Judging nudging: can nudging improve population health? BMJ. 2011;342:d228.
49. Hollands GJ, Shemilt I, Marteau TM, Jebb SA, Kelly MP, Nakamura R, et al. Altering micro-environments to change population health behaviour: towards an evidence base for choice architecture interventions. BMC Public Health. 2013;13(1):1218.
50. Thomas AM, Parkinson J, Moore P, Goodman A, Xhafa F, Barolli L. Nudging through technology: choice architectures and the mobile information revolution. In: Paper presented at the eighth international conference on P2P, parallel, grid, cloud and internet computing, 2013.

Aids, Equipment, and Treadmills

15

Edda Maria Capodaglio, Nicola Cau, Veronica Cimolin,
Manuela Galli, and Paolo Capodaglio

Key Points

- Discuss with administrations the appropriate technology to meet the safety and mobility needs of the patient and provide equipment training to the staff
- Presence of at least one floor-based lifting device to rescue patients up from the floor in areas not covered by a ceiling lift
- Presence of a ceiling lift above the parallels and traverse tracks above treatment tables in physiotherapy units
- Choice of treadmill focusing on weight capacity, ease of use, construction quality, ergonomics, exercise range, and user's safety

E. M. Capodaglio (✉)
Istituti Clinici Scientifici Maugeri IRCSS,
Occupational Therapy and Ergonomics Unit of Pavia Institute, Pavia, Italy
e-mail: edda.capodaglio@icsmaugeri.it

N. Cau · P. Capodaglio
Rehabilitation Unit and Clinical Lab for Gait Analysis and Posture,
Ospedale San Giuseppe, Istituto Auxologico Italiano, IRCCS, Piancavallo, Verbania, Italy
e-mail: n.cau@auxologico.it; p.capodaglio@auxologico.it

V. Cimolin · M. Galli
Department of Electronics, Information and Bioengineering,
Politecnico di Milano, Milan, Italy
e-mail: veronica.cimolin@polimi.it; manuela.galli@polimi.it

P. Capodaglio (ed.), *Rehabilitation Interventions in the Patient with Obesity*,
https://doi.org/10.1007/978-3-030-32274-8_15

15.1 Aids

Patient-handling equipment and technology describe equipment, devices, aids, and resources designed as alternative to manual handling, and inherent to lifting, transferring, repositioning, moving, and mobilizing of patients ensuring that patients are cared for safely, while maintaining a safe work environment for employees and preventing consequences of immobility associated with size. The Bariatric Safe Patient Handling and Mobility Guidebook [1] outlines management strategies that facilitate the use of patient-handling technology and foster a culture of safety in the patient care environment. First step is patient's needs assessment: individual physical, mental, cognitive, and medical conditions are important factors to consider, together with the required level of assistance, weight-bearing capability, height, weight, body circumference, and other conditions that will likely affect the patient's ability to participate in transfer or repositioning activities (i.e., hip and knee replacement, paralysis, amputations, contractures, osteoporosis, respiratory and cardiac conditions, skin/wound conditions, and spinal stability) [2]. An example to detect the type of assistance needed and to select the correct equipment is offered in Table 15.1 [3].

Also, algorithms have been proposed [4] to set standards for assistance and technology and guide the performance of high-risk handling/transferring tasks, and some evidence exists that their application can significantly reduce staff injuries. Patient benefits include prevention of falls, pressure ulcers, incontinence and hospital-acquired pneumonia, reduction in hospitalization and readmissions, and functional improvements [5, 6].

15.1.1 Handling and Mobility Equipment

Informed physiotherapists and nurses should discuss with administrations the appropriate technology to meet the safety and mobility needs of the patient and provide initial equipment training. Selection and purchase of equipment should occur after having identified the needs of the patient population and the physical environment where equipment is used. Convenience about buying or renting bariatric equipment should be rated against number, frequency, and type of bariatric admission; space needed when using/storing equipment; maintenance needs; and purchase/rental cost. The equipment categories for bariatric use [7] are the following:

Table 15.1 The bariatric mobility gallery

Bariatric gallery	Motor and behavioral patient's characteristics	Space requirements	Handling and mobility task	Aid/device
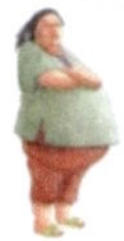	An independent patient who performs daily activities without assistance, walks with/without cane; may request monitoring. Early fatiguing may incur. One assistant may suffice	Allow space for ambulation accompanied by one caregiver beside and one behind with equipment. A 1.8 m/72 in. turning radius allows use of floor-based equipment. Suggested room dimension: 3.8 × 3.3 m/12.4 × 10.6 ft	Walking	Walking cane or walker
			Bed transfers	Friction-reducing device; separate bedside rails; trapeze
			Main supports	Chair/armchair
			Hygiene	In bathroom: Shower or hygiene chair/commode
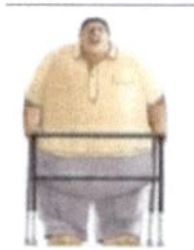	A cooperative patient who needs moderate assistance and support from nurse. Seating and standing devices requested	Allow space for ambulation accompanied by one caregiver beside and one behind with equipment/two caregivers on either side of the patient. Allow a 1.8 m/72 in. turning radius for floor-based equipment. Allow room for transfers between bed, chair, wheelchair, and commode. Frequently occurring are transport in a commode to the toilet, repositioning in bed, wound care in bed or chair, and assisted ambulation. Suggested room dimension: 3.8 × 5.3 m/12.4 × 17.5 ft	Walking with support	Walker
			Bed transfers	Active lifter (standing aid)
			Main supports	Chair/armchair/wheelchair
			Hygiene	In bathroom: Shower chair/commode
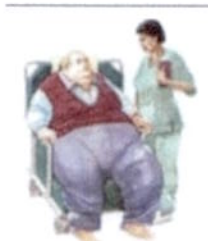	A partial-cooperative patient, seated. Cannot do daily activities without assistance. Partially able to support body weight. Potential of physically overloading of the nurse assistant	Three caregivers may be required to assist during use of floor lift or sit-to stand lift. Allow transfers between bed, chair, wheelchair, commode, or stretcher; recommended use of commode/shower chair for toileting. Frequently occurring repositioning in bed; wound care in bed. Suggested room dimension: 3.8 × 5.3 m/12.4 × 17.5 ft	Room transfers	Wheelchair; active lifter (standing aid)/ceiling hoist with walking sling
			Bed transfers	Ceiling lift/active lifter; air-assisted device
			Main supports	Wheelchair, bed
			Hygiene	In bathroom: Shower chair/easy chair; bedside commode

(continued)

Table 15.1 (continued)

Bariatric gallery	Motor and behavioral patient's characteristics	Space requirements	Handling and mobility task	Aid/device
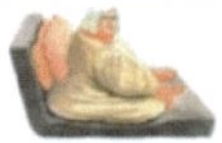	A dependent patient seated; cannot support body weight. Extensive assistance required. Physical overload is a real risk for the assisting nurse	Allow space at bedside for at least two assistants. An easy/convertible chair is convenient at bedside. Suggested room dimension: with mobile lift: 4.4 × 6.0 m/14.4 × 19.8 ft; with ceiling lift 4.0 × 5.0 m/13 × 16.4 ft	Room transfers	Convertible chair
			Bed transfers	Ceiling lift with whole body sling; air-assisted device
			Main supports	Convertible chair; fully equipped bed
			Hygiene	In bathroom: Shower chair. Sponge rinsing in bed
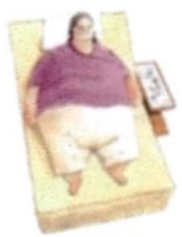	A passive bedridden dependent patient. Extensive assistance required. Prevention of bedsores and contractures recommended. Physical overload is a real risk for the nurse	Allow space at bedside for at least three assistants. A convertible chair is convenient at bedside. Suggested room dimension: with mobile lift/ceiling lift/lateral transfer 4.4 × 6.0 m/14.4 × 19.8 ft	Room transfers	Motorized bed
			Bed transfers	Ceiling lift with stretcher/full support; air-assisted device and bed adjustment for repositioning
			Main supports	Fully equipped bed
			Hygiene	Sponge rinsing in bed

- Ambulation/fall prevention/mobility aids (non-powered standing aids, walker)
- Patient transportation chair with motorized lift or transportation feature
- Lateral or vertical air-assisted transfer equipment
- Bed frames with repositioning and bariatric features (optional low bed feature)
- Specialty mattress, pressure redistribution surface, or support surface
- Bathing equipment aids
- Overhead lift (ceiling mounted, wall mounted, or portable lift)
- Floor-based sling lift or multipurpose portable mobile lift
- Sit-to-stand (stand assist or standing) lift
- Specialty slings
- Mechanical lateral transfer device
- Friction-reducing device (sliding board, roller board, slippery sheet, etc.)
- Transfer chairs
- Stretchers/gurneys
- Height-adjustable exam tables
- Patient evacuation device

Selection of technology should stem also from considerations of effectiveness of the device, its efficiency of use, acceptance by the intended users, potential safety and comfort associated with use, integration with other devices, and training needs that are all aspects to evaluate prior to purchase. Basic ergonomics design principles (facility, comfort, safety, and efficiency of use) should drive the choice of every device for maximal benefit and greatest usability for patients and operators. The term "extended capacity" defines those devices, equipment, supplies, furniture, and technology designed to accommodate a patient whose weight or weight distribution or size interferes with the use of standard-sized tools. Stickers denoting "EC" provide a quick identification of the right equipment (for example, an "EC 1000" label would indicate a weight capacity limit of 1000 lb/450 kg for the device).

15.1.2 Ambulation

Specially designed walkers are available to accommodate the unique needs of the bariatric patient and enhance safety (for example, supports for large abdominal pannus, or mechanism to attach a ventilator, chest tubes, catheters, and others) while supporting the goals of early progressive mobility. Active standing and transfer aids, for users with some arm strength and standing function, serve to test and train standing function, with removable footplate to work on ambulation. Space accommodation should be tested for use (i.e., door widths, extra space for the caregivers) (Table 15.2).

Table 15.2 The basic bariatric equipment

1. *Ambulation/mobility aids* Active transfer and transport aids: Ambulation belt, canes and crutches, motorized and nonmotorized stand and transfer aid, walker. For users with some arm strength and standing function. For standing function and ambulation training. Weight capacity 600–1000 lb (272–453 kg). Space encumbrance of a typical walker: 910–1060 mm/36–42 in. wide	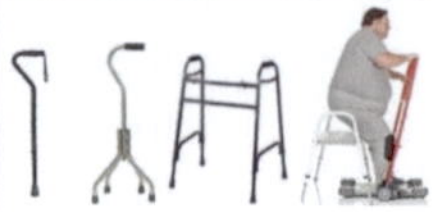
2. *Bed frame* Fully electric, multi-positioning, locking castors. Side rails, bed-mounted trapeze, scale w/digital display. Transforms into a chair for easy egress, cardiac chair position, Fowler. Power-drive system. Mechanical CPR release. Standing frame with tilt adjust from 0 to 180 degrees for early mobilization. Variable bed width (100–150 cm/40–61 in.) and length (200–270 cm/78–106 in.) dimensions, designed to accommodate comfortably different-size patients, or to make the transit easier. Extra low bed height reduces the risk from fall injuries. Many options available: Patient lockout features, head angle indicator, integrated scale with weight history; Braden Scale assessments, BMI calculator, integrated nurse protocol timer, bed exit alarm, anti-entrapment alarm; arrangement for active compression system for prevention of venous thromboembolism. Weight capacity up to 453 kg/1000 lb	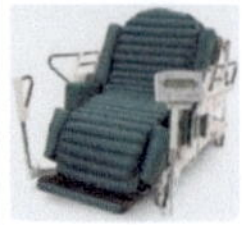
3. *Technology mattress* Technology that minimizes surface tension and reduces friction and shear. Range from low-risk (high memory viscoelastic foam, static or alternate low air loss) to high-risk systems (fluid immersion simulation, rotating/pulsating therapy) apt for patients with existing pressure ulcers. The non-powered self-adjusting technology allows pressure redistribution surface to automatically set in response to patient movements; zone control for different areas of the patient's body; lower safety cell remains inflated for up to 12 h in the event of power failure. The powered negative airflow technology implemented in a cover increases the effectiveness of prevention and care of bedsores, through the management of the moisture and warmth of the patient's skin. Pulsate feature increases patient comfort and pressure redistribution. Mattress dimensions vary in width and length. Weight capacity 1000–2000 lb (453–907 kg)	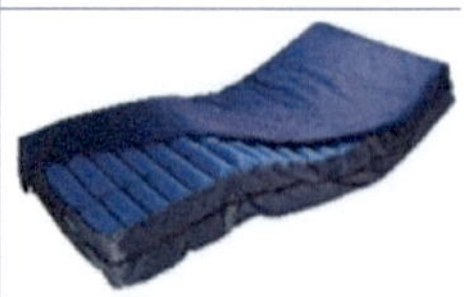
4. *Chairs, armchairs, wheelchairs, convertible chairs* Provide chairs without arms for individuals with lower body obesity (pear shape), and extra-wide seat depth chairs (with or without arms) for individuals with upper body obesity (apple-shaped bodies). A recliner is preferred in the room to facilitate respiratory function and comfort. For seated transfer aid, consider a chair with arms that recess or are removable. Wheelchair total dimensions reach up to 1200 × 1320 mm/48 × 52 in. A wheelchair mover could add up to 300 mm/12 in., to the length. Power chairs and electric scooters require additional front-to-back clearance (at least 1820 mm/72 in.), and even more convertible chairs especially if reclined to the stretcher position. Weight capacity 675–850 lb (300–385 kg).	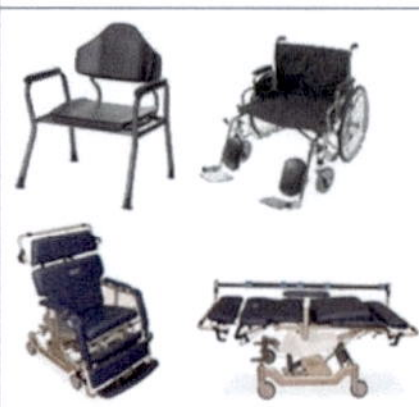

Table 15.2 (continued)

5. *Bathing/showering/toileting* Toilet supports and commodes are extra-wide toilet seat for bariatric and geriatric patients, to use either bedside or attached to a toilet with the added benefit of assisting the patient to standing. Powered version is available Shower chairs and trolleys are height adjustable and tilting; serve as shower, transport, and changing space; side rails for safety; welded steel or PVC construction, wheeled with brakes. Various bath benches or seats are available as heavy-duty models. Reclining and recumbent tubs along with a lift to assist with access could profit in special settings. Weight capacity up to 453 kg/1000 lb	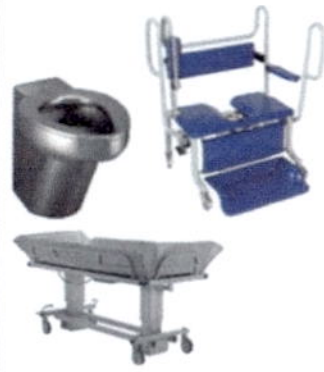
6. *Air-assisted lateral transfer devices* Air-assisted lateral transfer systems glide patients across a frictionless air surface for a smooth transition; turn also patient without manual power. Facilitate nursing care for hygiene, wound care, and linen changes. Wedge available, as inflatable positioning device. Inflatable battery-operated emergency lifting chairs and cushions serve to sit up and lift a fallen person from any location—indoors and outside. Weight limit: 180–454 kg/400–1000 lb. Combination air transfer and sling device reduces products required for lateral and vertical transfer of a patient; intended for use as a sling attached to a loop-style hanger bar with mobile hoist or stationary hoist. Weight limit: 1000 lb (454 kg)	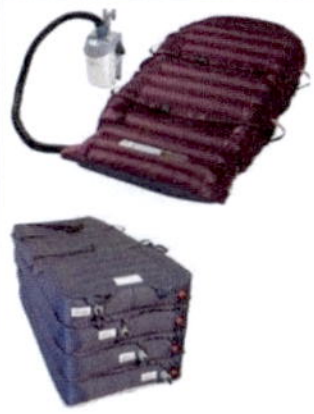
7. *Non-powered lateral transfer and repositioning devices* Bariatric transfer boards are nonmotorized lateral transfer devices assisting in slide transfer from wheelchair/bed to commode/stretcher. It comes as a foldable board, lightweight, and radiolucent for X-ray/MRI. Weight capacity 600 lb (272 kg). Friction-reducing slide sheets are sliding system that offers a wide range of patient-handling maneuvers. A friction-reducing device will also facilitate insertion and removal of a sling under a bariatric patient. Many assistants are required for a bariatric task. Variety of sheets and one-way slides for repositioning and transfer. Weight capacity 400 lb (180 kg) Mechanical lateral transfer devices are specially designed technology powered by an electric motor or manual crank. The device attaches to a draw sheet and moves the patient from one horizontal surface to another	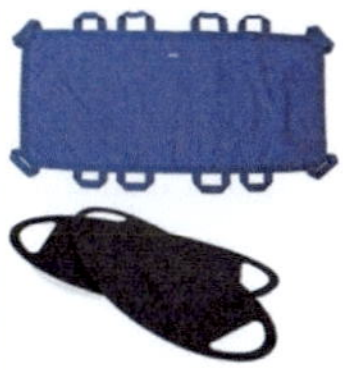
8. *Floor base, portable lift* Total body "passive" lift, for dependent patients, bedside use. Battery powered with internal charger. Four/six-point spreader bar with 360° rotation, tilts for comfort, foot pedal for leg opening, large easy grip handles for easy maneuvering, emergency lowering device, integrated scale. Sit-to-stand "active" lift, for cooperative patients, stand and transfer aid, for turn and pivots, rehabilitation, social reintegration, wheelchair repositioning, and car extraction; used with a safety belt. Many options in size, complexity, and weight capacity; portable version. Weight limit: 400–800 lb (180–360 kg)	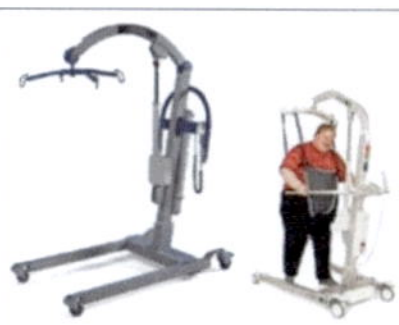

(continued)

Table 15.2 (continued)

9. *Overhead (ceiling, wall mounted, and portable gantries)* Many arrangements of the lift system (motor, track, hanger bar, and suspended sling) are possible according to the building characteristics and the patient handling needs, producing an all-around settlement. Free-standing room-covering rail systems are apt for temporary lifting needs, and tracks or motor retractable in the false ceiling or recessed in the wall allow for greater lifting vertical capacity and offer additional aesthetics. The operator can switch easily between spreader bars in complete range to meet each patient's specific care needs, for attachment from a corset to a stretcher support	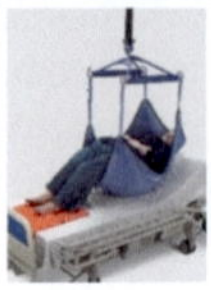 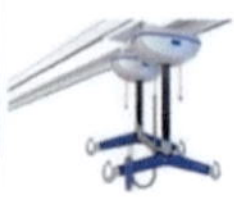
10. *Transport-assistive devices* Powered devices used to assist caregivers in moving patients from one location to another. If detachable motor, the device attaches onto handles of wheelchairs and/or beds and the caregiver simply guides the direction of the bed or wheelchair. Comprises bed movers, beds with power drive, motorized chairs, transfer and convertible-chairs, powered stretchers. Motorized transfer devices are necessary when frequent bariatric transports occur into the facility, since they significantly decrease effort, time, and personnel required in these tasks	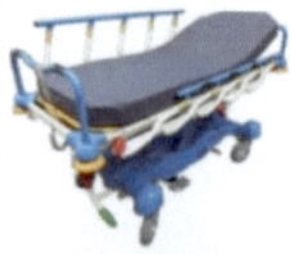 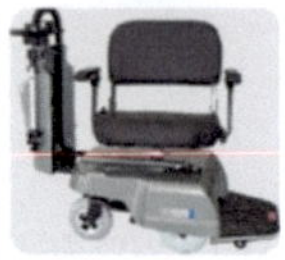
11. *Emergency devices* In case of quick evacuation of the bariatric dependent patient, the emergency crew can intervene with the reinforced rescue sheet (weight capacity 727 kg/1600 lb), or the cocooned mattress system (weight capacity 450 kg/992 lb) enables fast lowering onto the floor the patient and the mattress, and then sliding them or taking down stairs to safety. The stair chair (weight capacity 227 kg/500 lb) allows caregivers to transport seated patients downstairs without lifting. Manual height-adjustable bariatric cots or motorized highly configurable stretchers are available for load and transport of the patient on ambulance or for inhospital perioperative transport tasks	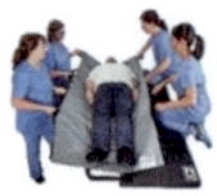 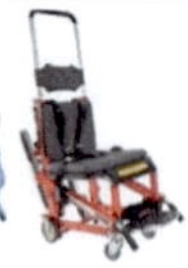
12. *Rehabilitation setting* Power-supplied bariatric Bobath tables are specially designed for patient examinations and treatments in training rooms, clinics, hospitals, and rehabs. They provide effective usage for patients who have a loss of sensation or poor balance, allowing postural exercises, rolling, turning, and balance training, but are also useful in treating neurological conditions For early mobilization, combination of ceiling lift with motor in locked positioning and a special training kit (elastic bands, strip slings, handles) allows the bedridden patient to exercise limbs and pelvis giving the chance to modulate the intensity of effort	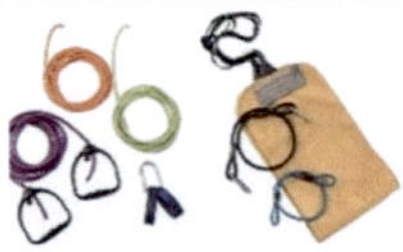 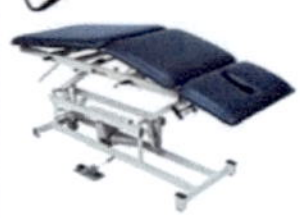

15.1.3 Beds

The characteristics of the hospital bed impact both the well-being of the patient and the physical burden of the operators. The features of the bariatric bed that allow a reduced effort and a minimum risk for the assistants, at the same time facilitating both bed mobilization and patient comfort, are the following:

- Weight capacity up to 450 kg/1000 lb
- Adjustability in bed's height, and frame dimensions
- Integrated scale
- Assisted patient's positioning (from lying to sitting, rotation)
- A therapeutic surface (low air-loss system)
- Side rails able to withstand weights to ensure patient independence and support during repositioning
- Powered transport device
- Easy maintenance and sanification

The resulting clinical benefits of adequate positioning of patient in a proper bariatric bed are skin pressure reduction, and improvement of respiratory, cardiac, gastrointestinal, genitourinary, and psychological functions. Integrated scale and power drive reduce effortful assistance [8]. Special bed structures aid in therapeutic activities, such as lateral rotation and percussion, and help reduce unnecessary transfer. Room design, floor surfaces, door widths, space available, and work practices are all important to the reduction of risk associated with bedside care (Table 15.3).

Table 15.3 Recommended workspaces for standard and bariatric patient-handling tasks

Working areas	Standard patient	Bariatric patient
1 assistant in front of patient	810–1000 mm/32–39 in.	1000–1300 mm/39–51 in.
1 assistant at bedside of patient	600–760 mm/24–30 in.	1000–1300 mm/39–51 in.
Workspace at the foot of the bed	900 mm/35 in.	1800 mm/71 in.
More staff at the side of bed	1200 mm/47 in.	2000–3600 mm/78–141 in.
Equipment use in critical areas; clear space at the bed perimeter	2000 mm/78 in.	4000–5000 mm/157–197 in.
Patient moving w/ walker, one nurse assisting at side	1700 mm/67 in.	2150 mm/85 in.
Patient seated on a chair, one nurse assisting at side	1300 mm/51 in.	2150 mm/85 in.
Wheelchair, 180° rotation, 1 assistant	1500 mm/59 in.	1900 mm/75 in.
Mobile lift, 180° rotation	1800 mm/71 in.	2500 mm/98 in.
Stretcher, 180° rotation	2400 mm/94 in.	3000 mm/118 in.

(continued)

Table 15.3 (continued)

Working areas	Standard patient	Bariatric patient
Devices' dimensions		
Bed	1060 mm × 1220 mm/42 × 48 in.	1000–1500 mm × 2000–2700 mm/40–61 in. × 78–106 in.
Wheelchair	560–780 mm × 880–1100 mm/22–30 in. × 34–43 in. Total height: 914–939 mm/36–37 in. *Seat: Width: 300–580 mm/12–23 in.; depth: 400 mm/16 in.; height: 495–520 mm/19.5–20.5 in.*	860–1210 mm × 940–1320 mm/34–48 in. × 37–52 in. (length up to 1880 mm/74 in. in convertible chair) Total height: 970 mm/38 in. *Seat: Width: 710 mm/28 in.; depth: 500 mm/20 in.; height: 470 mm/18.5 in.*
Shower chairs	650 mm × 940–1520 mm (reclining)/25.5 in. × 37–60 in.	960–1160 mm × 980–1900 mm/38–45 in. × 38.5–75 in.; turning diameter 1500 mm/59 in.
Stretcher	600–800 mm × 1100 mm/24–31 in. × 43 in.	700–990 mm × 1770–2080 mm/27–39 in. × 70–82 in.
Mobile lift	700-mm × 1300 mm/27 in. × 51 in.	1200 mm × 1820 mm/47 × 72 in.
Bedrooms' area	12 m^2/129 ft^2	14–28 m^2/150–300 ft^2; 5020 × 3990 mm/197 in. × 157 in.
Minimal space allowed for the bed	1000 mm × 2200 mm/39 in. × 86 in.	1560 mm × 2590 mm/61 in. × 102 in.
Bathrooms' area	3.8 m^2/41 ft^2	5 m^2/54 ft^2
Space allowed around the Wc	600–1000 mm/24–39 in.	1400–2100 mm/55–83 in.
Bathroom dimensions, to operate with a shower chair	4.8 m^2/51 ft^2	9 m^2/99 ft^2; 3135 × 2970 mm/123 × 117 in.
Central bathroom with use of shower stretcher	12 m^2/129 ft^2	14 m^2/150 ft^2
Door width (bedrooms, bathrooms, corridors, elevators)	850–1200 mm/33–47 in.	1300–1520 mm/51–60 in.
Elevators (weight capacity)	1200 kg/2645 lb	2721–2950 kg/6000–6500 lb
Elevator dimensions for an occupied bed, 2 staff, and any additional technology	1200 × 1400 mm/47 × 95 in.	1500 × 2700 mm/59 × 106 in.

15.1.4 Chairs, Wheelchairs, and Stretchers

Bariatric chairs and recliners allow for alternative seated rest and assisting in patient's independence. Features should include adjustability of seat height, back recline angle and foot rest angle, removable arms, and castors with locks/wheel brakes. Manually or electrically driven wheelchairs' dimensions are depicted in

Table 15.2. The convertible chair is a powered all-purpose chair, used as a stretcher or litter, and patient transport. A comprehensive selection of options and accessories provides a customizable transport and treatment platform on one piece of equipment.

15.1.5 Transferring Devices

Manual repositioning and lateral transfer devices include a variety of sheets and one-way slides (friction-reducing devices) for patients ideally weighing up to 180 kg/400 lb. The slippery material design reduces friction during manually applied sliding movements in the horizontal plan (an operator every 45 kg/100 pounds of weight of the patient is recommended), with the device previously positioned underneath the patient. For manual repositioning of the bariatric patient in bed, ceiling hoist with repositioning sling provides the safest method with two operators. Bariatric transfer boards are low-friction semirigid lateral transfer devices, for seated transfer from wheelchair to commode, or supine transfer from stretcher to bed. Special shaped smaller boards help also in sling placement. Air-inflatable devices in low-friction fabric add up the force of air to decrease friction and result in easy movement of patient in a supine position from one flat surface to another, reducing the force needed to move the patient by 80–90%. They also decrease shear forces on the skin of patients during lateral transfers, positioning, turning, and pronation. Contraindications exist for patients who are experiencing thoracic, cervical, or lumbar fractures deemed unstable, unless using in conjunction with a spinal board for lateral transfers. Two nurses are required during air-assisted patient transfers and additional caregivers when patient weighs over 340 kg/750 lb. Inflatable wedges or mattresses are available as positioning or emergency device. Air-inflatable special bariatric slings (disposable version too) are designed for vertical and lateral turning patient with a ceiling lift, targeted to the radiological area or specific for surgical, orthopedic, and delivery setting.

15.1.6 Commodes, Shower Chairs, and Stretchers

The wheeled bariatric commode is an important piece of furniture both at bedside and in the bathroom. Toilet supports attached to a standard toilet provide the extra capacity with the added benefit of assisting the patient to standing. Mobile commodes and shower chairs for toilet/shower transfers should have rubber wheels, brakes, removable arms and foot brackets, and a seat with a front or central space to allow toileting and washing. Some can be padded or specifically designed with support for a patient who has limited sitting balance, while others may be fully reclining and height adjustable for shower, transport, and undergarment change of dependent patients. Design for safe use of the commode chair should take into account the floor surface and the available workspace. The opportunity of having a bariatric shower stretcher in the ward depends on the mobility levels of the patients' majority, on the hygienic care and treatment planning, and on the space arrangement. While it is not generally recommended bathing bariatric patients in the tub, in some cases a spa-type bathroom with a ceiling lifter is preferred.

15.1.7 Scales

Weighing is a critical part of the bariatric patient assessment. In-floor scales provided with grab bars can be accessed by wheelchair-bounded patients, and scales built into the bed frame or in the lifting equipment allow monitoring weight avoiding unnecessary handling. Digital recording of data and trends are available.

15.1.8 Exam/Therapy Tables

Bariatric power tables for the rehabilitative and clinical/diagnostic setting are electrically adjustable in surface height and backrest angle, and large padded on the support area. Flexible chair-to-table design facilitates the powered patient's transfer. Safety grab bars and arm/leg brackets could support the patient while exercising, in special rehabilitative models.

15.1.9 Lifting

Lifting technology covers all mechanical equipment or devices used to assist caregivers in performing patient-handling tasks, including lifting, transferring, wound care, ambulation, and others. Powered bariatric lift devices serve the dependent or the cooperative patient, and comprehend floor-based and overhead/ceiling lifts. Usually two assistants are required, or more according to patient's conditions [4]. General standards indicate the type of devices needed to create a safe working environment, according to the patients assisted and the performed handling activities [9]. The floor-based total body lift assists tasks such as lifting-dependent patients from bed to chair, bed to trolley, and up from the floor. The lift motor functions to raise or lower the patient, but caregivers must manually push the lift on the wheeled base to the desired location. Turning and twisting of equipment under load entail a potential risk for push/pull injuries for assistants [10]. The standing lift raises and lowers a cooperative patient from a seated position to a standing one, and assists for turn-and-pivot transfer, rehabilitation, social reintegration, wheelchair repositioning, and car extraction. Wired by a safety belt, the patient must have some upper body strength, cognitive ability, weight-bearing capability, stability of the trunk, and ability to grasp with hands. Overhead lifts offer a superior alternative to the traditional mobile hoists, comparing organizational, physical, and safety aspects. Permanently installed ceiling lifts require fewer personnel and less space than floor-based lifts, and are easier and quicker in the use.

Their use is apt where dependent or semidependent people need assistance with transfers or movements, but their suitability ranges really through a variety of settings and tasks. Spreader bars switched in complete range for sling attachment meet each patient's specific care needs. The lift system is implementable in a variety of different models, up to full-room coverage and combined system leading and connecting to different areas. Dual-motor systems with wide-set four-point hanger bars can allow space for extra-wide body size.

The need of ceiling lift system coverage is equal to the sum of average percent total dependent patients and those requiring extensive assistance [1].

Overhead lifts not only allow the typical transfer tasks, but also assist in treatment-targeted and training activities in the rehabilitative sector, including:

- Over the bed, for on-bed movements and bed-to-chair/trolley transfers
- Rehabilitation exercise of the bedded patient, with elastic bands attached to the overhead motor in the locked position
- In the bathroom, on/off the toilet, in/out of the bath, assisting the patient in the standing position for independence in personal hygiene
- In therapy settings, for assisted walking, standing, balancing, and muscular reinforcement
- In water therapy, for ingress and egress of the swimming pool
- In specialist treatment or diagnostic settings, to get and hold specific positioning of the patient's limbs or body sector

The costs of installing overhead ceiling hoists are comparable to using traditional mobile lifting equipment when the productivity and space advantages are considered; moreover, they decrease the incidence of staff injuries.

The main advantages of ceiling lift are the following:

- They allow patients to be handled anywhere in the room.
- Do not present problems of space on the ground or for maneuvering the trolley.
- Require a shorter maneuvering time, and are accessible and practical.
- Substantially reduce the risk of biomechanical overload in the assistants.
- They allow good control and communication with the patient during use.

15.1.10 Slings

Slings used with mechanical lifts temporarily lift or suspend a patient or body part for handling task, but they also aid in rising, standing training, and gait training. Sling styles include seated, standing, ambulation, repositioning, turning, pannus holder, limb support/strap, supine, toileting, bathing, and others (Table 15.4). Criteria for choosing the right sling are patient's characteristics (size, shape, weight) and medical conditions, including head and trunk stability and muscle tone, beyond the task to be performed and the required patient's position [11].

Table 15.4 Sling selection criteria

Type of sling	Indication	Tasks	Patient's characteristics	Concerns	Sling features	Example
Seated sling (lifting capacity up to 500 kg/1100 lb)	Transfer and lift patients in a seated position. Matches with ceiling-mounted or floor-based lift	Vertical transfers to and from bed, chair or toilet, bathing/showering, repositioning in a chair, lifting off the floor	Sitting tolerance, hip and knee flexion	Wounds affecting transfer and positioning, head control, shoulder injury/surgery, thoracic injury/surgery	Back and leg support	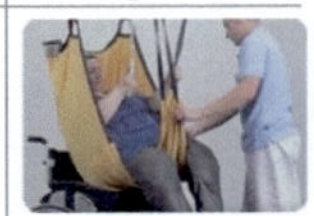
Standing sling (lifting capacity up to 205 kg/450 lb)	Provides assistance for standing upright and weight bearing. Matches with an active lift	Toileting, dressing, peri-care, vertical transfers to and from bed, chair or toilet, support during functional sit-to-stand training	Grasp and hold handles with at least one hand, upper body strength, partial weight-bearing capacity, cooperative, follow simple instructions	Wounds in area of sling, rib injuries, shoulder instability, orthostatic hypotension	Thoracic and pelvic support straps	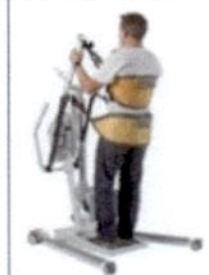
Ambulation sling, gait trainer (lifting capacity up to 500 kg/1100 lb)	Provides support during walking. Matches with ceiling-mounted or floor-based lift	Ambulation training, fall rescue, therapy pool	Partial weight-bearing capability, follow simple instructions, cooperative	Wounds/medical devices interfering with comfort and safety, rib injuries, ambulation readiness	Harness, vest	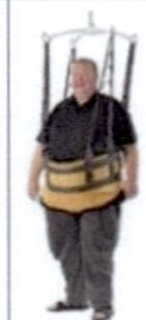
Strip sling, limb support sling (lifting capacity up to 255 kg/560 lb)	Sustained holding of any extremity. Matches with ceiling-mounted or floor-based lift	Wound care, dressing, bathing, bedside procedures, applying therapeutic devices, hygienic care	Tolerance to a prolonged position	Wounds in area of sling, risk of pressure ulcer, neurovascular issues, joint issues	Band	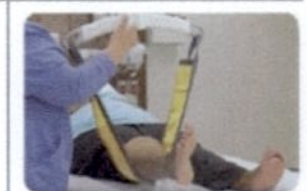

Multipurpose sling (lifting capacity up to 255 kg/560 lb)	Sustained holding of the trunk or pelvis, rotating on one side in the bed. Matches with ceiling-mounted or floor-based lift	Wound care, dressing, bathing, bedside and clinical procedures, turn in the bed, positioning for radiology exams, making an occupied bed, rehabilitation exercises	Tolerance to a prolonged position	Wounds affecting use of sling, respiratory difficulties in supine and on side position	Wide band	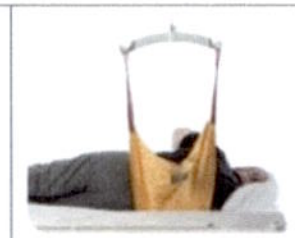
Pannus support (lifting capacity up to 255 kg/560 lb)	Assists in holding and supporting the abdomen; eliminates heavy manual lifting of the patient's pannus. Matches with ceiling-mounted or floor-based lift	Personal hygiene, skin care procedures (examination, treatment, and care); allow safe transfer tasks	Tolerance to a prolonged position	Wounds affecting use of sling, respiratory difficulties in supine and on side position	Pannus sling	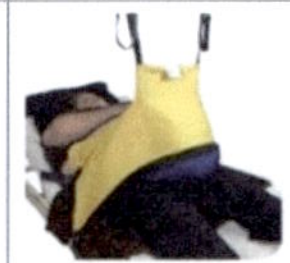
Supine lift/*repositioning* sling (lifting capacity up to 500 kg/1100 lb)	Provides full-body support in the supine position. Matches with ceiling-mounted or floor-based lift	Horizontal-lateral transfers, making an occupied bed, bathing, repositioning in bed, fall rescue from floor	Be able to lay in a flat position	Wounds affecting use of sling, respiratory difficulties in supine position	Hammock, stretcher, repositioning sling	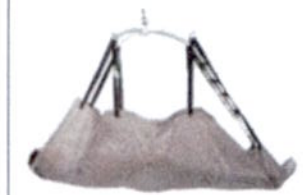

The effective application of patient-handling slings significantly impacts safety, comfort, and dignity, while ineffective sling use can lead to negative consequences, such as patient falls, discomfort, pressure ulcers, or even fear of lift device. Organizational gaps could interfere with effective application of patient-handling slings, such as defects in infection control, lack of inventory, or inadequate staff competency.

The sling's fabric is soft, breathable, and reinforced, and comes in different sizes and shapes. Relative to weight capacity, congruency must keep among all parts of the lifting system (track, motor, hanger bar, and sling) with the lowest weight limit applied if any difference exists. Slings' safety over time has to be checked regularly, and they are to be replaced when no longer safe. Disposable patient-specific slings are particularly effective for infection prevention.

Inserting the sling under the dependent bariatric patient is physically challenging, and requires competency and safety awareness; usually three caregivers are required, along with the use of some aiding devices and the adoption of a proper ergonomic technique.

Use of slings combined with bed adjustments and with other devices eases the regular mobilization and repositioning of the patient to avoid pressure ulcers, during nursing and hygiene procedures, and for rehabilitative purposes too.

In the rehabilitative setting, corset slings aid in the very first phases of motor recovery supporting standing, walking, and balancing functions exercised while standing or sitting. Combination of ceiling lift with elastic bands attached to the overhead motor in the locked position allows even the bedridden patient to perform early rehabilitative exercises, using handles for the upper limbs, the band sling for the lower limbs, and the multipurpose sling for the pelvis to mobilize.

15.1.11 Spaces

Adequate space both promotes the patient's mobility and supports nurses in the use of assistive technology [6, 8].

Given the general prevalence of obesity and the estimated one in rehabilitation units [12], 10–20% of the rooms of a rehabilitation unit should be able to accommodate bariatric patients. Ceiling lifts may reduce the space required for both caregivers and rehab equipment [13].

Any diagnostic/treatment or clinic setting will require a minimum clear area of 18.5 m^2/200 ft^2, with a minimum clear dimension of 1.5–3.6 m/5–12 ft on each side and at the foot of the electric tables/beds.

15.1.12 Emergencies

It is important to plan for emergencies that may occur during the patient admission, avoiding unexpected delays and unpreparedness. Emergency medical teams would benefit greatly from powered ambulance gurney loaders as well as powered ambulance gurneys. Air-assisted lateral transfer devices are apt for transferring the patient out of a bed and onto the gurney in the home setting too. Bariatric blood pressure cuffs, tracheostomy kit, and IV kit are required to manage the emergency.

15.1.13 Staff Training

All bariatric patient-handling and mobility tasks require specialized knowledge and training to ensure safe and effective care. A more advanced training should include information on the space and technology needs for safe bariatric care, an understanding of the comorbidities that occur in the bariatric patient, and assessment and decision-making tools, such as algorithms, with related hands-on technology training. Interactive and participatory style is to be preferred by providing an effective learning strategy and simulation training. Education and training should be provided for all healthcare workers who have direct clinical contact with bariatric patients (nurses, nursing assistants, health technicians, radiology technicians, and physical and occupational therapists). Training needs to be provided once a year, also because equipment and technology evolve.

15.2 Motor Rehabilitation Equipment

Treadmills are widely used for testing and training patients with different pathological conditions—obesity, cardiopulmonary, orthopedic, and neurological. They present wide differences in terms of structure and function that have a direct impact on specific rehabilitation protocols. Technological, therapeutic, and rehabilitative advances together with the pressure for reducing hospitalization costs have fostered in recent years the development of more sophisticated treadmill-based systems for rehabilitation of lower limbs. The purpose of this paragraph is to provide rehabilitation specialists a guide that may help in the selection of the most appropriate system for patients with obesity.

Commercially available treadmill models present with a wide range of products with notable differences in structure and functionality. Such differences make certain models more suitable for training specific kind of patients or adopting specific rehabilitative protocols.

In a previous paper dated 2008 [14], the criteria for a goal-oriented selection of treadmills for rehabilitation purposes were defined. Such criteria are to be based on specific clinical needs, on the anthropometrics of the patient, as well as on physiological, techno-structural, and economic considerations.

15.2.1 Treadmills

The structural characteristics to be considered for selecting an adequate rehabilitation treadmill are engine, structure, dimensions, weight, weight capacity, belt, platform, safety, and control panel. Technical factors include noise, speed, inclination, and resilience. Selection criteria must always be functional to the type of patients to be trained [15]. This means that we have to take into account how we use the treadmill during rehabilitation programs. Here is the guideline for the best treadmill choice for obese.

15.2.2 Technical and Structural Characteristics

15.2.2.1 Motor

The motor is a key component of the treadmill. Its power is expressed in horsepower, HP, or continuous horsepower (CHP). CHP is most useful because it indicates how much power a motor can put out continuously versus just at its peak. How much treadmill motor power is needed depends on the type of exercise and on the body weight. For people weighing up to 90 kg (around 200 lb), these general recommendations should be valid [16]:

- Walking: Choose 2.0 CHP or higher.
- Jogging: Choose 2.5 CHP or higher.
- Running: Choose 3.0 CHP or higher.

The use of treadmill for obese and bariatric patients is limited to walking (in some cases a light jogging) considering the high risk of injuries and morbidity conditions of these subjects.

For those subjects the engine power should be around 3–4 CHP.

15.2.2.2 Speed

We need to evaluate starting velocity, incremental interval, and peak velocity. The first one is the minimal velocity at which the belt moves when switching on the treadmill. Sometimes that is not the absolute minimal velocity, since velocity can be further reduced once the belt has started. Usually, the belt starts at 0.5 km/h, but for rehabilitation purposes a velocity of 0.1 km/h is often necessary which allows evaluation/training even in highly deconditioned patients. Starting velocities above 0.8 km/h may result dangerous for some patients. The incremental interval is the minimal delta between a velocity and its subsequently selected value. It usually ranges from 0.5 km/h in baseline models to smaller increments (0.1 km/h) in more refined models.

15.2.2.3 Inclination

Different mechanisms (electric, pneumatic, and manual) allow inclination of the treadmill. Electric elevation is nowadays the most common mechanism. It needs a separate engine that must have enough power to elevate the treadmill with its maximal load—for obese subjects it should have the proper power. Some models allow downhill gait at negative inclinations of 10–16%, with 1% increments. Some other may reach −25% negative inclinations.

15.2.2.4 Resilience and Track Cushioning

Resilience is the capacity of absorbing the elastic deformation energy determined by the impact of the foot on the belt. This is crucial in preventing articular stress on the lower limbs. Manufacturers have developed different systems for reducing the impact forces as flexible board or specific cushioning systems. Track (or belt) cushioning helps protect joints from the impact of exercise and the optimal resilience value is that one closer to the soft ground. In any case it is important to wear a pair of running shoes that protect feet during locomotion.

15.2.2.5 Weight Capacity

The weight capacity of the treadmill generally varies from 110 to 180 kg but in some cases up to 225 kg. Bariatric capacities up to 300 kg have to be considered for severely obese patients. It is recommended to choose a treadmill that can officially handle at least 30 kg more than the subject weight [16].

This will help ensure that the motor is not strained. Some manufacturers have developed treadmills with integrated partial body weight support to improve training.

Some treadmills are specially designed for rehabilitating gait-impaired patients. The redistribution of weight with the unloading system allows the patient to concentrate on coordination without running the risk of falling. This type of treadmill is indicated as body weight-supported treadmill (BWST).

15.2.2.6 Track Size

During walking, the step length is shorter than during running. The track has to be of enough length for this movement, but on the other hand, the longitudinal dimension is not of great importance during walking. Today's standards for treadmill track length are around 150 and 60 cm width, but for obese subjects the treadmill width should be larger. In general, a treadmill track is planar but recently treadmills with curve tracks are available. The particular shape allows walking and running without the use of an engine. The movement is created using the natural friction of the foot with the track itself. This innovative approach allows the patient to guide and regulate all the walking phases changing itself the speed. This solution seems to increase the metabolic intensity and muscle activation.

15.2.2.7 Structure

The structure's weight is generally correlated to maximal weight capacity, which is also related to the engine power. Steel structures have the characteristic of being more stable and durable, but at the same time they are heavier than those in aluminum. It is preferable to choose welded structures than screwed ones. Plastic structures should be avoided. A very useful accessory, especially if the treadmill has a high weight, is the wheels to allow treadmill handling. Dimensions range from 80 to 95 cm of width, from 185 to 218 cm of length, and from 135 to 150 cm of height.

15.2.2.8 Safety Systems

Treadmills are in general equipped with safety bars or handles mounted in the structure according to specific needs. Safety bars and handles can be placed frontally or to the side of the track. They are designed based on the pathological condition of the subject and the specific task (walking or running). Long handrails offer additional patient safety, especially for using the treadmill in rehabilitation. Thanks to their special shape, the handrails also serve as handgrips to access the treadmill. They must be solid and should not hinder the natural swing of the arms during the locomotion. They serve mainly at equilibrium, so they must be easily accessible and comfortable in the grip and have a length that covers almost the entire surface of the track surface.

The following infographic (Fig. 15.1) indicates the technical features to be taken into account for a treadmill suited for the patient with obesity. The number of stars is directly related to the importance of the specific aspect for patients with or without obesity.

In light of the fact that the market of the treadmill is dynamic and constantly expanding it is difficult to summarize in a table all of the treadmill models that meet all the technical features for the rehabilitation of the patient with obesity. We have therefore limited the search to specific queries. Among the main parameters of choice, we considered the user's maximum body weight, the power of the motor, and the width of the belt. The selection of models was made among the treadmill models produced over the last 5 years.

Table 15.5 shows a non-exhaustive list of treadmill with indication of use for subjects with obesity. In the first column (light green) the category of use is reported: medical, bariatric, and nonmedical. The dark gray columns are related to the technical characteristics of the motor. Those in light blue, on the other hand, are linked to the track speed, while those in yellow are related to its geometric characteristics. The light gray columns show information about the load capacity (related to the patient's weight). Within this group we have added a column relating to lifting systems that can be used in the rehabilitation phase. The treadmills with the "tip" are those that highlight this possibility in the data sheet. The last red column is related to safety. We took into account those treadmills which have, in addition to the front safety bar, at least two side bars running along the belt for at least 50% of its length.

Criteria for the treadmill's choice:

- Specific clinical needs
- Anthropometrics of the patient
- Type of exercise (walking or running)
- Technical aspects (track size, cushioning, safety)
- Costs

15.2.2.9 Treadmill-Based Systems

Advances in robotics have contributed to the development of new devices for the rehabilitation and evaluation of sensory-motor capacities. The line between treadmills and robotic devices has become fuzzier and we have examples of systems that finely integrate and merge those technologies in a unique device for

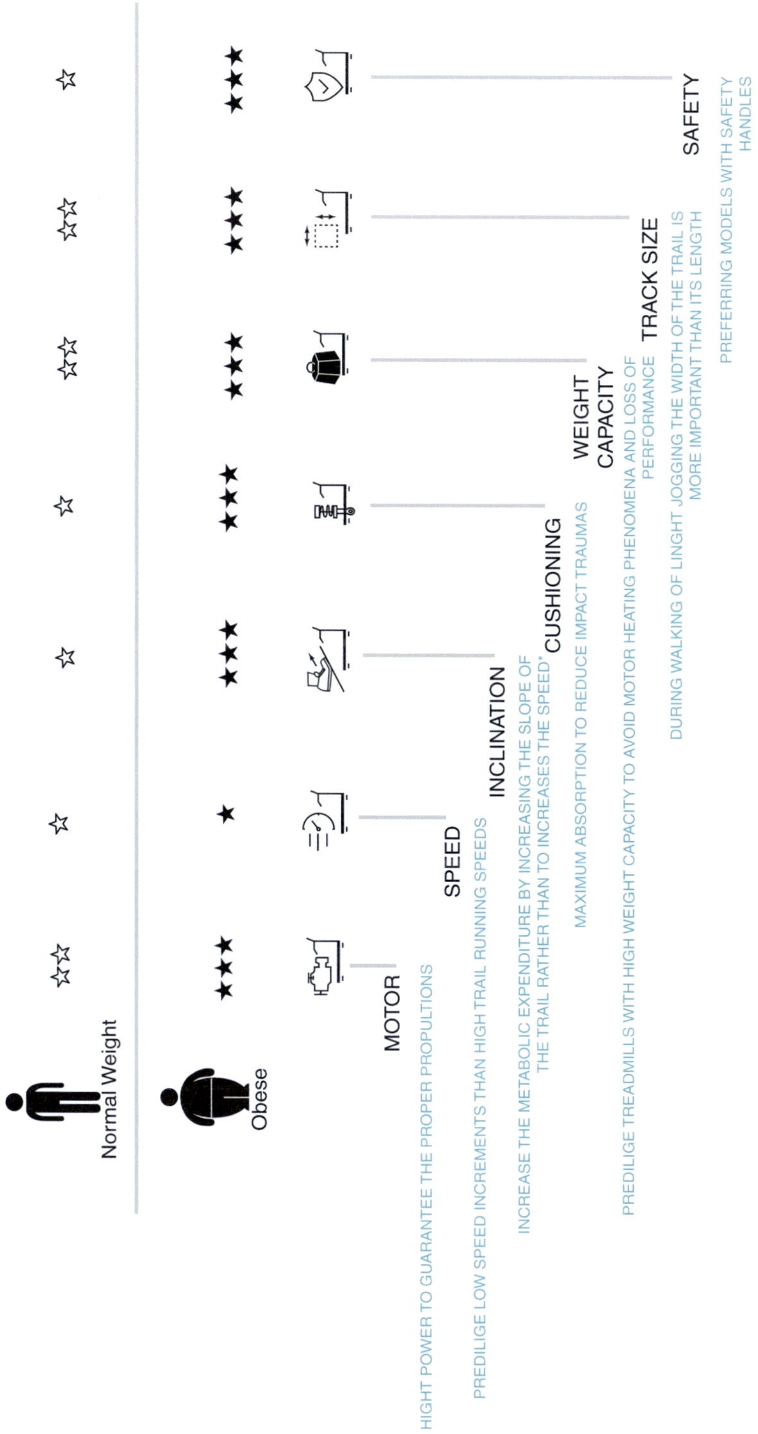

Fig. 15.1 Technical features for a treadmill suited for the patient with obesity

Table 15.5 Brand and treadmill model

	Treadmill use [–]	Motor power [HP]	Motor CHP [HP]	Speed [km/h]	Starting speed [km/h]	Speed increments [km/h]	Inclination [%]	Track shape [–]	Track dimension: width [cm]	Track dimension: length [cm]	Weight capacity [kg]	Weight support system [–]	Safety [–]
Brand and treadmill model													
Biodex RTM600	Medical	2	n.a.	0–17	0.16	n.a.	−3 to 12	Flat	51	160	181	OPT	OPT
Biodex New Gait Trainer™ 3	Medical	2	n.a.	0–16	0.48	n.a.	0 to 15	Flat	51	160	182	OPT	OPT
Cosmed T250MR	Medical	4.42	n.a.	0–40	0.1	n.a.	−35 to 35	Flat	100	250	210	✓	✓
Cosmed T170 DE Med	Medical	4.42	n.a.	0–25	0.1	n.a.	0 to 25	Flat	66	170	200	✗	OPT
Cybex R Series	Not medical	4	n.a.	0.8–20	n.a.	n.a.	0 to 15	Flat	56	152	181	✗	✗
Cybex V Series	Not medical	3	n.a.	0.8–19.3	n.a.	n.a.	0 to 15	Flat	51	152	181	✗	✗
Landice L7 rehab	Medical	4.	n.a.	0.16–19.2	n.a	n.a.	0 to 15	Flat	51	147	181	✗	✓
Landice L8 Rehab	Medical	4	n.a	0.16–19.2	n.a	n.a.	0 to 15	Flat	56	160	225	✗	✓
Ergo-FIT Xrcise Runner Med	Medical	n.a.	n.a.	0.2–25	n.a.	0.1	0 to 20	Flat	n.a.	n.a.	200	✗	OPT

Ergo-FIT TRAC 4000/4100 MED	Medical	n.a.	n.a.	0.2–25	n.a.	n.a.	0 to 20	Flat	n.a.	n.a.	200	✗	✓
Runner 7410 T	Medical	7 (max peak)	n.a.	0.1–25	n.a.	0.1	0.1 to 22	Flat	54	154.5	220	✗	✓
Runner RUN 7411/T-PC	Medical	7 (max peak)	n.a.	0.1–25	n.a.	0.1	0 to 20	Flat	54	204	220	✓	✓
Woodway Bari-mill	Bariatric	2	n.a	0–19.2	n.a		−25 to 25	Flat	55	173	360 (walking)	✓	✓
Woodway Curve XL	Medical	Nonmotorized	Non-motorized	0-no max	Indefinable	Inde-finable	Inde-finable	Curve	55	218	360 (walking)	✗	✓
SportsArt T653 M	Medical	3.2	n.a.	0.2–16	n.a.	n.a.	0 to 15	Flat	56	155	182	✗	✓
SportsArt T655MD	Medical	5	n.a.	0.2–20	n.a.	n.a.	0 to 22	Flat	56	155	227	✗	✓
Technogym Skillmill	No medical	Nonmotorized	Non-motorized	0–no max	n.a.	n.a.	0 to 20	Curve	n.a.	n.a.	200	✗	✓
Technogym Run 1000 Excite Med	Medical	6 (peak)	n.a.	0.4–20	n.a.	n.a.	0 to 15	Flat	52	152	220	✗	✓

lower limb rehabilitation. There are treadmill-based systems, developed to provide partial body-weight support (BWS) during treadmill training. BWS can be useful in the rehabilitation of patients with orthopedic or neurological conditions who are also obese, where unloading of the joints bearing weight is crucial in earlier stages.

These systems have embedded in the track a ground reaction force platform used for the spatiotemporal and kinetics parameter detection during the gait or running.

These systems can be considered as a combination of an exoskeleton and a treadmill [17, 18]. They execute conventional therapists' task of assisting legs and hip of the patient walking on a treadmill while patient's body weight is partially supported by an overhead support. No specific examples of robotic treadmills for patients with obesity are present in the literature, with the exception of the Biodex gait trainer. The Biodex Gait Trainer 2 is a device designed specifically for assessment, rehabilitation, and retraining of gait. It is the only treadmill with an instrumented deck that monitors and records step length, step speed, and right-to-left time distribution (step symmetry). It provides both audio and visual feedbacks to facilitate gait training. A high-resolution color touch screen LCD display is attached to the treadmill to control the device settings. Moreover, the Biodex Gait Trainer 2 is supplied by a serial interface that allows the download of patient data to a computer for archiving, reporting, or exporting data. In the assessment mode, the therapist is able to print out objective measurements about various components of the gait pattern [19]. This equipment has been used in obese children, nongenetically obese children, and genetically obese children with Down syndrome, with the aim of quantifying and comparing the spatiotemporal parameters of gait and comparing results with normal-weight control children [20]. In another study, the Biodex Gait Trainer 2 was used to investigate the effect of different categories of weight abnormalities on gait parameters in children [21].

References

1. VHA Center for Engineering & Occupational Safety and Health (CEOSH). Bariatric safe patient handling and mobility guidebook: a resource guide for care of persons of size, St. Louis, Missouri, July 2015.
2. Gallagher S. A practical guide to bariatric safe patient handling & mobility. Sarasota, FL: Visioning Publishers LLC; 2015.
3. Huntleigh A. Guidebook for architects and planners: functional design for mobilisation and ergonomics. 4th ed; 2015.
4. https://mobile.va.gov/app/safe-patient-handling
5. ANA, American Nurses Association. Safe patient handling and mobility: inter-professional national standards, 2013.
6. FGI, Facilities Guidelines Institutes. Guidelines for design and construction of hospitals and outpatient facilities, Chicago, IL, 2014. www.fgiguidelines.org.
7. Baptiste A, et al. VISN8 Patient Safety Center of Inquiry Technology resource guide for bariatric patients, Tampa, FL, 2015.
8. AIA: American Institute of Architects. Planning and design guidelines for bariatric healthcare spaces, 2006.

9. ISO/TR 12296:2012. Ergonomics—manual handling of people in the healthcare sector.
10. Marras WS, Knapik GG, Ferguson S. Lumbar spine forces during manoeuvring of ceiling-based and floor-based patient transfer devices. Ergonomics. 2009;52(3):384–97.
11. VISN8 Patient Safety Center of Inquiry & Arjo Inc. Patient care sling selection and usage toolkit, Tampa, FL, 2006.
12. Capodaglio P, Ventura G, Petroni ML, Cau N, Brunani A. Prevalence and burden of obesity in rehabilitation units in Italy: a survey. Eur J Phys Rehabil Med. 2018; https://doi.org/10.23736/S1973-9087.18.05393-5. [Epub ahead of print].
13. Muir M, Archer-Heese G. Essentials of a bariatric patient handling program. Online J Issues Nurs. 2009;14(1):5.
14. Capodaglio P, Vercelli S, Colombo R, Capodaglio EM, Mattai del Moro V, Franchignoni F. Il treadmill in medicina riabilitativa: caratteristiche tecniche e criteri di selezione. G Ital Med Lav Erg. 2008;30(2):169–77.
15. Wilson MS, Qureshy H, Protas EJ, Holmes SA, Krouskop TA, Sherwood AM. Equipment specifications for supported treadmill ambulation training. J Rehabil Res Dev. 2000;37(4):415–22.
16. https://www.treadmillreviews.net/treadmill-buyers-guide/
17. Dìaz I, Gil JJ, Sanchez E. Lower-limb robotic rehabilitation: literature review and challenges. J Robotics. 2011;2011:759764. https://doi.org/10.1155/2011/759764.
18. Poli P., Morone G., Rosati G., Masiero S Robotic technologies and rehabilitation: new tools for stroke patients' therapy BioMed Res Int. 2013, 153872, 8. https://doi.org/10.1155/2013/153872.
19. Tong RK, Ng MF, Li LS. Effectiveness of gait training using an electromechanical gait trainer, with and without functional electric stimulation, in subacute stroke: a randomized controlled trial. Arch Phys Med Rehab. 2006;87(10):1298–304.
20. Elshemy SA. Comparative study: parameters of gait in down syndrome versus matched obese and healthy children. Egypt J Med Hum Genet. 2013;14:285–91.
21. Heneidy, W. E. T. (2012). Gait parameters in children with different weight abnormalities. CU Theses.

MIX
Papier aus verantwortungsvollen Quellen
Paper from responsible sources
FSC® C105338

If you have any concerns about our products,
you can contact us on
ProductSafety@springernature.com

In case Publisher is established outside the EU,
the EU authorized representative is:
Springer Nature Customer Service Center GmbH
Europaplatz 3, 69115 Heidelberg, Germany

Printed by Libri Plureos GmbH
in Hamburg, Germany